The UKMLA Applied Knowledge Test

Are you a medical student preparing for the UKMLA exam? A practical companion to the textbook, *The UKMLA Applied Knowledge Test: Practice Questions* provides a comprehensive revision tool for any student looking to succeed in the exam. The book features over 500 multiple-choice questions (MCQs) covering all the clinical presentations and conditions required for the examination. Each MCQ includes five answer options, and explanations for both the correct and incorrect answers are provided, allowing readers to test the knowledge gained from the main textbook and to support student recall and comprehension. Conveniently organised into 18 areas of clinical practice, the book follows the General Medical Council's exam content map and is ideal for on-the-go revision. An essential preparation resource for UK-based medical students, and students sitting the PLAB examination.

Dr Ian Hodgins is a General Practitioner based in Buckfastleigh, South Dartmoor, Devon. He also holds the position of Lead for the Clinical Assessment Panel, Peninsula Medical School. Ian's medical career took him from five College, London (where he qualified in 1990) to Margate, Kent, and ultimately to Plymouth. Ian has great experience in creating, improving, mending and occasionally binning applied knowledge questions. He leads the local question writing panel and is an active participant in a national one.

Dr Elizabeth Drake is Director of Clinical Studies and Honorary Associate Professor at Peninsula Medical School. Currently she works as a Consultant Anaesthetist in Plymouth. She completed her masters in Clinical Education and is the Deputy Head of Peninsula Medical School. She has a vast experience of under- and post-graduate examinations from both an educator and examiner perspective. She graduated in medicine from the University of Southampton in 1998 and trained in anaesthesia in the Oxford region and Vancouver Canada. Highlights of her clinical career include being the anaesthetist for the safe delivery of conjoined twins and writing the first and widely quoted paper on training and reaching competency in epidural anaesthesia.

Steven Burr is Professor of Medical Education at Peninsula Medical School, University of Plymouth. Steven started as a university student in 1990. Having now graduated from five different ivory towers and having had a multitude of different roles in medical education, Steven thinks that he knows a thing or two about what students both want and need to know. Only now is he beginning to realise that these may actually have been two different things all along.

The UKMLA Applied Knowledge Test

Practice Questions

Edited by

Ian Hodgins
GP, Head of the Clinical Assessment Panel, Peninsula Medical School, Plymouth

Elizabeth Drake
Consultant Anaesthetist, University Hospitals Plymouth

Steven Burr
Professor of Medical Education, Peninsula Medical School, Plymouth

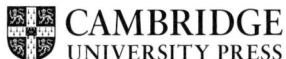

CAMBRIDGE
UNIVERSITY PRESS

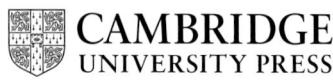

CAMBRIDGE
UNIVERSITY PRESS

Shaftesbury Road, Cambridge CB2 8EA, United Kingdom

One Liberty Plaza, 20th Floor, New York, NY 10006, USA

477 Williamstown Road, Port Melbourne, VIC 3207, Australia

314–321, 3rd Floor, Plot 3, Splendor Forum, Jasola District Centre,
New Delhi – 110025, India

103 Penang Road, #05–06/07, Visioncrest Commercial, Singapore 238467

Cambridge University Press is part of Cambridge University Press & Assessment,
a department of the University of Cambridge.

We share the University's mission to contribute to society through the pursuit of
education, learning and research at the highest international levels of excellence.

www.cambridge.org
Information on this title: www.cambridge.org/highereducation/isbn/9781009578011

DOI: 10.1017/9781009578059

First published 2025

Printed in the United Kingdom by CPI Group Ltd, Croydon CR0 4YY

A catalogue record for this publication is available from the British Library

Library of Congress Cataloging-in-Publication Data
Names: Hodgins, Ian, editor. | Drake, Elizabeth (Physician), editor. | Burr, Steven
(Professor of medicine), editor.
Title: The UKMLA applied knowledge test : practice questions / edited by Ian
Hodgins, Elizabeth Drake, Steven Burr.
Description: Cambridge ; New York, NY : Cambridge University Press, 2025. | Series:
Essential guides to the UKMLA | Includes bibliographical references and index.
Identifiers: LCCN 2025005425 | ISBN 9781009578011 (paperback) | ISBN
9781009578059 (ebook)
Subjects: LCSH: Physicians – Licenses – Great Britain – Examinations – Study guides
| General Medical Council (Great Britain) – Examinations – Study guides.
Classification: LCC RA396.A5 G7 2025 | DDC 616.0076–dc23/eng/20250421
LC record available at https://lccn.loc.gov/2025005425

ISBN 978-1-009-57801-1 Paperback

Contents

Contents

Preface

This work has brought together 368 specialist authors under 28 expert section editors to produce a resource to help those prospective doctors who will be taking the Medical Licensing Assessment Applied Knowledge Tests (MLA AKT) in the UK. The combined effort has been a 'not for profit' charitable enterprise, and all royalties from the sale of this publication will fund a scholarship at Peninsula Medical School.

This work comprises two linked books: one covers 'Clinical Presentations and Conditions', and the other covers 'Practice Questions'.

The content is intended to cover only what is needed for Foundation practice in the UK (equivalent to a resident doctor in the USA) and written at the level someone in Foundation practice should understand. We have not included a glossary as we expect you to be able to look up any unfamiliar term or abbreviation using the internet. Similarly, we have not included citations and references or lists for further reading, as these can interrupt the continuity of your reading, can go out of date, might not all be accessible to you, and you may prefer to read the style of other sources.

We have explicitly covered *all* the conditions and presentations specifically as listed *verbatim* by the General Medical Council (GMC) in the most recent available version of their content map for the MLA AKT (version 2, March 2021). Other topics that may be relevant to Foundation practice have not been included. We have covered each presentation or condition only once, as a single topic under a primary clinical area, to avoid overlap and enable ordering of the work. This means that some clinical areas listed by the GMC (e.g. Cancer, and Surgery) are not included as separate sections. For each topic, we have listed all the clinical areas in the GMC's MLA content map where that topic appears.

We have not included abstract or metaphorical images, preferring instead to source images from, or produce illustrations for, clinical practice. Consent has been obtained and confidentiality preserved wherever relevant. Our special thanks go to Susan Tyler for producing all of the illustrations, Kim Ingram for her remarkable persistence in tirelessly coordinating all of the content, Leigh Mueller for her attention to detail in the copy-editing, Charles Howell for coordinating the proofs, and Jessica Papworth for overseeing the publication process.

In photographic images, care has been taken to ensure gender balance where this is relevant to the presentation or condition. Similarly, any images of presentations or conditions showing skin are presented wherever possible with another example to aid recognition by showing variation with skin colour, and where possible also showing variation in stage of development. All statistics refer to the current UK population unless otherwise stated.

An important feature of this work is the inclusion of a separate book with practice questions covering all presentations and conditions. We intend that separating the knowledge from its application to practice questions will prevent the production of a single unwieldy book, while increasing flexibility. The two books can be used either: separately, for revision and practice purposes; or alongside each other, with both open at the same time for easier cross-referencing. We are fortunate to have inherited a long history of progress testing at Peninsula Medical School. One thousand questions, all rigorously set at the level of Foundation practice, have been delivered every year since the year 2000 to students in all years of study. We wish to thank all those whose expertise has refined our approach to question writing and remediation, so that we have been able to bring to you robustly refined example questions, covering every presentation and condition, along with advice for how to best prepare yourself to answer such questions.

We would be grateful to receive any constructive suggestions that could enable us to improve future editions.

Ian Hodgins
GP Principal, Buckfastleigh Medical Centre, Devon
MBBS AKC

Elizabeth Drake
Consultant Anaesthetist, University Hospitals Plymouth NHS Trust
Honorary Associate Professor of Education, Deputy Head of School, Peninsula Medical School, University of Plymouth
BM FRCA MClinEd SFHEA

Steven Burr
Professor of Medical Education,
Peninsula Medical School, University of Plymouth
BSc(Hons) MSc PGDE(FAHE) MMedSci(ClinEd) PhD FIBMS FAcadMEd FRSB PFHEA

Disclaimer

Every effort has been made in preparing this book to provide accurate and up-to-date information that is in accord with accepted standards and practice at the time of publication. Although case histories are drawn from actual cases, every effort has been made to disguise the identities of the individuals involved. Nevertheless, the authors, editors and publishers can make no warranties that the information contained herein is totally free from error, not least because clinical standards are constantly changing through research and regulation. The authors, editors and publishers therefore disclaim all liability for direct or consequential damages resulting from the use of material contained in this book. Readers are strongly advised to pay careful attention to information provided by the manufacturer of any drugs or equipment that they plan to use.

Guide to Taking the Medical Licensing Assessment Applied Knowledge Test

Christian Gray, BBiotech(Hons) PhD PGCert FHEA, Iain Robinson, BSc(JtHons) PhD PGCert FHEA and Alina Beltechi, MD PhD SFHEA

How to Use This Book

It is important that you prepare for the Medical Licensing Assessment (MLA) Applied Knowledge Test (AKT) using *The UKMLA Applied Knowledge Test: Clinical Presentations and Conditions* to support your learning within your medical curriculum. A comprehensive knowledge within the areas identified in this book will support your understanding of the content in MLA AKT questions. In addition, it will be important that you are 'exam ready' through supporting your physical and emotional health.

Whilst a working knowledge is crucial in understanding the content of the multiple-choice questions (MCQ) within the MLA AKT, an effective test-taking strategy is also important. Attempting formative MLA AKT-style questions will help you to develop an effective test-taking strategy and can allow you to evaluate how effectively you have achieved your learning goals. Most importantly, practice questions will help gauge your current level of knowledge and identify gaps that may require further learning. The MLA AKT-style questions included in this book align to the MLA content map that is used to prepare the MLA AKT.

Being Test-Wise

The questions used in the MLA AKT are not there to trick you through some obscure or exotic applied medical knowledge reported in a single medical journal. The content will be common and routine, or rare but important to know, in order to practise safely as a foundation doctor. Candidates who perform poorly often lack skills in taking the types of question represented within the MLA AKT. To be prepared for the test, you will need to strengthen your medical knowledge, have an effective study strategy and, most importantly, be 'test-wise'. Repetitive testing, supported by an effective test-taking strategy, can improve your confidence in achieving higher scores and reduce your anxiety. The MLA AKT is more than a test of medical knowledge – it is also a test of your ability to apply principles of clinical reasoning and understanding. When answering an MLA AKT question, imagine yourself taking a patient's history. This requires you to link your learning from different disciplines to understand the reasoning behind the correct answer. It may be possible that, within the MLA AKT, there will be clinical presentations or conditions with which you may not be familiar. Using information provided within the clinical vignette of a question may help you to narrow down the answer options and increase your chances of answering the question correctly. As there is no negative marking, you should answer all questions even when you cannot work out the correct answer option for a given question. Within this process, you are demonstrating your skill in clinical reasoning through narrowing down the potential diagnosis. Within the clinical environment, narrowing down the potential diagnoses will allow you to make better decisions regarding choosing appropriate tests and treatments for your patients.

Anatomy of a Single-Best-Answer Multiple-Choice Question

An example of a multiple-choice question of the type that will be used in the MLA AKT is described in *The UKMLA Applied Knowledge Test: Clinical Presentations and Conditions*. Each MLA AKT includes a short clinical vignette, the question to be answered and five answer options.

Approach to Answering Each MLA AKT Question

Read the question first and then the clinical vignette, carefully ensuring you understand what the question is asking. Use the question to inform you of the key information in the clinical vignette that you need to note. The current Medical Schools Council Assessment Alliance (MSCAA) examination software allows you to highlight keywords in the question to identify knowledge that may lead more clearly to the correct answer option. For example, are you being asked to diagnose or treat a condition? Is there any time sensitivity that means you must prioritise one approach over another for the patient in question, or do you need to deviate from a first-line approach for this particular patient?

There are many strategies used by candidates to guess answers, and these should all be avoided. When writing questions, examiners take steps to ensure these strategies can't benefit you. Such strategies include choosing the most scientific-sounding answer, choosing the longest answer, choosing the answer which is most different from other options, or avoiding the simplest answer. Identification of the most plausible answer should be made through eliminating incorrect answer options based on information within the vignette.

The Five-Step Approach to Answering MLA AKT Questions

1. What Is the Question About?

It is important to understand the type of question that is being asked. Which theme is the question asking about (core knowledge, a skill or a behaviour)? Understanding which domain the question is aligned to may also help you answer the question. Attempt to deduce the areas of clinical practice and professional knowledge, then the clinical presentation or condition that the question relates to, and whether the question is about diagnosis, management, investigations, assessing and managing risk, practical skills, patient signs, symptoms or pathophysiology.

2. Look For Key Concepts in the Clinical Vignette

Identifying the key concepts within the clinical vignette may help you decide the answer. It is important to look for the patient history, onset of symptoms, physical examinations, laboratory investigations and treatments the patient may have received.

3. Try to Answer the Question Before Looking at the Options

You may become confused by a list of options (or fall into the trap of picking the option you recognise, by pattern recognition). It is important to try to answer the question first *before* looking at the answer options. The distractors are designed to be plausible – however, they do not give the (most) correct answer. Answering the question before looking at the answer options may provide you with more confidence in your answer.

4. Rule Out Incorrect Answers

As medical knowledge continues to evolve and expand, it is impossible to be familiar with the answers for every clinical condition. However, you can often apply knowledge to arrive at the correct answer through clinical reasoning. If you are not sure of the correct answer option, clues within the vignette may help you to eliminate incorrect answer options. It is important that you justify why an option is incorrect rather than ruling it out because you don't understand it. For every option you eliminate correctly, you increase your statistical chances of guessing the correct answer.

5. Identify the Best Option

Choose the best answer option based on clinical reasoning methods described in steps 1–4. It is important that you answer every question, even if you resort to guessing. Through making a guess, you have a 1/5 chance of getting the correct option even if you have no knowledge about the question.

Developing an effective test-taking strategy is not easy and it will be important to work out which strategy works best for you through undertaking practice questions. Whilst the five-step approach is an effective strategy for many, it is important to identify what works most effectively for you. Some candidates find that reading the question and answers before reading the clinical vignette can help them to identify the answer more quickly – however, this method may confuse you or bias your answer. It is a good idea to practise questions under exam conditions, trying to answer questions in the same timeframe you will have in the MLA AKT.

Timing During the MLA AKT

Within an examination, some candidates find the steady approach of going through each question works best; other candidates review all questions through a quick first pass, answering easy questions and flagging more difficult ones (the current MSCAA examination software allows you to 'bookmark' questions, and to differentiate questions you have answered from those you have not). It is important that you spend time reading the clinical vignette and try not to rush answering the question. Set a 'time limit' for each question, including set 'check-points' for yourself (how many questions you need to have answered at different time points during the examination). If you are stuck on a question that may take more time to answer, you should answer it with your best educated guess and flag it to come back to before the end of the examination if there is time.

When to Change Your Answer?

As a clinician, it is important that you develop a gut feeling in clinical decision-making to avoid second-guessing yourself. This approach is also 'best practice' in answering MLA AKT questions. Whilst going with your gut feeling is useful, there are times when you may wish to change your answer. It is useful to develop your own criteria regarding when you may change your answer. For example, you may wish to consider changing your answer: if new information comes to mind that wasn't part of your thinking when you first answered the question; or if, on re-reading the question, it isn't the question you thought it was originally. Developing an effective test-taking strategy is not easy and it is important to work out which strategy is best for you through using practice questions. As a clinician, there may be times when you will change your decision – for example, about treatment options, based on further examination or progression of the patient's condition.

Take-Home Messages

There are several key steps which you can take in order to be prepared for the MLA AKT. These include:

- Be familiar with the clinical presentations and conditions that align to the MLA content map
- Develop an effective test-wise strategy
- Use practice MLA AKT-style questions to identify gaps in your knowledge
- Learn from your test-taking mistakes
- Analyse each question for clues within the clinical vignette that indicate why your answer was the correct or incorrect option
- Become familiar with the MSCAA examination software
- Practise taking formative MLA AKT-style questions under timed conditions
- Prepare yourself for the sustained effort of a real examination
- Believe in yourself

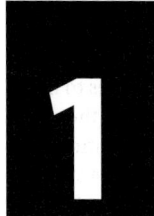

Cardiovascular

Q1

A 69 year old man arrives in the GP surgery with central chest pain and breathlessness. He is clammy, pale and looks unwell but is currently pain free. His temperature is 36.8 °C, pulse 105 bpm, BP 130/70 mmHg, respiratory rate 20 breaths per minute, oxygen saturation 96% breathing air. His ECG shows a sinus rhythm with ST elevation in leads II and III. Analgesia is given.

What therapy should be given immediately in the community?

1. Aspirin
2. Atorvastatin
3. Bisoprolol
4. Inhaled oxygen
5. Ramipril

Q2

An 85 year old man has a sudden onset of back and lower abdominal pain. His temperature is 36.5 °C, pulse 92 bpm, BP 130/80 mmHg, respiratory rate 16 breaths per minute. He has a pulsatile mass in his abdomen.

What is the most appropriate test for diagnosis?

1. CT angiogram
2. MRA
3. Non-contrast CT
4. PET scan
5. Ultrasound

Q3

A 78 year old man has a sudden onset of severe new abdominal pain. He had a myocardial infarction 3 days ago, after which he went into atrial fibrillation. He is tachycardic and is tender to examine across his central abdomen, with rebound and guarding.

What is the most likely diagnosis?

1. Acute mesenteric ischaemia
2. Aortic dissection
3. Colitis
4. Duodenal ulceration
5. Pancreatitis

Q4

A 76 year old woman has 10 weeks of breathlessness on exertion. She has hypertension and type 2 diabetes mellitus. Her pulse is 86 bpm, BP 152/49 mmHg, and oxygen saturation 98% breathing air. Her JVP is 7 cm above the sternal angle. She has an early diastolic murmur at the left sternal edge and a low-pitched diastolic rumble at the apex. Her first and second heart sounds are normal. Her lungs are clear. She has no peripheral oedema.

Which is the most likely diagnosis?

1. Aortic regurgitation
2. Hypertrophic obstructive cardiomyopathy
3. Mitral stenosis
4. Pulmonary regurgitation
5. Tricuspid stenosis

Q5

A 68 year old man has an ulcer on his left leg. It has been present for the last 4 weeks, gradually increasing in size. He has hypertension. He is an ex-smoker with a 50 pack year history. The ulcer is over the lateral malleolus; it is deep, revealing the underlying tendons.

What is the likely most significant cause of the ulcer?

1. Arterial insufficiency
2. Lymphatic stasis
3. Peripheral neuropathy

4. Venous insufficiency
5. Vitamin B12 deficiency

Q6

A 50 year old man has a routine diabetic review. He is otherwise well and asymptomatic, and his type 2 diabetes is controlled with diet only. He takes amlodipine 10 mg. His BP is 184/97 mmHg. He has brought a week of home BP readings (morning and night) averaging 147/89 mmHg. Blood tests two weeks ago showed normal renal function.

Which of the following would be the best plan of action?

1. Offer ACE inhibitors and check renal function in 2 weeks' time
2. Offer diuretics and check renal function in 2 weeks' time
3. Refer to specialist for further investigations and therapy
4. Request 24-hour ambulatory BP monitoring
5. Review BP in 2 weeks and then offer ACE inhibitors

Q7

A 52 year old man has central crushing chest pain radiating to the jaw associated with breathlessness and diaphoresis. He is a smoker and has high cholesterol. He has recently fractured his ankle and is in a boot. His pulse is 90 bpm, BP 110/60 mmHg, oxygen saturation 99% breathing air.

What is the most likely diagnosis?

1. Acute myocardial infarction
2. Aortic dissection
3. Pericarditis
4. Precordial catch syndrome
5. Pulmonary embolus

Q8

A 63 year old man has a cramping left calf pain that occurs after walking 50 metres on the flat. He has diabetes and mild hypertension. He takes metformin and atorvastatin. He smokes 100 g of tobacco a week. On examination his pulse is 82 bpm, BP 156/82 mmHg. His ankle brachial pressure indexes are 0.6 and 0.65, there is no tissue loss.

His bloods are as follows:

Serum sodium 138 mmol/L (137–144)

Serum potassium 3.5 mmol/L (3.5–4.9)

Serum creatinine 86 μmol.L (60–110)

eGFR 83 mL/min (> 60)

HbA1c 56 mmol/mol (20–41)

Serum cholesterol 7.2 mmol/L (< 5)

What intervention will have the most significant effect on his prognosis?

1. Change diet to include more potassium
2. Optimise cholesterol control
3. Optimise diabetes control
4. Optimise hypertension control
5. Patient to stop smoking

Q9

A 66 year old man has 2 days of pain and swelling in the back of his right leg. This has made walking more difficult. He has had congestive heart failure for 12 months and had a myocardial infarction 3 years ago. His temperature is 37.2 °C, pulse 86 bpm, BP 140/70 mmHg, respiratory rate 16 breaths per minute, his left calf is swollen and tender to palpation.

Investigations:

D-dimer 2.4 mcg/mL (< 0.4)

What is the most appropriate next investigation?

1. CT venography
2. Direct venography
3. Duplex ultrasonography
4. Magnetic resonance imaging
5. Plethysmography

Q10

An 87 year old man has leg swelling and ongoing shortness of breath. He is a heavy smoker and uses inhalers several times a day. On examination, he has a soft pansystolic murmur, which is loudest in inspiration.

What is the most likely cause of the murmur?

1. Mitral regurgitation due to a pacing lead
2. Mitral regurgitation due to age-related degeneration
3. Pulmonary regurgitation due to lung disease

4. Tricuspid regurgitation due to rheumatic fever as a child
5. Tricuspid regurgitation due to right ventricular dysfunction

Q11

A 35 year old lady presents with large varicose veins on her left leg. She has no skin changes but gets occasional aching sensations at the end of the day after being at work.

What would be an appropriate initial intervention to manage her symptoms?

1. Compression hosiery
2. Duplex ultrasound
3. Laser therapy
4. Lifestyle advice
5. Vein stripping

Q12

A 58 year old man has 3 months of malaise, loss of appetite and weight loss. On examination he looks well, his temperature is 37.1 °C, pulse 68 bpm, BP 130/75 mmHg, and you can hear a decrescendo blowing diastolic murmur best at the left lower sternal border grade 2/6. He is not septic and looks well from the end of the bed.

Routine bloods are normal except:

Haemoglobin 112 g/L (130–180)

CRP 34 mg/L (< 6)

Which is the most likely diagnosis?

1. Ascending aortic dissection
2. Bacterial endocarditis
3. Cardiac tamponade
4. Rheumatic fever
5. Ruptured papillary muscle

Q13

A 25 year old woman has a syncopal episode. Witnesses described her collapsing after standing in a queue at a theme park on a hot day. She remembers feeling nauseated and dizzy before the blackout and took several minutes to recover after the episode. She has no past history of note, she is not pregnant. Examination and electrocardiogram are normal.

What management is required?

1. Admission for cardiac monitoring and an echocardiogram
2. Cardiology referral for further assessment and consideration of midodrine or fludrocortisone
3. Discharge with education about the importance of hydration and avoidance of triggers
4. Discharge with outpatient Holter monitoring and echocardiogram
5. Referral to neurologists for exclusion of epilepsy

Q14

A 74 year old woman has 6 months of worsening breathlessness on exertion. On auscultation, an ejection systolic murmur is heard at the upper right sternal edge and is loudest on expiration.

What is the most likely heart valve problem?

1. Aortic incompetence
2. Aortic stenosis
3. Innocent flow murmur
4. Mitral incompetence
5. Mitral stenosis

Q15

A 72 year old woman has an ulcer on her right leg. It has been present for the last 6 weeks, gradually increasing in size. She has hypercholesterolaemia. She is an ex-smoker with a 30 pack year history. The ulcer is proximal to medial malleolus, it is shallow and sloughy, there is a brown discolouration to the surrounding skin.

What is the likely most significant cause of the ulcer?

1. Arterial insufficiency
2. Lymphatic stasis
3. Peripheral neuropathy
4. Venous insufficiency
5. Vitamin B12 deficiency

Q16

A 60 year old man has severe epigastric pain for the last 40 minutes. It is associated with nausea and sweating. He is pale. His pulse is 105 bpm, BP 100/60 mmHg, and respiratory rate is 18 breaths per minute.

Which is the most likely diagnosis?

1. Aortic coarctation
2. Aortic dissection
3. Myocardial infarction
4. Pericarditis
5. Right-sided pneumonia

Q17

An 84 year old man has a cold painful left leg. The leg is painful even at rest. He has atrial fibrillation. He is not known to the vascular team and has never had any problems in this leg prior to this. His left shin is hairless, his pedal pulses are not palpable, there is fixed mottling of the shin. The hallux nail is yellow and thickened.

Which of the following suggests irreversible ischaemia has occurred?

1. Absence of pedal pulses
2. Fixed mottling of the skin
3. Hair loss over the shin
4. Pain at rest
5. Yellow discolouration with thickening of the nail of the hallux

Q18

A 45 year old man with diabetes has a hypertension review. The clinic BP shows readings of 140/85 mmHg and matches the patient's home recordings. He takes amlodipine 5 mg. Blood tests are normal. He has some microalbuminuria. He is given appropriate lifestyle advice.

What is the appropriate next step?

1. Add a thiazide diuretic
2. Add an ACE inhibitor
3. Change the amlodipine to another calcium antagonist
4. Continue with the present medication and dose and review in 3 months
5. Increase amlodipine to 10 mg

Q19

A 20 year old man attends the emergency department complaining of palpitations. These occur two or three times per week, develop suddenly and persist for up to 10 minutes before resolving. On this occasion, they have not resolved. He describes them as regular and rapid. They are associated with shortness of breath and light-headedness. He feels otherwise well between episodes and has no prior medical problems.

You perform a 12-lead electrocardiogram (Figure 1.1).

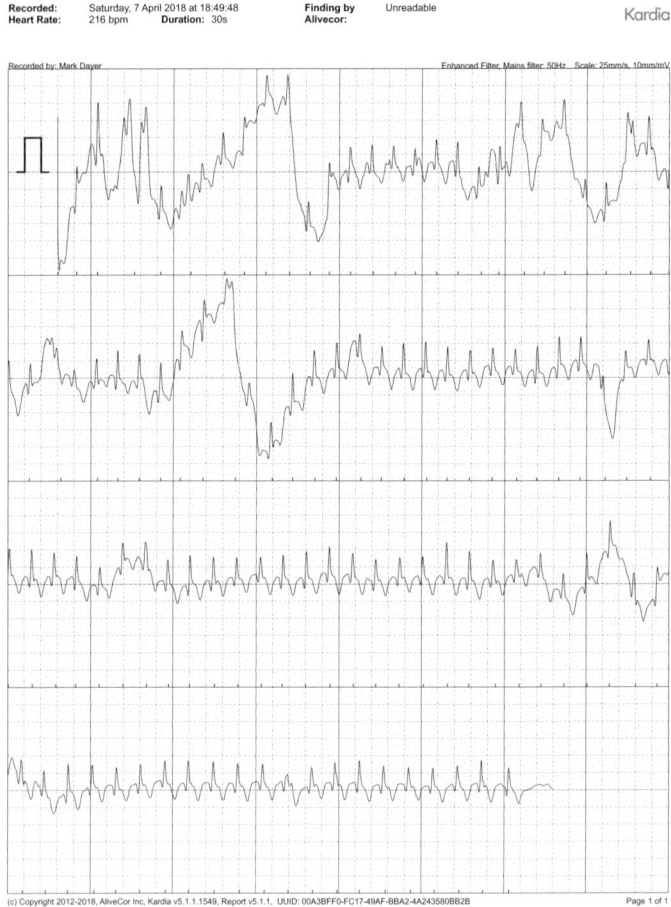

| Recorded: | Saturday, 7 April 2018 at 18:49:48 | Finding by Alivecor: | Unreadable | Kardia |

Recorded by: Mark Dayer   Enhanced Filter, Mains filter: 50Hz   Scale: 25mm/s, 10mm/mV

(c) Copyright 2012-2018, AliveCor Inc, Kardia v5.1.1.1549, Report v5.1.1, UUID: 00A3BFF0-FC17-49AF-BBA2-4A243580BB2B   Page 1 of 1

Figure 1.1 Electrocardiogram

What is the finding?

1. Atrial fibrillation
2. Atrial flutter
3. Sinus tachycardia
4. Supraventricular tachycardia
5. Ventricular tachycardia

Q20

A 64 year old man has severe pain in his left foot. This follows 8 weeks of pain in the back of his left knee associated with swelling. He has hypertension and hyperlipidaemia. He smokes 10 cigarettes/day, does not drink and is a retired factory worker.

On examination he has a cold and dusky left foot with absent pulses.

What is the most appropriate investigation in this patient?

1. Bilateral ABPIs
2. CT angiography lower limbs
3. Transcutaneous oxygen pressures in both feet
4. USS arterial duplex
5. X-ray left leg

Q21

A 70 year old man presents to the emergency department following an episode of tearing chest pain of sudden onset. The pain was 9/10 for severity when it started and gradually settled to a 2/10. He has a history of hypertension but takes no medication and has never smoked. His temperature is 37.1 °C, pulse 94 bpm, BP 174/64 mmHg, respiratory rate 18 breaths per minute, oxygen saturation 98% breathing air, he has a murmur at the left sternal edge.

His electrocardiogram shows no ischaemic changes but some evidence of left ventricular hypertrophy. Chest X-ray is normal.

D-dimer 0.56 mcg/mL < 0.4 mcg/mL

Troponin is also mildly elevated.

He has been started on treatment for acute coronary syndrome by the emergency department physician.

What is the next most appropriate step?

1. Arrange CT angiogram of aorta
2. Arrange CT pulmonary angiogram
3. Continue treatment for acute coronary syndrome
4. Discharge with medical management for NSTEMI
5. Echocardiogram

Q22

A 16 year old boy presents to the emergency department with his heart pounding in his chest. He had to stop running because he felt breathless. He has not lost consciousness. His pulse was 220 bpm, BP 105/60 mmHg, and respiratory rate 24 breaths per minute. An electrocardiogram shows a narrow complex tachycardia.

Which is the most likely diagnosis?

1. Atrial fibrillation
2. Complete heart block
3. Panic attack
4. Supraventricular tachycardia
5. Ventricular tachycardia

Q23

A 52 year old man was admitted to the critical care unit after having suffered a cardiac arrest. Pre-hospital team reported return of spontaneous circulation after 45-minute down time at scene. Patient has been receiving intensive care post-cardiac arrest treatment and support since admission. On day 3 of his ICU stay, the patient's Glasgow Motor Score remains M2 after having been off sedation for 36 hours.

Which one of the following is associated with a poor neurological outcome in this patient?

1. Bilaterally absent N20 Somatosensory Evoked Potential
2. EEG showing partial complex seizure activity
3. Neuron Specific Enolase > 30 mcg
4. Not opening eyes to voice or painful stimuli
5. Ongoing need for respiratory and cardiovascular support

Q24

A 77 year old woman has four days of tightness in her left leg. This is associated with slight swelling, moderate pain and erythema. She has a history of hypertension and nothing else of note.

On examination, the leg circumference in the thigh is 38.2 cm on the left, 38.4 cm on the right. At 10 cm below the tibial tuberosity, it is 24 cm on the left compared to 20.5 cm on the right; there is symmetrical pitting oedema. There is no localised tenderness or conspicuous superficial veins.

Using the table, calculate the Wells' score.

1. Score = 0
2. Score = 1
3. Score = 2
4. Score = 3
5. Score = 4

Wells' Score criteria description	Points
Active cancer (treatment within last 6 months or palliative)	+1 point
Calf swelling ≥ 3 cm compared to asymptomatic calf (measured 10 cm below tibial tuberosity)	+1 point
Swollen unilateral superficial veins (non-varicose, in symptomatic leg)	+1 point
Unilateral pitting oedema (in symptomatic leg)	+1 point
Previous documented deep vein thrombosis	+1 point
Swelling of entire leg	+1 point
Localised tenderness along the deep venous system	+1 point
Paralysis, paresis or recent cast immobilisation of lower extremities	+1 point
Recently bedridden ≥ 3 days, or major surgery requiring regional or general anaesthetic in the past 12 weeks	+1 point
Alternative diagnosis at least as likely	−2 points

Q25

A 76 year old woman has 3 months of an ulcer on the medial aspect of her left forefoot. She has hypertension and type 2 diabetes mellitus with peripheral neuropathy. Her temperature is 37.3 °C, pulse 94 bpm, BP 120/76 mmHg, pulses to both feet are present and normal. The surrounding skin is erythematous and swollen and the ulcer exudes a small amount of pus. X-ray of the left foot shows periosteal reaction and cortical thinning at the first metatarsal base.

Which is the most appropriate next course of action?

1. Intravenous antibiotics
2. Oral antibiotics
3. Silver sulfadiazine dressing
4. Surgical intervention
5. Topical antibiotics

Q26

A 55 year old man presents with a 2-hour history of severe central crushing chest pain radiating into his left arm and jaw after lifting heavy boxes. He has hypertension and diabetes and has smoked 20 cigarettes a day for the last 35 years.

His pulse is 82 bpm, BP 156/82 mmHg, oxygen saturation 95% breathing air.

His chest is clear and heart sounds normal on auscultation. An electrocardiogram shows a normal sinus rhythm and ST elevation in the inferior leads.

What is the most likely diagnosis?

1. COPD
2. Musculoskeletal pain
3. Myocardial infarction
4. Pericarditis
5. Pulmonary embolism

Q27

A 32 year old Pakistani woman presents with chest pain. She complains of increasing shortness of breath and is coughing clear sputum. She is 20 weeks pregnant. Her temperature is 36.5 °C, pulse 130 bpm, BP 135/80 mmHg, respiratory rate 24 breaths per minute, oxygen saturation 94% breathing 60% oxygen. Auscultation reveals a mid-diastolic murmur. She has bi-basal crepitations and a mild pedal oedema. Her chest X-ray shows diffuse opacifications in both lungs.

What is the most likely explanation?

1. Aortic dissection
2. Asthma exacerbation
3. Mitral regurgitation
4. Mitral stenosis
5. Pulmonary embolism

Q28

A 69 year old man has 6 weeks of worsening ankle and leg swelling associated with breathlessness on exertion. He had a myocardial infarct 5 years ago. He is an ex-smoker (20 pack year history). There is no significant family history. His pulse is 70 bpm, BP 119/78 mmHg, respiratory rate 18 breaths per minute, oxygen saturation 94% breathing air.

A urine dip showed proteinuria. He has an NT-proBNP of 7598 ng/L (< 200).

His electrocardiogram demonstrates sinus rhythm with small QRS complexes. His echocardiogram is reported as showing severe left ventricular hypertrophy with an ejection fraction of 59%, biatrial dilatation and a speckled appearance to the myocardium.

What is the most likely diagnosis?

1. Cardiac amyloid
2. Dilated cardiomyopathy
3. Hypertensive heart disease
4. Hypertrophic cardiomyopathy
5. Ischaemic cardiomyopathy

Q29

A 27 year old man presents with breathlessness and chest pain. He is normally fit and well and takes no regular medications. He recently had coryzal symptoms in the last week. His bloods show a troponin of 1563 ng/L (normal < 14 ng/L), with an elevated CRP of 189 (< 6 mg/L). A D-dimer is negative. His electrocardiogram shows a sinus tachycardia with no specific ST changes. His observations are otherwise normal.

What is the likely diagnosis?

1. Acute coronary syndrome
2. Myocarditis
3. Pericarditis
4. Pneumonia
5. Pulmonary embolism

Q30

A 32 year old man presents to the emergency department with 3 days of slowly worsening sharp chest pain in the centre of his chest that is helped by sitting up. Five days ago, he had coryzal symptoms and mild cough. His pulse is 90 bpm, BP 110/60 mmHg. He has quiet heart sounds. Blood tests revealed a raised CRP and white blood cells. Electrocardiogram showed concave ST elevation across most leads. Chest X-ray was normal.

What is the best initial management strategy?

1. Admit, request CT scan, start corticosteroids and colchicine
2. Admit, request echocardiogram, start colchicine and ibuprofen
3. Admit, request echocardiogram, start corticosteroids and colchicine
4. Discharge with colchicine and follow up in 1 month with echo
5. Discharge with ibuprofen and safety-netted

Q31

A 68 year old man has a new-onset, severe angina at rest. His cardio-vascular risk factors include type 2 diabetes, current smoking and a family history of heart disease. Serial troponins at 3 and 6 hours post-chest pain onset are within normal reference ranges. Electrocardiogram shows dynamic T wave inversion in lateral leads I, V5 and V6.

What feature of this case would not be an indication for admission and an early invasive strategy in the management of unstable angina?

1. Age
2. Cardiovascular risk factors
3. Dynamic electrocardiogram changes
4. History of highly suspicious cardiac angina
5. Normal troponin cardiac biomarkers

Q32

A 27 year old man is found collapsed at the side of the road. He had been competing in a 50-mile endurance race. When he is found, there is no cardiac effort, and he is pronounced dead after 30 minutes of unsuccessful cardiopulmonary resuscitation. Which of the following is the most likely cause of sudden cardiac death in this young athlete?

1. Aortic dissection
2. Brugada syndrome
3. Dilated cardiomyopathy

4. Hypertrophic cardiomyopathy
5. Long QT syndrome

Q33

An 80 year old patient appears unresponsive on an orthopaedic ward. He is unresponsive to painful stimuli with agonal breathing efforts, and there is no palpable carotid pulse.

What is the most appropriate next step?

1. Put out an emergency arrest call
2. Start chest compressions
3. Start rescue breaths
4. Try to clarify the CPR status of this patient
5. Try to find a monitor / ECG device to check the cardiac rhythm as soon as possible

Q34

A 68 year old man has bilateral intermittent claudication at 300 metres. He is a smoker with a 20 pack year history.
  The BPs in his upper and lower limbs are listed below.

Right brachial: 150 mmHg

Left brachial: 140 mmHg

Right anterior tibial: 135 mmHg

Right posterior tibial: 120 mmHg

Left anterior tibial: 105 mmHg

Left posterior tibial: 90 mmHg

What is his left leg ankle brachial pressure index?

1. 90/140
2. 90/150
3. 105/135
4. 105/140
5. 105/150

Q35

A 60 year old man has a high MEWS score following routine observations on the ward. He was admitted under the orthopaedic team and underwent an elective right total hip replacement for osteoarthritis

3 days ago. The operation was uncomplicated, and he has been recovering well. He is normally fit and well with no significant past medical history and does not take any regular medications. On systems review, he describes feeling short of breath with right-sided pleuritic chest pain. His temperature is 37.2 °C, pulse 112 bpm, BP 82/60 mmHg, respiratory rate 24 breaths per minute, oxygen saturation 92% breathing air; his chest is clear on auscultation. An electrocardiogram shows sinus tachycardia.

What is the most likely diagnosis?

1. Acute coronary syndrome
2. Haemorrhage
3. Pneumonia
4. Pneumothorax
5. Pulmonary embolus

Q36

A 63 year old man presents to the emergency department with painful swelling of his left leg. Examination shows significant unilateral pitting oedema (width of left calf 4 cm greater than the right), redness, prominent superficial veins, and tenderness to palpation. The patient has no history of cardiovascular disease and is not complaining of shortness of breath or chest pain.

What is the most likely cause of the oedema?

1. Acute heart failure
2. Chronic congestive heart failure
3. Deep vein thrombosis
4. Nephrotic syndrome
5. Sepsis

Q37

A 42 year old woman is brought into the emergency department following a motorcycle road traffic accident. She had needle decompression of tension pneumothorax at the side of the road.

Her temperature is 36.5 °C, pulse 120 bpm, BP 90/60 mmHg and respiratory rate 20 breaths per minute. She is anxious and shouting at the nurse to be discharged.

Which is the most appropriate next step in the management of this patient?

1. Allow her to discharge herself
2. Insert a chest drain
3. Order a chest X-ray to check for resolution of the pneumothorax
4. Start 2 L of oxygen via nasal cannula
5. Start vasopressors to improve BP

Child Health

Q38

A 7 year old boy is brought by his mother to the GP. He is fidgety, cannot seem to concentrate, and has been like this since he was a toddler. It is affecting his progress at school, and he is getting into fights in the lunch queue. His hearing and vision have been tested and there is no other medical history.

What is the most likely diagnosis?

1. ADHD
2. Autism spectrum disorder
3. Dyspraxia
4. Lead toxicity
5. Tourette syndrome

Q39

An 11 year old girl is brought by her mother to the GP. The girl has struggled starting at her new senior school and is now refusing to go to school at all. She seems very anxious and distressed. She has always been bright at her lessons but has never been comfortable in groups and has always found it difficult to make friends. She has only rarely been invited to birthday parties. Her mother states that she was very similar when she was that age.

Her mother is concerned that she may have autism spectrum disorder.

Which traits does she have that conform to the diagnostic criteria?

1. A qualitative impairment in reciprocal social interaction
2. Abnormal behaviour at the transition between primary and secondary school

3. Emotionally determined selectivity in verbal communication
4. Intellectual impairment
5. The presence of challenging behaviour

Q40

A 2 year old boy has delayed walking and early hand preference. He was born at term following prolonged labour, and needed resuscitation. Examination shows increased tone in left arm and left leg with brisk reflexes, right arm and right leg examines normally.

Which of the following is the most likely diagnosis?

1. Ataxic cerebral palsy
2. Athetoid cerebral palsy
3. Spastic diplegic cerebral palsy
4. Spastic hemiplegic cerebral palsy
5. Spastic paraplegic cerebral palsy

Q41

A 2 year old girl is admitted by ambulance with noisy breathing. She has had a runny nose and mild fever for the last 2 days. Overnight, she developed very noisy breathing and a harsh cough. She has been previously well and is up to date with her vaccinations.

Her temperature is 38 °C, pulse 160 bpm, respiratory rate 36 breaths per minute, oxygen saturation 98% breathing air, capillary refill 2 seconds. She is clingy with mum and a bit miserable, but is alert and is not drooling. She has a barking cough and inspiratory stridor at rest. There is some moderate intercostal recession but her air entry is good bilaterally.

What would be an appropriate management strategy?

1. Arrange an urgent neck and chest X-ray to look for foreign body inhalation leading to stridor
2. Arrange for urgent senior paediatric, anaesthetic and ENT review and plan how best to secure her airway and administer intravenous antibiotics
3. Do a thorough throat examination to look for evidence of inflammation and consider starting oral antibiotics
4. Give her a dose of prednisolone and allow her home with safety netting

5. Keep her settled with mum and administer an oral dose of dexamethasone and antipyretics before admitting for close observation

Q42

A 7 year old boy has presented with his mother after continually getting into trouble at school. He is often blurting out answers, fidgeting and constantly being loud. They are struggling to continue to manage his behavioural challenges both at school and at home. He has a background history of being born preterm and has epilepsy. His observations are all normal and during the examination you notice him constantly fidgeting on the chair and making infrequent eye contact.

What is the most appropriate next management step?

1. Make a diagnosis of ADHD
2. Offer parents a referral to group-based ADHD-focused support
3. Send an urgent referral to secondary care for assessment
4. Start methylphenidate
5. Tell the parents not to worry

Q43

A 34 year old woman requests genetic advice. She is homozygous for p.Phe508del cystic fibrosis-causing mutation. Her proposed partner is heterozygous, being phenotypically normal, with one copy of the p. Phe508del allele and one wild-type allele.

What is the probability that any child they have would have cystic fibrosis disease?

1. 0%
2. 25%
3. 50%
4. 75%
5. Impossible to tell without more information

Q44

A 4 year old boy is brought by his mother as she is concerned regarding his behaviour and speech. His mother describes him as very impulsive, restless and easily distractible. This is also corroborated by his school. On examination he has a long narrow face and slightly prominent ears. There are no other abnormalities on physical examination. His speech has poor articulation with only two-word sentences and often his mother has to tell you what he is saying.

Which investigation is most likely to give you the diagnosis?

1. Fragile X genetic testing
2. Microarray-based comparative genomic hybridisation
3. MRI brain
4. Thyroid function tests
5. Urine organic acids

Q45

A 32 year old woman presents for advice. She is in her 11th week of pregnancy has been told that there is a 1 in 50 chance that her baby has Down syndrome. She would like to know definitively whether her child has Down syndrome

What is the most appropriate investigation to offer her?

1. A blood test for Robertsonian translocation
2. A choice of amniocentesis or chorionic villus sampling
3. A fetal echocardiogram
4. A nuchal translucency scan
5. MRI pelvis

Q46

A 28 year old woman is concerned about possible spina bifida in her unborn child. She is 9 weeks pregnant. The pregnancy was unplanned and she has not been taking any folate supplements. There is no family history of neural tube defects.

Which routine investigation will provide the most accurate assessment of a neural tube defect in her baby?

1. 12-week ultrasound scan
2. 20-week ultrasound scan
3. Combined test
4. Nuchal translucency measurement
5. Quadruple test

Q47

A 5 year old boy is brought into the emergency department by his mother, looking very unwell. He was very hot on waking this morning and complained of a sore throat. As the day went on, he developed noisy breathing and was reluctant to talk or swallow. He was previously well but has not received any vaccinations.

On examination, he sits on his mother's knee leaning forwards and breathing rapidly with a high-pitched noise on inspiration. He looks scared and is drooling. His temperature is 39.2 °C, pulse 162 bpm, respiratory rate 36 breaths per minute, oxygen saturation 94% breathing air, capillary refill 1 second.

What is your next step in management?

1. Discussing with his mother the importance of vaccinating children
2. Examining his throat to identify the cause of his symptoms
3. Inserting a cannula in order to administer a third-generation cephalosporin
4. Moving him onto the examination couch in order to do a full assessment
5. Urgently assembling an appropriate team to manage him, including an experienced anaesthetist, ENT surgeon and paediatrician

Q48

An 18 month old girl has a 4-minute tonic clonic seizure in the emergency department, which resolves spontaneously without treatment. She was brought to the department following a similar event 2 hours ago. Her temperature is 38.8 °C; all other observations and examination are normal. Her temperature quickly normalises with oral paracetamol. Mum reports that following this she is back to her normal self and wants to go home.

What would be the most appropriate next management step?

1. Admit to paediatrics
2. Continue observations in the emergency department for further 2 hours, then discharge
3. Discharge home now with appropriate advice leaflet and safety netting

4. Obtain a mid stream urine and prescribe best-guess antibiotics before results

5. Refer for routine follow-up in paediatric outpatients

Q49

A 6 year old girl has been unwell for the last 2 days with a high temperature and earache. She and her family have recently returned home from a tour of Eastern Europe. She has had no immunisations.

Her temperature is 40.4 °C, pulse is 124 bpm, respiratory rate is 17 breaths per minute, capillary refill time is < 2 seconds. She has small pinpoint ulceration in her mouth on the buccal surface at the level of the first upper right molar.

What is the most likely cause of this illness?

1. Chickenpox
2. Measles
3. Mumps
4. Rubella
5. Toxoplasmosis

Q50

A 6 year old boy has 2 days of diffuse crampy abdominal pain around his umbilicus. He is nauseous but denies vomiting or diarrhoea. His temperature is 37.2 °C, and there is tenderness in the right lower quadrant without guarding or rebound tenderness.

What is the most likely diagnosis?

1. Appendicitis
2. Crohn's disease
3. Irritable bowel syndrome
4. Meckel's diverticulitis
5. Mesenteric adenitis

Q51

A 3 year old boy is brought into the emergency department with 4 days of diarrhoea and vomiting. He is pale, floppy and lethargic but responding to his father and able to tell you his name. He weighs 15 kg. His temperature is 36.6 °C, pulse 163 bpm, BP 75/55 mmHg, respiratory rate 42 breaths per minute, oxygen saturation 99% breathing air. His airway is patent, with no added sounds, and he has no increased work of breathing or central cyanosis. He is pale, cool at the peripheries, has dry lips and mouth and has poor skin turgor. His eyes are not sunken. His pupils are equal and reactive to light, and he is responsive to voice. His blood glucose level is 3.2 mmol/L. A cannula is inserted.

What are the first fluids he should receive?

1. 30 ml 10% dextrose
2. 150 ml bolus of 0.9% saline
3. 150 ml bolus of 0.9% saline + 5% dextrose
4. 300 ml bolus of 0.9% saline
5. 500 ml 0.9% saline + 5% dextrose at 52 ml/hour

Q52

A boy is born at term in the UK. His parents have both lived in the UK all their lives. The child has no neonatal complications and is fit and well. The parents wish for their child to have his vaccinations as per the recommended guidelines in the UK.

At what age should he receive his first MMR vaccination?

1. 2 months
2. 3 months
3. 6 months
4. 12 months
5. 3 years and 4 months

Q53

A 2 month old girl attends the children's assessment unit with a mark on her left lower leg. She was born at full term and has no medical history. Her observations are normal and she has no fever. On examination she has a 3 mm x 1 mm linear purple mark on her left lower leg. No other marks or clinical findings are detected on full examination. Her mother has not seen this mark before but thinks it might have happened during a nappy change.

What is the most likely diagnosis?

1. Accidental bruising
2. Birthmark
3. Henoch–Schönlein purpura

4. Meningococcal sepsis

5. Non-accidental injury

Q54

A 9 year old girl has been unwell for 2 days with a fever, sore throat and tiredness. This is associated with three tender nodes on the back of her neck and a macular pink-red rash. She is not vaccinated. She returned from a holiday to India 3 weeks ago. Her mum is currently pregnant. The GP is concerned about rubella.

Which of the following is the typical pattern of spread for the rubella rash?

1. Affects the hands and feet only

2. Causes Koplik spots in the mouth prior to the main rash developing

3. Causes painful lesions in the mouth and genitals

4. Starts behind the ears and on the face, then spreads over the whole body

5. Starts on the trunk and spreads to the extremities

Q55

An 8 year old boy has a runny nose and low-grade fever for 10 days. In the last 2 days he has developed a short hacking cough with brief 'whoop' sounds between coughs, where he struggles to get his breath at times. He is normally fit and well and has no drug allergies. The GP suspects whooping cough and prescribes clarithromycin for this.

How long does the patient need to be excluded from school according to the UK Health Security Agency?

1. 2 days

2. 5 days

3. 14 days

4. 21 days

5. No exclusion needed

Q56

A 10 week old baby boy is brought in by his mother to paediatric outpatient clinic with jaundice, vomiting and a fever. He has not been feeding well and has been passing clay-coloured stools. He shows no signs of sepsis. An urgent ultrasound scan of the liver is suggestive of biliary atresia.

What is the most appropriate next step in the management?

1. CT scan
2. Endoscopic retrograde cholangiopancreatography
3. Phototherapy
4. Refer to a specialist centre for operation
5. Refer to a transplant unit for liver transplantation

Q57

A 5 year old boy has 1 week of abdominal pain, arthralgia and palpable purpura of the legs. A diagnosis of Henoch-Schönlein purpura is made. Urinalysis and BP readings are sufficiently reassuring that the child does not require immediate referral to hospital. Analgesia is provided and appropriate follow-up is arranged.

Within what timeframe would you expect his symptoms to resolve?

1. 4–6 days
2. 24–48 hours
3. 4–6 weeks
4. 8–12 weeks
5. 4–6 months

Q58

A 3 year old boy has 6 days of fever that doesn't resolve with paracetamol or ibuprofen. This was initially associated with bilateral conjunctivitis without discharge. He is normally fit and well and up to date with the UK vaccination schedule.

He is miserable and irritable. His temperature is 39.1 °C, pulse 148 bpm, respiratory rate 38 breaths per minute, oxygen saturation 98% breathing air. He has cervical lymphadenopathy, a widespread erythematous rash on his hands and soles. Examination does not reveal a clear source of infection. Kawasaki disease is considered.

What is the most significant potential complication of this disorder?

1. Coronary arteritis
2. Glomerulonephritis
3. Liver failure

4. Meningoencephalitis
5. Myocarditis

Q59

A 3 week old, full-term male infant has increasingly forceful vomiting after feeding. He was initially diagnosed as having formula intolerance, but there has been no relief in his symptoms despite multiple changes to his formula. His vomit is non-bilious.

What is the most likely blood biochemistry result?

1. Hyperchloraemic hyperkalaemic metabolic acidosis
2. Hypochloraemic hyperkalaemic metabolic acidosis
3. Hypochloraemic hyperkalaemic metabolic alkalosis
4. Hypochloraemic hypokalaemic metabolic acidosis
5. Hypochloraemic hypokalaemic metabolic alkalosis

Q60

A 3 year old boy has a temperature of 38.9 °C. You diagnose a viral upper respiratory tract infection. On examination you have noticed he is very unkempt, has dirty fingernails, poor dental hygiene and dirty clothing. Mum is very tearful as her partner has been away working for the past 2 weeks and she is finding it difficult to manage the patient and her other child, a 6 month old girl. She has a history of depression.

What constitute the recognised triad of risk factors for child abuse?

1. Mental health, substance misuse, domestic violence
2. Mental health, substance misuse, low income
3. Mental health, substance misuse, single parent
4. Substance misuse, domestic violence, single parent
5. Substance misuse, low income, domestic violence

Q61

A 2 month old baby boy has been crying continuously for the last 2 hours. His parents describe him as a 'colicky' baby who is difficult to put down. He has been started on alginate raft-forming oral suspension by his GP due to vomiting after feeds. The pregnancy was unremarkable. He is breastfed and gaining weight, remaining on the 50th centile. He has regular wet and dirty nappies, with normal stool.

His temperature is 36.4 °C, pulse 120 bpm, respiratory rate 36 breaths per minute, oxygen saturation 98% breathing air. Examination is entirely unremarkable, and since being in the department he has stopped crying and taken a good breastfeed, after which he has a small posset but otherwise seems content.

What is the most appropriate course of action?

1. Commence dairy- and soya-free trial for mum
2. Commence omeprazole
3. CT head
4. Parental reassurance with consideration of prolonged period of observation
5. Partial septic screen and commence intravenous antibiotics

Q62

A 28 year old woman is 9 weeks pregnant. She is concerned because her sister died aged 14 years with cystic fibrosis. She and her parents are well and show no signs of the disease. The background chance of being a carrier in her community is 1 in 25.

What is the chance that she is a carrier for cystic fibrosis?

1. 1 (i.e. a certainty)
2. 1 in 2
3. 1 in 4
4. 1 in 25
5. 2 in 3

Q63

A 3 month old baby boy is taken by his parents to see his GP with a history of frequent vomiting occurring after every feed. He is breastfed and the vomits are mostly digested milk and are non-forceful. He sometimes seems a little uncomfortable after feeds but has no other symptoms. Examination shows he is gaining weight well, and appears developmentally normal.

What is the most appropriate management?

1. Advise changing to formula feeding with thickener
2. Advise mother to try a soya- and dairy-free diet
3. Commence omeprazole and refer for paediatric opinion

4. Reassure parents and advise his symptoms should improve with age
5. Request a barium swallow

Q64

An 8 week old baby girl is declared dead in her home. She was found unresponsive by her mother who was sleeping on the same bed as her 3 year old sibling. She was breastfed, was in good health with no preceding illness and was a second-born term baby. Her mother had an uncomplicated pregnancy, is a non-smoker and the family is not known to social services.

What is a risk factor for sudden unexpected death of this infant that you can identify from the information provided in the scenario?

1. Bed sharing
2. Breastfeeding
3. Room sharing
4. Second-born infant
5. Uncomplicated pregnancy

Q65

A 10 year old boy is brought to the GP by his parents. He has social anxiety, repetitive behaviours, and intellectual disability. He has a long face and large ears (a feature that neither the mother nor his father has).

What is the most likely diagnosis for this patient?

1. Attention deficit hyperactivity disorder (ADHD)
2. Autism spectrum disorder (ASD)
3. Down syndrome
4. Fragile X syndrome
5. Williams syndrome

Q66

A baby girl is delivered at 29-week gestation by caesarean section due to tailing growth with abnormal maternal dopplers. The anticipated birthweight is on the 2nd centile, and the mother has been given steroids and magnesium sulphate.

Which of the following approaches is most appropriate for very preterm (28–32 week) stabilisation?

1. Avoidance of optimal cord clamping, but non-invasive ventilatory support
2. Immediate intubation to administer surfactant
3. Non-invasive ventilatory support to ensure lung inflation, and withdrawal of active care if baby fails to respond
4. Optimal cord clamping, gentle ventilatory support, maintain normothermia, and consider surfactant administration
5. Prompt cardiopulmonary resuscitation for bradycardia, avoidance of hypothermia, early administration of resuscitation drugs

Q67

A 15 year old boy is concerned that he is shorter than his friends and has few signs of pubertal development.

He has occasional headaches which have been quite longstanding and unchanged. He sometimes associates these with exam stress or fatigue. They do not wake him at night and he has no associated vomiting. There has been no weight loss. He does well in school.

His height is on the 2nd centile for age, with expected weight for height; 4 years ago, he was between 25th and 50th centile for height. Systems examination including neurology are normal. His testicular volume is 3.5 ml.

What is the most likely diagnosis?

1. Acquired gonadal defect
2. CNS tumour
3. Constitutional delay of growth and puberty
4. Delayed puberty secondary to an underlying medical condition
5. Kleinfelter's syndrome

Q68

A 15 year old girl was brought to the GP as she has not yet started having periods. She has no other medical problems but does have additional support at school for learning difficulties. On examination she is short for her age, plotting below the 0.4th centile. She has a broad neck and widely spaced nipples with Tanner stage 1 breast development and Tanner stage 3 for pubic hair development, but an otherwise unremarkable examination.

What is the most likely diagnosis?

1. Congenital hypothyroidism
2. DiGeorge syndrome
3. Down syndrome
4. Klinefelter syndrome
5. Turner syndrome

Q69

An 8 month old girl has nausea and vomiting when she eats egg or egg products: 2 hours after ingestion, she develops an itchy area on her torso with occasional hives; this resolves after 1 hour. She has no previous medical history and is reaching her developmental milestones. Her father is concerned about immunisations considering her egg allergy.

What immunisations are appropriate to give her?

1. All of them
2. All of them, but MMR should be given as separate vaccines
3. All of them except MMR
4. All of them except nasal flu vaccination
5. No immunisations should be given

Dermatology

3

Q70

A 6 month old girl is brought to her general practitioner with a rash. She has been irritable and is refusing feeds. There is no significant past medical history, and she is fully immunised.

The child is drowsy, her temperature is 38.4 °C; she has a dark rash over her abdomen and on her right arm. The rash does not blanch.

You ask your receptionist to call for an emergency ambulance.

What is the most appropriate next course of action?

1. Administer intramuscular antibiotics
2. Administer rectal diazepam
3. Cannulate and set up fluids
4. Give oral paracetamol to bring down the temperature
5. Reassure the parents and wait for the ambulance

Q71

A 15 year old girl presents to dermatology outpatients. She has multiple comedones, papules and scarring acne over her face and upper back, which has been present for the last 2 years. This is affecting her confidence and self-esteem. She has taken adapalene and oral lymecycline with minimal improvement noted. She takes the combined oral contraceptive pill. Examination reveals severe acne.

Which treatment would be appropriate to start after careful counselling?

1. Isotretinoin
2. Laser treatment
3. Oral doxycycline
4. Topical azelaic acid
5. Topical benzoyl peroxide

Q72

A 22 year old man attends the dermatology outpatient clinic for severe atopic dermatitis, which he has had for the last 15 years. He has experienced numerous flares, with the last two resulting in hospital admissions for treatment of erythroderma. His mother suffers from asthma and his younger brother also has atopic dermatitis. Treatment with methotrexate is considered.

Which class of drug is methotrexate?

1. Alkylating agent
2. Anthracycline
3. Antimetabolite
4. Vinca alkaloid
5. Xanthine oxidase inhibitor

Q73

A 46 year old woman has abnormal thickening and opacification of most of her toe nails. She has treated this with over-the-counter medication but the appearance has not improved.

Which is the most appropriate diagnostic test?

1. Beta-D-mannan antigen test
2. Blood culture
3. Skin culture
4. Skin scraping and microscopy using KOH
5. Urease test

Q74

A 37 year old woman has a 2 mm ulcerated lesion in the right supra alar crease for the last 5 months. She works as a catalogue model in the Caribbean and is Fitzpatrick skin type 1. A nodular basal cell carcinoma is suspected.

What is the most appropriate treatment?

1. CO_2 laser
2. Curettage and cautery
3. Mohs micrographic surgery

4. Reassure and discharge
5. Two cycles of cryotherapy

Q75

A 32 year old woman has 6 months of an enlarging lump on her left earlobe. The lump is now 1.5 x 1.5 x 2 cm, hard and rubbery in texture, with no breaks in the overlying skin (see Figure 3.1). She had a similar lump surgically removed from the same ear 2 years ago.

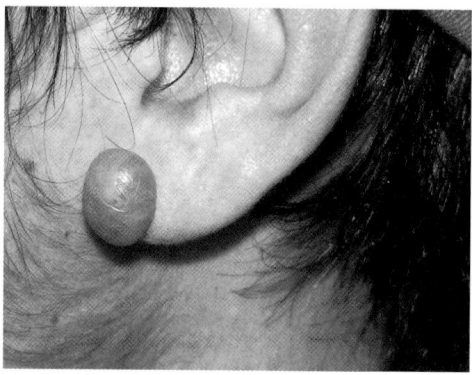

Figure 3.1 Image reproduced with permission from ©DermNet www.derm netnz.org.

Which is the most likely diagnosis?
1. Keloid scarring
2. Keratoacanthoma
3. Lipoma
4. Sebaceous cyst
5. Squamous cell carcinoma

Q76

A 45 year old man has 4 days of a swollen erythematous right calf. The redness started just above his ankle and is now tracking towards his knee. He has poorly controlled type 2 diabetes.

He looks systemically well. His temperature is 37.9 °C, pulse 94 bpm, BP130/70 mmHg, respiratory rate 16 breaths per minute, oxygen saturation 98% breathing air. The affected calf is erythematous, tender and warm to touch.

What is the most appropriate next management?

1. Admit for a fasciotomy
2. Commence appropriate oral antibiotics
3. CT pulmonary angiogram
4. Reassure
5. Ventilation/perfusion lung scan

Q77

A 22 year old woman has a new painful vesicular erythematous rash over the palmar aspect of both hands, with patchy dermatitis over the dorsum. She started a new job as a hair stylist and colourist in a salon 4 weeks ago. She is usually fit and well but suffered with atopic dermatitis as a child. Patch testing reveals a contact allergy to the paraphenylene-diamine (PPD) chemical found in hair dyes or irritants in shampoos/conditioners.

Which kind of hypersensitivity reaction is she most likely to be suffering from?

1. Complex mediated
2. Type I
3. Type II
4. Type III
5. Type IV

Q78

A 16 year old boy has common warts on both his hands. He is embarrassed about them and has stopped going into school due to fear of his warts being noticed.

What is the first-line treatment in managing this boy's warts?

1. Cryotherapy
2. Immunotherapy
3. Recommend topical salicylic acid paints
4. Surgical excision under local anaesthetic
5. Watch and wait

Q79

An 18 year old woman has 6 weeks of an intermittent self-resolving pruritic, asymmetrical rash, which she describes as non-tender 'bumps' typically appearing over her torso and limbs. The rash resolves after a few hours. She denies any facial/oropharyngeal oedema. Today her skin is clear. There are no other comorbidities of note, and no allergies. She is currently completing her A-level exams. The history and clinical images indicate a diagnosis of urticaria. She has been taking one 180 mg fexofenadine a day without any relief.

What treatment would be indicated next?

1. Advise a dairy-free diet
2. Increase fexofenadine to 180 mg four times a day
3. Start flucloxacillin 1 g four times a day for 7 days
4. Start ibuprofen 400 mg three times a day
5. Start prednisolone 30 mg daily for 10 days

Q80

An 8 year old girl has itchiness and irritation in her scalp for the last 2 months. There are small 1 mm white grains on the shaft of some of her hairs.

What is the most likely diagnosis?

1. Atopic dermatitis
2. Head lice
3. Scalp folliculitis
4. Scalp psoriasis
5. Tinea capitis

Q81

A 60 year old man has a changed mole on his mid back which his wife noticed had increased in size and pigmentation over the preceding 6 months. There is a pigmented macular lesion on the mid back with varying pigmentation and blue-white veil on dermoscopy. There is an enlarged lymph node in the left axilla. There is no hepatosplenomegaly.

Which malignant melanoma subtype has the patient presented with?

1. Acral lentiginous melanoma
2. Amelanotic melanoma

3. Lentigo maligna melanoma
4. Nodular melanoma
5. Superficial spreading melanoma

Q82

A 3 year old boy has 5 days of a golden, crusting, oozing lesion over the left malar region of his face, associated with a flare of facial atopic dermatitis. He is eating and drinking normally. He is irritable but observations are normal. A skin swab is taken.

What is the most appropriate management?

1. Hospitalisation for intravenous antibiotics
2. Mildly potent topical steroid applied to the area
3. No treatment
4. Oral flucloxacillin
5. Topical application of fusidic acid

Q83

A 17 year old woman has evolving, widespread and bilateral pinpoint scaly plaques over her upper/lower limbs and torso with no nail involvement. This has been present for 2 weeks; 3 weeks ago she had a sore throat and non-productive cough. Her ASO titre is positive for group A streptococcal infection.

What is the most likely diagnosis?

1. Chronic plaque psoriasis
2. Erythrodermic psoriasis
3. Flexural psoriasis
4. Guttate psoriasis
5. Palmoplantar psoriasis

Q84

A 54 year old man has 3 weeks of generalised pruritis, particularly worse at night. He has been frequently applying a topical emollient which has made no difference to his symptoms. There is no past medical history of comorbidities or dermatological illness. On examination, there are several excoriation marks over the torso and groin and widespread erythematous papules. In the interdigital web spaces, there are burrows.

What is the most appropriate management?

1. Oral B12 and folate supplementation to continue for life
2. Oral fexofenadine for 4 weeks
3. Oral flucloxacillin for 1 week
4. Oral prednisolone for 1 week
5. Topical permethrin 5% cream once weekly for 2 weeks

Q85

A 5 year old girl has a dark rash for 48 hours. She is clinically well, having had an upper respiratory infection a few weeks ago. There is no history of pain, diarrhoeal illness or abdominal or joint symptoms. Her temperature is 36.4 °C, pulse 104 bpm, oxygen saturation 98% breathing air. There are widespread non-blanching petechiae over her torso and extremities. There is no hepatosplenomegaly nor signs of anaemia. Investigations:

Isolated low platelet count

What is the most likely diagnosis?

1. Acute leukaemia
2. Haemolytic uraemic syndrome
3. Henoch-Schönlein purpura
4. Immune thrombocytopenia
5. Sepsis

Q86

A 55 year old man has a tender ulcerating keratotic lesion on his left forearm, which he noticed 3 weeks ago. He underwent a renal transplant over 10 years ago for glomerulonephritis. He works as a crop farmer but generally covers up when outside. His mother died of malignant melanoma, aged 43 years. He is a smoker with a 30 pack year history. He denies ever living abroad. He takes azathioprine. He is Fitzpatrick skin type 3.

Which risk factor from the patient's history most contributes to his risk for the development of further skin cancers?

1. Excessive sun exposure
2. Family history
3. Immunosuppression

4. Pesticide exposure
5. Smoking

Q87

A 6 year old boy has a fever and rash for 3 days. On examination, he has erythematous rashes on both cheeks with sparing of nasal ridge, which is followed by a pink lace-like or network-pattern rash on the limbs.

Which of the following is the most likely diagnosis?

1. Chickenpox
2. Erythema infectiosum
3. Herpes virus infection
4. Pityriasis rosea
5. Scabies

Q88

A 24 year old woman is stung by a bee on her arm. She experiences intense pain.

After a few minutes, she develops an itchy rash all over her trunk, face and arms. 15 minutes later, she has a 'tight' feeling in her throat and is breathing heavily. She has hayfever and takes antihistamines when required. Her temperature is 37.2 °C, pulse 108 bpm, BP 110/85 mmHg. She is given intramuscular adrenaline with improvement in her symptoms.

What is the most appropriate next step in her management?

1. Administer oral antihistamine and send patient home
2. Admit to a general medical ward for observation and referral to immunology specialist
3. Admit to ITU for close observation
4. Send patient home and advise to attend the emergency department if she feels unwell again
5. Send patient home and advise to see her GP for follow-up with an EpiPen prescription

Q89

A 62 year old man is admitted, having been burnt in a house fire. He has a mixture of superficial and deep dermal burns over an estimated 36% of his total body surface area.

He is normally fit and well. His weight is 75 kg.

How much fluid should he receive in the first 8 hours of his hospital stay?

1. 270 mLs
2. 1000 mLs
3. 2700 mLs
4. 5400 mLs
5. As much as he wants to drink

Q90

A 15 year old boy has a solitary nodule on his right shoulder. His temperature is 36.4 °C. The nodule is raised 0.7 mm and has central core of pus. The surrounding skin appears red and is tender to the touch.

What is the most appropriate management of this condition?

1. Incision and drainage
2. No management needed
3. Oral flucloxacillin
4. Surgical excision
5. Topical benzoyl peroxide

Q91

A 42 year old woman has 4 months of erythema and pruritus of her hands associated with stinging, burning and pain. She has asthma but seldom uses her inhalers. Her observations are normal. She has areas of weeping, discharge and crusting on her hands. She denies changes to her daily routine – more specifically, she has not used new detergents. She does not have pets. She works as a hairdresser. What is the most relevant investigation?

1. Patch test
2. Radioallergoabsorbance test
3. Serum IgE
4. Skin biopsy
5. Skin swab for MC&S

Q92

A 60 year old black man has 4 weeks of a new pigmentation in the right ring finger. He is a retired farmer. He denies any pain at the site or bleeding. On examination there is black/ purple streak extending to the proximal nail fold. Hutchinson's sign is positive.

What would be your next management step?

1. Multiple site biopsy followed by surgical excision
2. Obtain a nail clipping
3. Reassure and discharge
4. Treat with cryotherapy
5. Treat with penicillin-based antibiotics

Q93

An 89 year old woman develops a grade 4 pressure ulcer over her right buttock. She is housebound and immobile. She has type 2 diabetes.

What is the definition of a grade 4 ulcer?

1. Exposure of deep structures, e.g. bones or tendons
2. Formation of eschars
3. Full-thickness skin loss exposing subcutaneous fat
4. Non-blanchable erythema of intact skin
5. Partial-thickness skin loss which involves the epidermis

Q94

A 70 year old man has a generalised itch for 2 years, with no rash or other associated symptoms. An initial screen could find no obvious underlying cause for the itch and he was diagnosed with idiopathic generalised pruritus.

What is the best first-line treatment for this patient?

1. A course of oral prednisolone
2. Aqueous menthol 1% cream and non-sedating antihistamines
3. Referral to dermatology for consideration of UVB therapy
4. Topical capsaicin cream
5. Topical steroids and an emollient

Q95

A 36 year old man has a swelling in his back which is 3 x 2 cm in size. It is fixed to his skin.

What is the most likely diagnosis?

1. Dermoid cyst
2. Melanoma
3. Sebaceous cyst
4. Seborrhoeic keratosis
5. Wart

Q96

A 70 year old man has a 4 x 5 cm ulceration on his left lower calf from a gardening injury. The resulting ulcer has increased in size and is now very tender. On examination, the ulcer has undermined edges and violaceous hue.

What is the likely diagnosis?

1. Basal cell carcinoma
2. Pyoderma gangrenosum
3. Squamous cell carcinoma
4. Vasculitis
5. Venous ulceration

Q97

A 47 year old woman has a swelling at the back of the neck for 6 years' duration. On examination, it is a 2 x 2 cm, soft, mobile, rubbery, non-tender swelling. There is no lymphadenopathy.

What is the likely diagnosis?

1. Abscess
2. Epidermoid cyst
3. Ganglion
4. Lipoma
5. Skin abscess

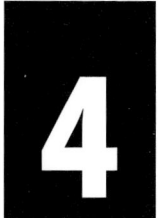

Ear, Nose and Throat

Q98

A 3 year old boy attends the emergency department with inspiratory stridor. He has been unwell for the last 12 hours and has avoided eating and drinking. He has had no routine childhood immunisations.

On examination, the child is sat upright, looks unwell, his temperature is 39.5 °C, pulse 154 bpm, respiratory rate 32 breaths per minute. He is drooling and is agitated by any attempts to examine him or administer treatment.

What is the next most appropriate step?

1. Administer high-flow oxygen via reservoir mask
2. Bloods for FBC, U&E, CRP
3. Chest X-ray
4. Examine pharynx using tongue depressor
5. Urgent ENT and ITU involvement

Q99

A 35 year old man has 12 weeks of reduction in his sense of smell. He has had pain and pressure in his left ear for the last 8 weeks, nasal blockage and facial pain for the last 6 weeks, and postnasal drip for 4 weeks.

Which of the above is considered a part of the diagnostic criteria for chronic rhinosinusitis?

1. Facial pain or pressure lasting 6 weeks
2. Nasal blockage lasting 6 weeks
3. Otalgia lasting 8 weeks
4. Postnasal drip for 4 weeks
5. Reduction or loss of sense of smell lasting 12 weeks

Q100

A 65 year old man is referred to ENT with ongoing episodes of epistaxis which have failed to resolve with simple measures at home. He takes warfarin. On examination, you find the source is Little's area / Kiesselbach's plexus in the left nostril.

Which of the following arteries contribute to this area?

1. Anterior ethmoid artery
2. Anterior sphenopalatine artery
3. Lateral nasal artery
4. Ophthalmic artery
5. Superficial temporal artery

Q101

A 47 year old woman has acute vertigo lasting 30–40 minutes. It is associated with the sensation of losing balance and she has tinnitus.

Which of the following signs would suggest that this is cerebellar disease rather than Ménière's disease?

1. Aural fullness
2. Dysdiadochokinesia
3. Hearing loss
4. Tinnitus
5. Vertigo

Q102

A 56 year old woman is tired all the time and has difficulty concentrating. She falls asleep when watching TV at home and snores loudly. She drives a lorry for work and almost fell asleep whilst driving 2 weeks ago. She is asthmatic, obese and had a thyroidectomy 5 years ago.

Which is her most significant risk factor for obstructive sleep apnoea?

1. Asthma
2. Female sex
3. Obesity
4. Sleeping prone
5. Thyroidectomy

Q103

A 2 year old boy has otalgia, fevers and lethargy. On otoscopy, the tympanic membrane is erythematous with loss of light reflex.

Which of the following is a complication associated with this condition?

1. Mastoiditis
2. Paralysis
3. Parapharyngeal abscess
4. Stroke
5. Visual loss

Q104

An 18 year old woman presents to the emergency department with fever, headaches and difficulty swallowing due to a sore throat. Her tonsils are enlarged with a whitish membrane. She has bilateral cervical lymphadenopathy. There is no trismus or any sign of an upper airway obstruction.

What is the most appropriate investigation?

1. Arterial blood gases
2. Chlamydia screen
3. Full blood count and Monospot test
4. Throat swab
5. Ultrasound of the neck

Q105

A 38 year old man has 3 days of earache and muffled hearing on his right side. His observations are normal; the right ear canal is erythematous and exudes clear fluid; the left canal appears normal.

What is the most likely microbiological cause of his otitis externa?

1. Aspergillus niger
2. Haemophilus influenza B
3. Staphylococcus aureus
4. Streptococcus pyogenes
5. Treponema pallidum

Q106

A 62 year old man is brought into the emergency department with a sudden-onset dizziness, nausea, vomiting and unsteadiness that morning. He has atrial fibrillation and poorly controlled type 2 diabetes mellitus.

His basic observations are normal; he has diplopia, homonymous hemianopia and nystagmus. He is also generally ataxic; he has dysdiadochokinesia and dysmetria.

What is the most likely diagnosis?

1. Benign paroxysmal positional vertigo
2. Ménière's disease
3. Posterior circulation ischaemia
4. Postural hypotension
5. Vestibular neuritis

Q107

A 75 year old man has 6 weeks of severe otalgia with copious otorrhoea. He has tried topical drops but his symptoms are worsening and he feels feverish. He has COPD, type 2 diabetes mellitus and hypertension.

His temperature is 38.9 °C, pulse 102 bpm, BP 110/70 mmHg, oxygen saturation 98% breathing air. He is extremely tender on palpation of the mastoid process region. Otoscopy shows an erythematous auditory canal with significant granulation tissue on the right.

What is the most likely causative organism?

1. Haemophilus influenzae
2. Herpes simplex
3. Pseudomonas aeruginosa
4. Staphylococcus aureus
5. Streptococcus pneumoniae

Q108

A 25 year old man has 3 days of a sore throat, myalgia and fever. On examination, he has enlarged tonsils and cervical lymphadenopathy.

Which of the following viruses is most commonly associated with his condition?

1. Epstein–Barr virus
2. Hepatitis A virus
3. Herpes zoster virus
4. Paramyxovirus
5. Parvovirus B19

Q109

A 25 year old woman presents to the ENT clinic with gradual increase in hearing loss in her left ear, following the birth of her son a year ago. This is associated with tinnitus but not vertigo. She has no history of recurrent ear infections. She gives a family history of her mother having similar hearing loss. She is worried that she will become completely deaf in her left ear. Pure tone audiogram shows mild to moderate degree of conductive hearing loss, especially in low frequencies.

What is the most likely diagnosis?

1. Congenital cholesteatoma
2. Impacted wax
3. Otosclerosis
4. Superior semi-circular canal dehiscence
5. Traumatic perforation of the tympanic membrane

Q110

A 60 year old man has a hoarse voice and neck lump. He has had progressive dysphonia over 6 months with otalgia and breathlessness. He takes alginate raft-forming oral suspension intermittently for reflux but otherwise no medications. He has a 50 pack year history and drinks half a bottle of whisky per day.

What is the next most appropriate step?

1. 2-week-wait referral to ENT
2. Antireflux treatment
3. MR scan of the neck
4. Thyroplasty
5. Voice therapy

Q111

A 51 year old man has an acute-onset sore throat. He has a history of ulcerative colitis and takes weekly methotrexate. He has tried self-care in form of gargles and pain relief. His temperature is 36.7 °C. He has enlarged tonsils with white exudate.

What is the most likely diagnosis?

1. Glandular fever
2. Herpes simplex infection
3. Laryngitis
4. Pharyngitis
5. Streptococcal tonsillitis

Q112

A 77 year old man has 4 weeks of persistent right-sided nasal obstruction and mucous discharge. He has had four episodes of unilateral epistaxis, always from the right nasal cavity. His sense of smell is intact, he has had no headaches, numbness, or any ocular symptoms. He is an ex-smoker (20 years ago).

A nasal examination with an otoscope revealed a fleshy mass in the right nasal cavity.

Which is the most appropriate management for this patient?

1. 2-week fast-track referral to ENT
2. Nasal douching
3. No treatment, but review in another 2 weeks if not better
4. Oral antibiotic
5. Steroid nasal spray

Q113

A 42 year old woman has a slowly progressive hearing loss in her right ear. For the last 4 weeks she has had episodes of vertigo and tinnitus. She is known to have neurofibromatosis type 2. An acoustic neuroma is suspected.

What is the most appropriate investigation for acoustic neuroma?

1. Computed tomography
2. Flexible nasoendoscopy
3. Magnetic resonance imaging

4. Nerve function tests

5. Pure tone audiometry

Q114

A 42 year old woman has 10 days of intermittent dizziness. This is typified by profound dizziness lasting approximately 30 seconds on each occasion. The episodes occur when she sits up in bed and on looking up to the sky. Benign paroxysmal positional vertigo (BPPV) is suspected.

Which of the following tests is useful in diagnosing BPPV?

1. Active compression test

2. Allen's test

3. Buerger's test

4. Dix–Hallpike test

5. Ortolani's test

Q115

A 65 year old woman presents to general practice with a sudden-onset left ear pain, headache and blurred vision. The eardrum and canal are normal with normal light reflex.

A diagnosis of giant cell arteritis is considered.

What would be the best plan of action?

1. Routine referral to ophthalmologist

2. Routine referral to rheumatology

3. Treat with steroids and review in 1 week's time

4. Urgent referral to ophthalmologist

5. Urgent referral to rheumatology

Q116

A 34 year old man presents to his general practitioner with more than 6 months of snoring. This is associated with tiredness in the morning, headaches, daytime sleepiness. His wife has mentioned to him that he stops breathing sometimes while snoring. He does not smoke. He drinks approximately 16 units of alcohol in a week. His BMI is 33 kg/m^2. His neck collar size is 44 cm. His Epworth Sleepiness Scale score is 18/24.

What is the most likely next step in the management of this patient?

1. Prescribe sleeping tablets for him and his wife
2. Reassure the patient that no treatment is needed
3. Referral for gastric bypass surgery
4. Referral to sleep apnoea clinic
5. Urgent ENT referral

Q117

A 54 year old man has an irritation and a lump in his throat for the last 4 months. He tends to get a sore throat on the right side and has experienced some hoarseness and right earache on swallowing. He has started to choke on his food recently. He has smoked 15 cigarettes per day for the last 30 years, and drinks on average 20 units of alcohol per week.

What is the single most appropriate management for this patient?

1. 2-week-wait referral to ENT
2. Adequate hydration and vocal tract hygiene
3. Arrange CT scan of head and neck
4. Refer urgently to a speech and language therapist
5. Start omeprazole

Q118

A 17 year old girl has 1 day of acute dysphagia associated with sore throat, pyrexia and hoarse voice. There is no stridor. She is not managing to keep fluids down. She has no previous medical history, is on the oral contraceptive pill and there is no significant family history. She has palpable lymphadenopathy. There is significant trismus.

What is the likely diagnosis?

1. Foreign body
2. Glandular fever
3. Malignancy
4. Peritonsillar abscess
5. Supraglottitis

Q119

A 36 year old woman is seen in the ENT clinic with 6 months of episodes of rotatory dizziness, associated with nausea and vomiting.

Each episode lasts from 1 to 3 hours. In each of these episodes, she goes to bed and cannot do her work for the rest of the day. In addition, she also has fluctuating hearing loss in her right ear, with tinnitus and feeling of fullness. Otoscopic examination revealed normal external auditory canals and tympanic membranes.

What is the most likely diagnosis?

1. Acoustic neuroma
2. Benign paroxysmal positional vertigo
3. Ménière's disease
4. Otitis media
5. Vestibular labyrinthitis

Q120

A 55 year old man has unilateral right-ear tinnitus for 6 months. He denies hearing loss or vertigo. MRI of the internal acoustic meatus reveals a 10 mm-sized vestibular schwannoma.

Which of the following options is the most appropriate management?

1. Repeat the scan in 9 months' time
2. Stage the tumour by extending the MRI to whole of the CNS
3. Stereotactic radiosurgery
4. Surgical resection via retrosigmoid approach
5. Surgical resection via translabyrinthine approach

Q121

A 55 year old woman has 4 weeks of reduced smell. She has hayfever, Raynaud's and hypertension. She takes lisinopril, nifedipine and loratadine, and has recently received doxycycline and nasal steroid for sinusitis, which has now resolved. There is no sign of congestion.

Which of her recent medications is a possible cause of her anosmia?

1. Doxycycline
2. Intranasal steroids
3. Lisinopril
4. Loratadine
5. Nifedipine

Endocrine

5

Q122

A 52 year old woman has 3 months of weight loss, nausea and abdominal pain. This has been associated with general malaise, fatigue and occasional dizziness when getting up. She has a past history of tuberculosis 20 years ago.

Her temperature is 36.6 °C, BP 85/63 mmHg, pulse 56 bpm. Her skin has hyperpigmentation on her waist, hands and neck.

Investigations:

Na+ 132 mmol/L (135–146)

K+ 4.5 mmol/L (3.5–5.0)

eGFR 52 ml/min (> 60)

Cortisol serum level at 9 a.m., 68 nmol/L (138–635)

ACTH 56 nmol/L (1.3–16.7)

Glucose (fasting) 2.5 mmol/L (4.0–5.9)

TFTs were normal

What is the first line of management of this patient?

1. Admit to hospital urgently
2. Adrenal biopsy
3. Adrenocorticotropic hormone stimulation test
4. Prescribe hydrocortisone
5. Prescribe tuberculostatic medication

Q123

A 78 year old woman presented to the emergency department with 2 days of uncontrolled diarrhoea and vomiting. She has heart failure.

Her pulse is 106 bpm, BP 95/62 mmHg. She looks pale and drowsy, she weighs 65 kg.

Investigations:

Hb 162 (130–180 g/L)

WCC 9.2 (4–10 x 10^9/L)

Urea 17 (2.5–7.8 mmol/L)

Creatinine 172 (59–104 µmol/L)

Sodium 152 (133–146 mmol/L)

Potassium 2.9 (3.5–5.3 mmol/L)

Lactate 3.2 (0.63–2.44 mmol/L)

What would be the appropriate fluid treatment in this patient?

1. 2.5 L Hartmann's prescribed over 48 hours
2. Encourage oral fluids
3. Immediate 1 litre of 0.9% NaCl with 40 mmol KCl
4. Immediate 250 ml Hartmann's and reassessment
5. Immediate 500 ml 0.9% NaCl followed by 1 L Hartmann's over 2 hours

Q124

A 45 year old man has 2 months of excessive urination and nocturia. Despite frequent drinking, he is very thirsty all the time. He has bipolar disorder treated with lithium. He has no family history of diabetes mellitus. His BMI is 26 kg/m^2.

Investigations:

Serum sodium 146 mmol/L (135–145)

Urine output 4.2 L/day

Plasma osmolality 315 mosm/kg

Urine osmolality 270 mosm/kg

Plasma copeptin 23.5 pmol/L (< 21.4)

What is the likely diagnosis?

1. Complete central diabetes insipidus
2. Complete nephrogenic diabetes insipidus
3. Partial central diabetes insipidus
4. Partial nephrogenic diabetes insipidus
5. Primary polydipsia

Q125

A 46 year old woman has 4 months of poor mental health, weight gain and loss of libido. At the same time, she noticed persistent bruising and prolonged healing. Her BP is 145/95 mmHg, pulse 86 bpm, temperature normal. She does not take any medication. Her face appears to be puffy and there is visible central obesity.

Reference values for free serum cortisol level at 6–8 a.m. is 140 to 690 nmol/L; salivary cortisol concentration, 15.5 +/− 0.8 nmol/L; urinary free cortisol 120–384 nmol/day.

Which of the following results is most indicative of Cushing's syndrome?

1. Dexamethasone suppression test (1 mg) shows serum free cortisol 35 nmol/L at 8 a.m. next morning
2. Morning salivary cortisol level is normal, but at midnight is low
3. Random serum (at 16.00) cortisol level 96 nmol/L
4. Serum 9 a.m. cortisol 600 nmol/L
5. Urinary free cortisol 2765 nmol/day

Q126

A 38 year old man has a 2 month history of tiredness, weight loss and polydipsia. He has vomited in the waiting room and appears dehydrated. His pulse is 80 bpm, BP 110/80 mmHg, BMI is 28 kg/m^2. Random capillary glucose is 18.4 mmol/L.

Which of the following is the most appropriate next step?

1. Arrange urgent plasma C-peptide
2. Check urgent HbA1c
3. Measurement of capillary blood ketones
4. Refer to diabetes team
5. Start metformin

Q127

A 55 year old woman has fatigue, generalised body ache and abdominal pain. She has a history of non-obstructing renal stones and has recently been commenced on sertraline for low mood. She had a recent DEXA scan which suggested osteoporosis.

Investigations:

Haemoglobin 136 g/L (130–175)

White blood cells 5.6 x 10^9/l (3.6–9.2)

Sodium 132 mmol/L (133–146)

Potassium 5.1 mmol/L (3.5–5.3)

Magnesium 0.72 mmol/L (0.7–1)

Calcium 2.66 mmol/L (2.1–2.55)

Parathyroid hormone 7.0 pmol/L (1.6–7.2)

Phosphate mmol/L 0.6 (0.8–1.5)

Liver function tests normal

eGFR 70 ml/min/1.73 m^2 (> 90)

Ultrasound abdomen showed a non-obstructing renal calculus in left kidney.

What is the likely unifying diagnosis?

1. Hypercalcaemia secondary to primary hyperparathyroidism
2. Hyperkalaemia
3. Hypophosphatemia
4. Hypovolaemic hyponatraemia
5. Renal failure secondary to renal stones

Q128

A 27 year old man with known type 1 diabetes has been unwell for a few days and has been brought to hospital by his partner as he is very drowsy and has been vomiting and is unable to give his own insulin. He is too drowsy to give any further history and is able to follow commands. His BP is 110/65 mmHg, heart rate 110 bpm and respiratory rate 28 breaths per minute. His capillary blood glucose is 26 mmol/L, blood ketones 7 mmol/L, and venous blood gas show a pH of 7.1.

What is the best next step in management?

1. Prescribe intravenous fluid and give his usual subcutaneous insulin
2. Prescribe 0.9% normal saline along with a fixed-rate intravenous insulin infusion
3. Prescribe 0.9% normal saline along with a variable-rate intra-venous insulin infusion
4. Give a bolus of intravenous insulin followed by his usual sub-cutaneous insulin

5. Give a bolus of intravenous insulin followed by a fixed-rate intravenous insulin infusion

Q129

A 75 year old man presents to his general practitioner with a history of fatigue and general malaise. His appetite has been poor and he has lost a stone in weight over the previous 6 weeks. He has a blood test, the results of which are shown below, and is referred urgently to hospital.

Investigations:

Sodium	140 mmol/L (133–146)
Potassium	4.5 mmol/L (3.5–5.3)
Urea	8.2 mmol/L (2.5–7.8)
Creatinine	135 mmol/L (45–84)
Parathyroid hormone	0.8 pmol/L (1.6–6.9)

What is the most appropriate initial treatment?

1. Give zolendronate 4 mg IV
2. Give pamidronate 60 mg IV
3. Rehydrate with intravenous fluids for 24 hours
4. Start calcitonin 100 units sc every 8 hours
5. Treat with intravenous fluids and a loop diuretic

Q130

A 50 year old woman has a sudden-onset epigastric pain radiating through to the back, associated with nausea and vomiting. She is a non-smoker; she drinks approximately 12–14 units alcohol per week. On examination, she is obese (BMI is 34 kg/m^2), there are eruptive xanthomas over the extensor surface of the arms and epigastric tenderness on palpation of the abdomen. Electrocardiogram and chest X-ray are normal. An abdominal ultrasound shows changes consistent with fatty liver and normal appearance of the biliary tree.

Investigations:

Random blood glucose 23 mmol/L (3–7.8 mmol/L)

HbA1c 100 mmol/mol

TSH 1.06 mIU/L (normal range 0.35–4.5 mIU/L)

Cholesterol 9.0 mmol/L (normal range 0–5 mmol/L)

Triglycerides 25.9 mmol/L (normal range 0–2.3 mmol/L)

Troponin 5.9 ng/L (normal range 0–14ng/L)

Amylase 1500 IU/L (normal range 28–100 IU/L)

CRP 60 mg/L (normal < 6 mg/L)

What is the most likely diagnosis?

1. Cholecystitis
2. Hypertriglyceridemia-induced pancreatitis
3. Myocardial infarction
4. Pneumonia
5. Ruptured aortic aneurysm

Q131

A 72 year old man has been sweaty and agitated for the last 20 minutes. He has congestive cardiac failure, chronic kidney disease and type 1 diabetes. He is an inpatient after being admitted with a cough. He is conscious, alert and compliant. His temperature is 37.9 °C, pulse 94 bpm, BP 136/60 mmHg. He has scattered crepitations in his chest. His capillary blood sugar is 2.9 mmol/L.

What is the most appropriate next step in the management of this patient?

1. Administer intramuscular 1 mg glucagon
2. Administer intravenous 10% glucose at 200 ml over 15 minutes
3. Administer orally 15–20 g fast-acting carbohydrate
4. Arrange urgent chest X-ray
5. Urgently take blood cultures and administer paracetamol

Q132

An 83 year old woman is brought to the emergency department by ambulance having been found collapsed at home by her family. She has hypertension, ischaemic heart disease and type 2 diabetes that is usually well managed with diet. She responds to voice, and has a temperature of 35.1 °C, heart rate 150 bpm, BP 100/60 mmHg. Her capillary blood glucose is too high to measure.

Investigations:

Na 154 mmol/L (137–144)

K 4.6 mmol/L (3.5–4.9)

Urea 22 mmol/L (2.5–7.5)

Creatinine 190 μmol/L (60–110)

Plasma glucose 45 mmol/L (3.0–7.8)

Which of the following is the most appropriate management plan?

1. Prescribe 0.45% sodium chloride along with a fixed-rate intravenous insulin infusion

2. Prescribe 0.45% sodium chloride and give 10 units of actrapid subcutaneously

3. Prescribe 0.9% sodium chloride and give 10 units of actrapid subcutaneously

4. Prescribe 0.9% sodium chloride over 1 hour along with a fixed-rate intravenous insulin infusion

5. Prescribe 0.9% sodium chloride over 1 hour along with a variable-rate intravenous insulin infusion

Q133

A 68 year old man has 3 weeks of excessive thirst, associated with increased frequency of urination which is now disrupting his sleep. He has also noticed general fatigue, and unintentional loss of about 1 stone in weight over the past month despite a good appetite. He has no past medical history of note and is on no medication. He occasionally consumes up to 2 pints of cider at the weekend. He has a family history of heart disease and diabetes mellitus. His temperature and other parameters are normal.

Investigations:

Normal blood counts

Serum sodium 131 mmol/l (137–144)

Potassium 3.8 mmol/l (3.5–4.9)

eGFR 76

Random glucose 14 mmol/l (3.0–7.8)

Ketones 0.3 mmol/L (< 0.6)

What is the most likely cause for his excessive thirst and fatigue?

1. Alcohol excess

2. Diabetes mellitus

3. Diabetes insipidus

4. Hyponatremia

5. Psychogenic polydipsia

Q134

A 65 year old woman has a routine blood test, the results of which are shown below. She has a history of hypertension and diabetes and takes a combination of metformin, lisinopril and amlodipine tablets.

sodium	136 mmol/L (133–146)
potassium	4.5 mmol/L (3.5–5.3)
urea	5.4 mmol/L (2.5–7.8)
creatinine	69 μmol/L (45–84)
calcium	2.65 mmol/L (2.2–2.6)

A repeat calcium is 2.7.

What is the next most appropriate investigation?

1. CT thorax, abdomen and pelvis

2. Myeloma screen

3. Parathyroid hormone

4. Serum ACE

5. Vitamin D

Q135

An 88 year old woman is admitted to the emergency department with extensive bruising and confusion. She sustained a fall with a long lie of up to 14 hours. Her daughter saw her earlier the same day and reported she was well. She takes sertraline for depression.

Her temperature is 30.8 °C, pulse 42 bpm, BP 116/60 mmHg, respiratory rate 13 breaths per minute, oxygen saturation 87% breathing air. There is no obvious internal injury, spinal fracture or acute intracranial pathology.

What is the most appropriate initial management?

1. Assess the patient using an ABCDE approach, and consider whether this could be serotonin syndrome or neuroleptic malignant syndrome

2. Assess the patient using an ABCDE approach, apply blankets and a bear hugger, commence warmed intravenous infusion, and consider sepsis six treatment and analgesia

3. Assess the patient using an ABCDE approach, give paracetamol, perform an electrocardiogram and give a stat dose of atropine
4. No immediate action required; admit patient to the medical ward for monitoring
5. Start intravenous antibiotics immediately without further assessment

Q136

A 35 year old woman has 3 months of generalised tiredness, dry skin and feeling cold. She has been finding it difficult to concentrate lately and has gained 7 kg in weight. Primary hypothyroidism is suspected and blood tests requested.

Which of the following results is most likely?

1. High thyroid-stimulating hormone (TSH) and low T4
2. High TSH and high T4
3. Low TSH and high T4
4. Low TSH and low T4
5. Normal TSH, normal T4

Q137

A 33 year old woman requests a prescription for orlistat to help with weight loss. She has been trying to exercise more but finds it difficult and recently her weight has plateaued. She has a history of cholestasis, hypercholesterolaemia, non-alcoholic fatty liver disease, polycystic ovary syndrome (PCOS) and type 2 diabetes mellitus. Her BMI is now 34 kg/m^2.

Which of her conditions would be a contraindication for orlistat use?

1. Cholestasis
2. Hypercholesterolaemia
3. Non-alcoholic fatty liver disease
4. PCOS
5. Type 2 diabetes mellitus

Q138

A 65 year old woman presents to the emergency department following a seizure. She has a history of dyspepsia and hypertension. She takes atorvastatin, bendroflumethiazide, bisoprolol, lisinopril and omeprazole.

Investigations:

Serum sodium 143 mmol/L (133–146)

Potassium 3.8 mmol/L (NR 3.5–5.3)

Urea 5.4 mmol/L (2.5–7.8)

Creatinine 79 μmol/L (59–104)

Adjusted calcium 1.6 mmol/L (2.1–2.55)

Phosphate 1.56 mmol/L (0.8–1.5)

Magnesium 0.33 mmol/L (0.7–1.0)

Parathyroid hormone 7.9 pmol/L (1.6–6.9)

What drug is likely to be the cause of her metabolic abnormalities?

1. Atorvastatin
2. Bendroflumethiazide
3. Bisoprolol
4. Lisinopril
5. Omeprazole

Q139

A 36 year old woman has received radioactive iodine for thyrotoxicosis 2 weeks ago. Now, she and her new partner plan to start a family, but she is unsure when she can try for a baby.

How long should the patient wait before becoming pregnant?

1. No need to wait
2. 1–3 weeks
3. 1–2 months
4. 3 months
5. At least 6 months

Q140

A 37 year old woman has a severe headache with vomiting. She has a macroprolactinoma (15 mm) diagnosed 2 years ago. She admits poor compliance with bromocriptine. Her pulse is 110 bpm, BP 75/45 mmHg, and she has generalised non-specific abdominal tenderness.

Investigations:

Sodium 129 mmol/L (137–144)

Potassium 5.6 mmol/L (3.5–4.9)

Urea 15 mmol/L (2.5–7.5)

Creatinine 130 mmol/L(60–110)

CRP is normal and blood count shows mild leukocytosis. Random cortisol is still pending.

What is the best next management step?

1. Intravenous hydrocortisone and aggressive fluid resuscitation
2. Refer to neurosurgeons for urgent transfer
3. Urgent MRI of the head
4. Urgent visual field perimetry
5. Wait for the cortisol level before management can be decided

Q141

A 55 year old woman goes to her general practitioner after finding a lump in her neck the previous week. She says the lump has increased in size over time, so you decide to perform a physical examination of the thyroid starting with the isthmus.

Where would you palpate the isthmus of the thyroid?

1. Inferior to the cricoid cartilage
2. Inferior to the hyoid bone
3. Inferior to the sternum
4. Inferior to the thyroid cartilage
5. Lateral to the thyroid cartilage

Q142

A 27 year old woman presents to her general practitioner with 5 months of new, persistent fatigue and reduced activity, which is characterised by post-exertional malaise and slow recovery. She also describes unrefreshing sleep, painful lymph nodes, an inability to concentrate for long periods of time and intermittent nausea. She reports no recent weight loss or fevers.

Examination is normal, no lymphadenopathy or masses. She has no joint tenderness or swelling.

Bloods including Monospot and Borreliosis are normal.

What is the most likely diagnosis?

1. Chronic fatigue syndrome
2. Depression

3. Infectious mononucleosis

4. Lyme disease

5. Lymphoma

Q143

A 57 year old man has weight gain (4 kg in 1 year) despite no significant change to his diet. He was diagnosed with type 2 diabetes 1 year ago and takes gliclazide and dapagliflozin. He also takes atenolol, atorvastatin and ramipril. He is centrally obese, has acanthosis nigricans in his axillae. There is no evidence of abdominal striae or proximal myopathy.

Investigations:

Urea and electrolytes normal

HbA1c 55 mmol/mol (20–41)

TSH 1.35 mIU/L (0.35 to 4.5)

Which of his medications is most likely to be contributing to his weight gain?

1. Atenolol

2. Atorvastatin

3. Dapagliflozin

4. Gliclazide

5. Ramipril

Q144

A 55 year old man has the sensation of lumpiness over the right side of his chest different to the left side. He first noticed this 2 weeks ago. There is no nipple discharge. He is a non-smoker and drinks 2 pints of beer a week.

His BMI is 29 kg/m^2. There is a firm mass in the right breast with puckering around the right nipple. Examination of the left nipple is normal.

What is the most appropriate next step in management?

1. Advise weight loss

2. Ask the patient to return in 2 weeks to review any changes in the mass or breast tissue before deciding which would be the best management plan

3. Make an urgent referral to the 2-week-wait clinic for suspected breast cancer

4. Take bloods for prolactin and the gonadotrophins

5. Urgent MRI

Q145

A 40 year old woman has 3 months of fatigue, night sweats, palpitations and weight loss in spite of adequate food intake. She runs for 20 minutes twice weekly. Her temperature is 37.3 °C, pulse 102 bpm, BP 136/60 mmHg. She has a fine tremor and a diffuse symmetric enlargement of the neck. She has mild proptosis with lid retraction.

What is the most likely cause of her weight loss?

1. Addison's disease

2. Fibromyalgia

3. Hyperthyroidism

4. Lymphoma

5. Underlying infection

Gastrointestinal

6

Q146

A 17 year old boy has lethargy and fatigue for 4 weeks. He has been nauseous and has lost weight; his skin is slightly jaundiced. There has been no change in the colour of his stools or urine. He has been a strict vegan since the age of 13 and has never travelled outside of the UK. His examination is normal.

His MCV is elevated at 121 fL and a blood film reveals the presence of hypersegmented neutrophils, macrocytosis and poikilocytes.

Which deficiency is the most likely cause of his symptoms?

1. Vitamin A
2. Vitamin B5
3. Vitamin B12
4. Vitamin C
5. Vitamin E

Q147

A 42 year old woman has a day of upper abdominal pain, dark urine and pale stools. Her temperature is 38.4 °C, pulse 90 bpm, respiratory rate 20 breaths per minute, oxygen saturation 99% breathing air.

Investigations:

High bilirubin and alkaline phosphatase and normal clotting

What imaging should be performed?

1. Contrast-enhanced CT abdomen and pelvis
2. Endoscopic retrograde cholangiopancreatography
3. Magnetic resonance cholangiopancreatography
4. Non-contrast CT abdomen and pelvis
5. Ultrasound abdomen

Q148

A 61 year old man is brought to the emergency department by his daughter with mild delirium, jaundice, abdominal pain and nausea. He was found surrounded by bottles of alcohol. Examination reveals tender hepatomegaly, ascites and spider naevi. You suspect hepatitis and so take bloods to run a liver function test.

Which of the following is the strongest indicator of alcoholic hepatitis?

1. A Maddrey discriminant function ≤ 13
2. Aspartate transferase : alanine transaminase (AST:ALT) ratio ≥ 2
3. Jaundice
4. Spider naevi
5. Tender hepatomegaly

Q149

A 40 year old man has a sudden-onset abdominal pain which initially started as epigastric discomfort and is now generalised. He has type 2 diabetes and chronic knee pain. He takes metformin and ibuprofen. He drinks 14 units of alcohol every week. His temperature is 38 °C, pulse 112 bpm, BP 105/71 mmHg; he has severe abdominal pain, and his abdomen is rigid and tender on palpation.

What is the most likely diagnosis?

1. Acute pancreatitis
2. Decompensated liver cirrhosis
3. Ischaemic colitis
4. Metformin sensitivity
5. Perforated peptic ulcer

Q150

A 35 year old man has pain after defaecation and blood on wiping. He has a low-fibre diet and is often constipated. Examination reveals a linear tear of the distal anal canal. He is given topical lidocaine for pain.

What would the most appropriate next steps in management?

1. Abdominal ultrasound
2. Botox injection
3. CT colonography scan

4. Fibre supplement with stool softener

5. No further management needed

Q151

A 53 year old man has 5 days of increasing fatigue, shortness of breath when lying down and worsening abdominal distension. This has been associated with abdominal pain and a fever in the last 2 days. He has gout but takes no regular medications. He drinks 12 units of alcohol per day.

He is haemodynamically stable and has a tender, distended abdomen with scleral icterus, caput medusae and spider naevi. Renal function is normal. An ultrasound reveals ascites and an ascitic tap is performed:

Appearance: clear, straw-coloured

White cell count: 342 x 10^6/L (95% neutrophils) (normal ascitic neutrophil count < 250 x 10^6/L)

Albumin: 13 g/l (serum albumin = 28)

What is the most appropriate initial management plan?

1. Broad-spectrum intravenous antibiotics and spironolactone

2. Give ACE inhibitor + spironolactone

3. Intravenous 0.9% saline infusion + analgesia (paracetamol + codeine)

4. Pabrinex infusion

5. Therapeutic paracentesis

Q152

A 56 year old man has severe epigastric pain that radiates to his back. The pain was sudden in onset and progressively worsening over the past few hours. He admits to heavy alcohol consumption over the last weekend. He is obese, his temperature is 38.4 °C, pulse 110 bpm, BP 120/70 mmHg, respiratory rate 22 breaths per minute. He is in obvious pain with tenderness to palpation in the epigastric region, with guarding and rigidity.

What investigation would most support the likely diagnosis?

1. Arterial blood gas

2. Magnetic resonance cholangiopancreatogram

3. Serum amylase or lipase

4. Ultrasound scan of abdomen
5. X-ray of abdomen

Q153

A 42 year old woman has a right upper quadrant pain – she is known to have gall stones. Her temperature is 37.2 °C, pulse 86 bpm, BP 120/70 mmHg, BMI 30 kg/m², abdomen is soft, with a positive Murphy's sign.

Bloods are sent for white cell count, CRP, LFT, serum lipase or amylase.

What investigations should be requested or carried out?

1. CT abdomen
2. Erect chest X-ray
3. Magnetic resonance cholangiopancreatography
4. No further investigation
5. Ultrasound scan

Q154

A 78 year old woman has a right-sided pneumonia. She has hypertension. She lives with her husband and both are independent. She denies any recent weight loss.

What is the most appropriate next step in management regarding her nutrition status?

1. Calculate her BMI and complete a Malnutrition Universal Screening Tool (MUST) score
2. Commence enteral nutrition via a nasogastric tube
3. Prescribe oral food supplements
4. Switch to fortified meals
5. Take blood tests to assess for micronutrient deficiency

Q155

A 45 year old woman has itching and fatigue for the last 3 weeks. She has longstanding rheumatoid arthritis.

Investigations:

Serum total bilirubin 35 μmol/L (1–22)

Serum alkaline phosphatase 552 U/L (45–105)

Primary biliary cirrhosis is considered.

What would be the most appropriate test to check for primary biliary cirrhosis?

1. Anti-mitochondrial antibodies
2. Anti-smooth muscle antibodies
3. Ceruloplasmin level
4. Hepatitis B surface antigen
5. Serum ferritin level

Q156

A 32 year old woman has 2 months of loose motions associated with occasional abdominal pain. She has seen no blood or mucus in the motion. Her father died at the age of 48 from bowel cancer; her paternal grandmother died at a similar age (she does not know the cause). Observations and examination of the abdomen (including a rectal examination) are all normal.

Routine bloods are taken (including CA125). A qFIT is requested.

What is the next step in management?

1. CT colonoscopy
2. Genetic markers
3. Proctoscopy
4. Refer for colonoscopy as part of 2-week-wait
5. Watch and wait, reviewing the patient in 2 months' time if still symptomatic

Q157

A 32 year old woman has fatigue, recurrent abdominal pain and intermittent diarrhoea for the past 3 months. She has unintentionally lost 4 kg. She is pale, her temperature is 36.6 °C, pulse 80 bpm, BP 127/70 mmHg. Her arms and legs are covered in red blistery lesions. Coeliac disease is suspected.

Which test should be used first in clinical suspicion of coeliac disease?

1. Anti-gliadin antibody
2. Endomysial antibody
3. Full blood count
4. Human leukocyte antigen
5. Tissue transglutaminase 2

Q158

A 94 year old woman has 5 days of constipation, with infrequent passage of type 1 stools. She was discharged to a nursing home 2 weeks ago after a hip fracture and insertion of hip screw. She takes 15 mg of codeine, 4 times daily, for the last month. Her treatment escalation plan suggests full treatment and resuscitation. Her observations are normal. Abdominal examination is unremarkable, and rectal examination reveals hard stool only. A blood test taken 2 days ago is normal.

She is prescribed faecal softeners and glycerol suppositories.

What would be an appropriate ongoing management?

1. Admission to hospital for administration of intravenous fluids
2. Arrange CT colonoscopy scan
3. Change her treatment escalation plan to avoid future admission
4. No other management needed at the moment
5. Urgent referral to colorectal surgeon

Q159

An 18 year old woman has 18 hours of nausea, anorexia and worsening generalised abdominal pain. Her temperature is 37.5 °C, pulse 86 bpm. She has generalised abdominal pain radiating into her right lower quadrant.

Investigations:

White cell count	4.6 x 10^9/L (4–11)
CRP	4 mg/L (< 6)
Serum	hCG is 3 (< 5)

Her ultrasound is normal.

Which feature is most reassuring that this is not an appendicitis?

1. Absence of vomiting
2. Low-grade fever
3. Normal pulse
4. Normal white cell count and CRP
5. Normal ultrasound

Q160

A 67 year old man has 2 days of worsening generalised abdominal pain and fever. He has known diverticular disease that was detected at colonoscopy 4 years ago. The colonoscopy was otherwise normal.

His temperature is 38.4 °C, pulse 135 bpm, BP 110/70 mmHg, respiratory rate 25 breaths per minute

His abdomen is rigid with guarding and rebound tenderness.

Bloods are sent and the sepsis six guidelines are followed.

What is the next investigation of choice?

1. Blood cultures
2. Chest X-ray
3. Contrast CT abdomen
4. MRI abdomen
5. Ultrasound scan

Q161

A 42 year old woman has spasmodic right upper quadrant pain for 2 days, which radiates to her back, becoming more constant. This was associated with nausea and 3 episodes of vomiting. She weighs 52 kg, her temperature is 36.5 °C, pulse 96 bpm, and she is not jaundiced. She has severe tenderness in the right hypochondriac region. Her bloods are taken for FBC and liver function tests.

What is the most appropriate next investigation?

1. CT scan of abdomen
2. Intraoperative cholangiogram
3. Magnetic resonance cholangiopancreatography
4. Plain abdomen radiograph
5. Ultrasound abdomen

Q162

A 65 year old man has 4 weeks of dark urine and pale stools, associated with 10 kg unintentional weight loss over 2 months. He has type 2 diabetes. He is a current smoker and drinks a bottle of cider/day. He is keen to be managed as actively as possible. His observations are within normal range. He is clinically jaundiced.

Investigations:

Bilirubin 280 (1–22)

Alkaline phosphatase 1100 (45–105)

Alanine transaminase 110 (7–55)

CT TAP shows appearances consistent with metastatic pancreatic cancer with common bile duct dilatation.

What is the next management step?

1. Antibiotics
2. Biliary stent
3. Cholecystectomy
4. Commence chemotherapy
5. Whipple procedure (pancreaticoduodenectomy)

Q163

A 68 year old man has 3 months of nausea, anorexia, weight loss and iron deficiency anaemia. He smokes 20 cigarettes per day. He has no other symptoms and no significant past medical history. He has a solitary palpable supraclavicular lymph node.

Which is the most likely diagnosis?

1. Atrophic gastritis
2. Duodenal ulcer
3. Gastric carcinoma
4. Oesophageal carcinoma
5. Pancreatic carcinoma

Q164

A 45 year old woman has occasional retrosternal burning pain, which is worse when lying down in bed. She also noticed occasional acidic taste in her mouth. She smokes 10 cigarettes per day and drinks 2 glasses of wine on most days. Her BMI is 35.2 kg/m^2. Clinical examination was normal.

What is the most likely diagnosis?

1. Cardiac ischaemia
2. Costochondritis
3. Gastric cancer
4. Gastro-oesophageal reflux disease
5. Sinus congestion

Q165

A 48 year old woman has rectal bleeding after defaecation for the last month. This is associated with the sensation of a lump coming down.

She has six children, all from normal vaginal deliveries. Initial examination is normal; however, following valsalva manoeuvre, an internal haemorrhoid prolapses to cross the dentate line. The haemorrhoid requires finger pressure to reduce.

What is the classification grading of her internal haemorrhoid?

1. Grade 0
2. Grade I
3. Grade II
4. Grade III
5. Grade IV

Q166

A 27 year old man has diarrhoea for the last 2 months. The stools contain mucus and occasionally a small amount of blood. He also complains of abdominal discomfort and weight loss of 4 kg. He is afebrile and has mild tenderness and distended abdomen. He is a non-smoker and doesn't have a history of travelling or changes in diet during this time. Investigations:

CRP 36 (< 6)

Other routine blood tests are insignificant. Stool MC&S was negative. Anti-endomysial and tissue transglutaminase antibodies are negative and faecal calprotectin level is positive.

What is the most likely diagnosis?

1. Coeliac disease
2. Crohn's disease
3. Diverticulosis
4. Gastroenteritis
5. Ulcerative colitis

Q167

A 20 year old woman has a generalised fatigue, yellowing in skin colour, and dark brown urine. Her observations are normal; she has right upper quadrant tenderness. Investigations:

ALT 1035 U/L (8–20)

What is the most likely diagnosis?

1. Acute viral hepatitis
2. Crigler–Najjar syndrome
3. Gilbert's syndrome

4. Haemolysis secondary to glucose-6-phosphate dehydrogenase deficiency

5. Liver cirrhosis

Q168

A 64 year old man is admitted in the emergency department with abdominal pain and vomiting. He is a smoker. He has visited his GP previously with complaints of heartburn, following which the GP prescribed proton pump inhibitors.

Investigations:

Chest X-ray: shadow behind his heart with gas fluid level.

What is the probable diagnosis?

1. Emphysema
2. Gastric cancer
3. Haemomediastinum
4. Hiatus hernia
5. Lung abscess

Q169

A 45 year old man has a right-sided groin mass, which he noticed 2 days ago. This mass is not painful and disappears on lying flat. He is normally fit and well and has no other complaints.

Which of the following is a cardinal sign of groin hernias on clinical examination?

1. Firm consistency
2. Multiple palpable lumps
3. Positive cough impulse
4. Previous surgical scar over the mass
5. Rebound tenderness

Q170

A 28 year old woman has long-standing symptoms of constipation-dominant irritable bowel disease. She has been attempting to manage her symptoms by increasing exercise and by reducing insoluble fibre in her diet. However, she is still frequently bothered by abdominal pain.

What would be an appropriate first-line pharmacological treatment for this patient?

1. Amitriptyline
2. Citalopram
3. Hyoscine
4. Linaclotide
5. Loperamide

Q171

A 35 year old man has a splenectomy to control abdominal bleeding following a road traffic accident.

To which types of infection will he be particularly prone?

1. Covid-19
2. Encapsulated bacterial
3. Fungal
4. Helminth
5. Protozoal

Q172

A 56 year old man has 2 days of increasing abdominal pain radiating to his back. This has been associated with reduced appetite. He had a high-speed road traffic collision 5 days ago. His temperature is 38.5 °C, pulse 110 bpm, BP 110/60 mmHg, respiratory rate 22 breaths per minute. His abdomen is tender with guarding. Bowel sounds are absent.

A perforated bowel is suspected.

What is the most likely to have perforated?

1. Anus
2. Appendix
3. Hypopharynx
4. Oesophagus
5. Small or large bowel

Q173

A 45 year old man has a progressive abdominal distension and ankle swelling for the past 2 weeks. He drinks 2–3 litres of vodka a week. His pulse is 90 bpm, BP 98/68 mmHg; he has scleral icterus, multiple spider naevi on his chest and abdomen and pitting oedema of his legs. His abdomen is distended, but soft and non-tender. Shifting dullness was present. Other system examinations were normal.

What is the most likely diagnosis?

1. Colorectal cancer
2. Decompensated liver disease
3. Functional bloating
4. Small bowel obstruction
5. Small intestinal bacterial overgrowth

Q174

A 45 year old man has severe abdominal pain, watery diarrhoea and fever for the past 2 days. He recently returned from rural India. His abdomen is tender on palpation and there are hyperactive bowel sounds. Stool analysis reveals leukocytes and red blood cells.

What pathogen is the most likely cause of this patient's infectious colitis?

1. Campylobacter jejuni
2. Clostridium difficile
3. Coxiella burnetii
4. Escherichia coli
5. Norovirus

Q175

A 45 year old woman has had 3 days of fever, vomiting and diarrhoea after returning from a business trip in South Asia. She has familial hypercholesterolaemia and takes 40 mg simvastatin. Her temperature is 38.0 °C, pulse 78 bpm, BP 130/68 mmHg, oxygen saturation 98% breathing air.

What is the most appropriate management plan?

1. Admit to the hospital
2. Advise patient to stay home, drink fluid and get plenty of rest
3. Collect a faecal sample and send for microbiological culture
4. Isolate the patient
5. Prescribe broad-spectrum antibiotics

Q176

A 79 year old woman presents to the emergency department 3 hours after the sudden onset of severe and diffuse abdominal pain. She has had a large episode of diarrhoea; prior to this her bowel habits have been normal.

She is visibly distressed, clutching her abdomen. Her temperature is 38.0 °C, pulse 112 bpm (irregularly irregular), BP 100/60 mmHg, oxygen saturation 96% breathing air. Her abdomen is soft with mild tenderness. Venous blood gases show a metabolic acidosis with high lactate.

You suspect intestinal ischaemia.

Which is the most likely cause of intestinal ischaemia in her case?

1. Chronic colonic ischaemia
2. Mesenteric artery embolus
3. Mesenteric artery thrombosis
4. Mesenteric vein thrombosis
5. Non-occlusive ischaemia

Q177

A 52 year old woman has lower abdominal pain for 1 day. This is associated with nausea, vomiting, abdominal distention and tachycardia. Her temperature is 37.3 °C, pulse 112 bpm, BP 110/60 mmHg, oxygen saturation 96% breathing air. Her abdomen is diffusely tender. There are no masses palpable. Abdominal X-ray shows grossly dilated bowel loops. Her pregnancy test is negative. Fluid replacement is commenced intravenously.

How would you initially manage this patient?

1. Abdominal angiogram
2. Colonoscopy
3. Direct straight to the theatre for bowel resection
4. Nasogastric tube insertion and observe on ward
5. Reassure the patient and send her home following fluid replacement

Q178

A 75 year old woman has 6 weeks of change in bowel habit. She is obese and uses a wheelchair to mobilise. She has chronic obstructive pulmonary disease and atrial fibrillation. She drinks approximately 10 units of alcohol per week. Abdominal examination is normal. She is referred under a 2-week-wait cancer referral.

Investigations:

Iron deficient anaemia

qFIT is 20 (< 10)

What would be the most appropriate investigation for this patient?

1. Capsule colonoscopy
2. Colonoscopy
3. CT colonography
4. Flexible sigmoidoscopy
5. Water-soluble enema

Q179

An 18 month old boy is brought into the emergency department with crying and curling up into a ball every half-hour. He has had faeces like redcurrant jelly. His abdomen is soft with a sausage-shaped mass palpable in the right iliac fossa. You are concerned that this may be intussusception.

What would be the most appropriate first-line investigation?

1. Abdominal ultrasound
2. CT chest, abdomen and pelvis
3. Chest X-ray
4. Diagnostic peritoneal lavage
5. Gastroscopy

Q180

A 38 year old woman has persistent watery stools. She has Crohn's disease, and had a terminal resection for a long fibrotic stricture 6 months ago. She feels well and has put on 5 kg since the operation.

Investigations:

Hb 133 g/L (112–155)

Platelets 220 x10^9/L (150–400)

CRP 1 (< 6)

Faecal calprotectin: < 50 mcg/g (low)

Colonoscopy: normal to neoterminal ileum

Which of the following is most likely to help her loose stools?

1. Colestyramine
2. Gluten-free diet trial
3. Infliximab
4. Mesalazine
5. Pancreatic enzyme replacement

Q181

A 58 year old woman presents to the emergency department after being found unconscious in the street. Upon examination, she is clearly jaundiced, and has right upper quadrant tenderness. She is disorientated and her Glasgow Coma Score is 11/15. Her temperature is 36.5 °C, pulse 120 bpm, BP 90/60 mmHg.

Investigations:

liver function tests show hyperbilirubinaemia, a significantly raised aspartate transferase (AST) with AST: alanine transamine (ALT) ratio > 2, and slightly raised alkaline phosphatase and gamma-glutamyl transferase. Prothrombin time 22 sec (control 11).

What is the most likely cause of her acute liver failure?

1. Alcoholic hepatitis
2. Ascending cholangitis
3. Biliary obstruction
4. Hepatitis C
5. Paracetamol overdose

Q182

A 10 day old girl is brought to the emergency department with increased crying, vomiting and food intolerance for the last 48 hours. For the last 6 hours, she has rectal bleeding with loose stools and her breathing has been erratic. She was born at 34 weeks' gestation. Her temperature is 36.7 °C, pulse 165 bpm, BP 50/25 mmHg, respiratory rate 55 breaths per minute, oxygen saturation 94% breathing air, capillary refill 3 seconds. She appears dehydrated, pale and lethargic. Abdomen is hard and tender to touch with no erythema.

What is the most appropriate next step in management?

1. Abdominal X-ray
2. Blood gases
3. Haemodynamic resuscitation

4. Intravenous antibiotics

5. Surgical review

Q183

A 54 year old woman has severe abdominal pain and intermittent bloody diarrhoea, over the last 5 days. She is able to drink fluids. Her temperature is 38.2 °C, pulse 106 bpm, BP 110/62 mmHg, respiratory rate 22 breaths per minute, oxygen saturation 98% breathing air. She is tender in the left iliac fossa and is guarding.

What is the next most appropriate step in her management?

1. 2-week-wait referral to the colorectal team

2. Oral co-amoxiclav

3. Oral loperamide

4. Stool culture

5. Urgent transfer to the surgical assessment unit

Q184

A 72 year old man is 5 days post-operative following an Ivor–Lewis procedure for adenocarcinoma of the oesophagus. He is pyrexial.

Investigations:

CRP 58 (< 6)

What is the most likely early post-operative complication?

1. Anastomotic leak

2. Anastomotic stricture

3. Conduit necrosis

4. Dumping syndrome

5. Pneumonia

Q185

A 60 year old man has 2 weeks of epigastric pain, particularly after meals. He drinks 3–5 units of whisky a day. He came back from Asia 4 weeks ago. His temperature is 36.7 °C, pulse 82 bpm, BP 140/70 mmHg, respiratory rate 16 breaths per minute. He has epigastric tenderness on palpation and a jaundiced tinge in his eyes. His full blood count, urea electrolytes and liver function tests are normal. Helicobacter pylori faecal antigen test is negative.

What is the next management step?

1. 1 month PPI trial and review after 4 weeks
2. Abdominal CT scan
3. Bloods, including hepatitis screening and serum lipase
4. Referral for upper GI endoscopy
5. Send him home with antacids and lifestyle advice and review after 4 weeks

Q186

A 45 year old woman presents with 3-day history of colicky right upper quadrant pain, fever and jaundice. Her past medical history includes high body mass index and asthma.

What is the most likely diagnosis?

1. Acute cholecystitis
2. Ascending cholangitis
3. Fatty liver disease
4. Gilbert's disease
5. Pancreatic carcinoma

Q187

A 40 year old man has severe pain in his perineum, associated with fever with chills. His temperature is 37.6 °C. On examination, lateral to the anal opening, an area of severe tenderness and fluctuation was noted.

What is the best initial modality of treatment?

1. Antibiotics
2. Fistulectomy
3. Incision and drainage
4. Laxatives
5. Topical glyceryl trinitrate ointment

Q188

An 82 year old woman has 48 hours of a sudden onset of violent vomiting and diarrhoea. She has not passed urine for 24 hours. She has a history of hypertension, congestive cardiac failure (with an ejection fraction of 35%) and chronic kidney disease stage 3. She lives in a residential home where two other residents have a similar condition. Her temperature is 37.9 °C, pulse 108 bpm (irregularly irregular), BP 98/60 mmHg, respiratory rate 19 breaths per minute, oxygen saturation 95% on room air.

What is your next step in this patient's management?

1. Arrange emergency admission to hospital
2. Collect a stool culture
3. Commence a beta-blocker and anti-coagulation for atrial fibrillation
4. Commence loperamide to stop diarrhoea
5. Place the patient into isolation, encourage oral intake and review in 24 hours

Q189

A 56 year old man has a raised alanine transaminase detected on routine diabetic blood tests. His hepatitis B serology shows:

HBsAg	Negative
Anti-core antigen	Positive
Anti-HBsAg	Positive

How is his hepatitis B serology best described?

1. He has a chronic hepatitis B infection
2. He has a current acute hepatitis B infection
3. He has never had a hepatitis B infection, but has been vaccinated against hepatitis B
4. He has never had a hepatitis B infection or been vaccinated against hepatitis B
5. He has previously had a hepatitis B infection, which has resolved

Q190

An 84 year old man presents to the emergency department with lower abdominal pain and distension. His bowels have not opened for 5 days. An abdominal X-ray confirms your suspicion of sigmoid volvulus.

What is the most appropriate immediate management?

1. Analgesia and antibiotics
2. Flexible sigmoidoscopy and flatus tube
3. Needle decompression of the obstructed bowel

4. NG tube and bowel rest

5. Strong laxatives and an enema

Q191

A 28 year old woman has 4 days of lower right-sided abdominal pain, associated with nausea and vomiting and reduced appetite. She is normally fit and well. Her observations are normal.

Which of the following is an essential initial investigation in this patient?

1. Liver function tests

2. Pregnancy test

3. Troponin

4. Ultrasound

5. Urinalysis

Q192

A 65 year old man passed large amounts of blood when he went to open his bowels. He has atrial fibrillation and takes apixaban. His temperature is 36 °C, pulse 110 bpm, BP 90/60 mmHg, respiratory rate 20 breaths per minute, oxygen saturation 97% breathing air.

What is the most appropriate initial investigation?

1. Colonoscopy

2. CT angiogram

3. Laparotomy

4. Plain CT

5. Sigmoidoscopy

Q193

A 72 year old man has 72 hours of vomiting of brown offensive-smelling vomitus, associated with abdominal pain. He has not opened his bowels or passed flatus for 48 hours. His temperature is 37.4 °C, pulse 110 bpm, BP 100/60 mmHg, respiratory rate 22 breaths per minute, oxygen saturation 95% breathing air. He has dry mucous membranes and reduced skin turgor. He has a distended tympanic abdomen with a painful mass in the right inguinal region. Intravenous fluids are set up.

What intervention should be performed first?

1. Administration of metoclopramide
2. Blood transfusion
3. Immediate transfer to theatre
4. Intravenous antibiotics
5. Nasogastric tube insertion

Q194

A 43 year old man has a large-volume haematemesis. He has cirrhosis and alcohol excess. After 2 L rapid intravenous resuscitation with crystalloid, his pulse is 126 bpm, BP 72/33 mmHg.

What is the most important next step in his management?

1. CT angiogram
2. Further 1 L intravenous crystalloid
3. Gastroscopy within 24 hours
4. Immediate activation of the major haemorrhage protocol
5. Intravenous vitamin K 10 mg

Q195

A 73 year old woman has a black diarrhoea, lethargy and shortness of breath which has been worsening over the last week. She has had black stools for the last 3 months having been started on iron tablets for iron deficiency anaemia. She has osteoarthritis, and diverticular disease.

Investigations:

Haemoglobin	63 g/L	(120–150)
Serum urea	17.4 mmol/L	(2.5–7.5)
Serum creatinine	67 μmol/L	(60–110)
Ferritin	8 ng/mL	(10–300)

Which test is most likely to reveal the cause of her symptoms?

1. Colonoscopy
2. Faecal calprotectin
3. Flexible sigmoidoscopy
4. Oesophagogastroduodenoscopy
5. Stool culture

Q196

An 8 year old boy has 2 weeks of erythema and pruritus to the face and chest with associated tongue swelling. This has been with colicky abdominal pain. He has eczema but is otherwise well with no regular medications. His mother is concerned that he may have a food allergy as his symptoms develop soon after eating fish and nuts. His observations are stable, and there are no abnormal examination findings. You consider providing an adrenalin (epinephrine) auto-injector pen.

What is the next most appropriate step in his management?

1. Oral food challenge
2. Provide reassurance and discharge home
3. Review in 2 weeks with a food diary
4. Serum IgE blood test
5. Trial elimination diet

Q197

A 40 year old man has 4 months of gradual onset of cramping lower abdominal pain with occasional loose stools. He has lost 1 kg. There are no urinary symptoms. He is normally fit and well, has no family history or recent travel, smokes 5–10 cigarettes per day, and has a diet which reportedly 'could be better'.

His observations are normal. There is mild lower abdominal tenderness on palpation, but the abdomen is soft with no masses or organomegaly, and bowel sounds are present. C-reactive protein is 46 (< 6) but all other routine bloods, including full blood count, liver function and urea and electrolytes, are unremarkable. His stool FIT test = 18 ug Hb/g stool (positive).

What is the most appropriate next step in the management?

1. Prescribe an antispasmodic
2. Recommend dietary modifications and lifestyle changes
3. Refer the patient for a 2-week-wait colonoscopy
4. Stool microscopy
5. Urinalysis

Q198

A 30 year old woman has 24 hours of decreased appetite, nausea, multiple episodes of vomiting, and generalised abdominal pain. For the past 2 weeks, she has had frequent urination, blurred vision and occasional rapid breathing.

Her temperature is 36.5 °C, pulse 115 bpm, BP 100/55 mmHg, respiratory rate 27 breaths per minute. She is sweaty and clammy. There is no abdominal tenderness.

Investigations:

Sodium 140 mmol/L (137–144)

Chloride 100 mmol/L (95–107)

Potassium 4.6 mmol/L (3.5–4.9)

Bicarbonate 18 mmol/L (20–28)

Random glucose 44.6 mmol/L (3.0–7.8)

Urine ketones = positive

Urine HCG negative

What is the most likely diagnosis?

1. Acute mesenteric ischaemia
2. Acute pancreatitis
3. Diabetic ketoacidosis
4. Infectious gastroenteritis
5. Ureteric colic

Q199

A 48 year old woman has stress incontinence of urine and occasional faecal incontinence. She has had two vaginal deliveries, each resulting in a third-degree tear.

What is the most likely cause of her faecal incontinence?

1. Damage to the external anal sphincter
2. Damage to the internal anal sphincter
3. Damage to the puborectalis
4. Damage to the rectoanal inhibitory reflex
5. Rectocele

Q200

A 67 year old man has 3 days of a lump within the groin. The lump has been increasingly painful in the last day. He has had no fever. His bowels are regular but were loose this morning. He has dropped one clothes size in the past year. He returned from Malaysia 2 weeks ago, where he received unprotected oral sex 3 weeks ago. He is obese (BMI 30 kg/m^2). He is apyrexial; he has a tender, non-reducible, smooth lump above the pubic tubercle. There are no superficial skin changes. There is no other lymphadenopathy present.

What would be the most appropriate first management step?

1. Reassure and safety-net to return if symptoms do not settle in 24 hours
2. Refer to the sexual health clinic
3. Request a screen for blood-borne viruses
4. Request an ultrasound scan with doppler study
5. Request an urgent surgical review

Q201

A 60 year old woman is admitted to the emergency department after passing a large amount of black stool and feeling faint. She has type 2 diabetes and obesity. She drinks 18 units per week. While waiting to be reviewed by the emergency department triage nurse, she vomits 500 ml of bright red blood and collapses. Her pulse is 105 bpm, BP 100/60 mmHg lying down (75/52 sitting), capillary refill 3 seconds. Electrocardiogram shows sinus tachycardia.

Investigations:

Haemoglobin – 120 g/L (120–155)

Platelets 58 x 10^9/L (150–400)

Urea 12 mmol/L (2.5 – 6.7)

What is the most likely diagnosis?

1. Bleeding oesophageal varices
2. Colonic carcinoma
3. Gastric carcinoma
4. Haemorrhoids
5. Mallory–Weiss tear

Q202

A 7 month old boy is screaming and drawing his knees to his chest. He passed one episode of bloody stool and vomited this morning. He had a fever 5 days ago, which is now subsided. Abdominal examination reveals a mass palpable in right upper quadrant. What is the most likely diagnosis?

1. Choledochal cyst
2. Hydronephrosis
3. Intussusception
4. Viral hepatitis
5. Wilms tumour

Q203

A 56 year old man has 3 months of unintentional weight loss (20 kg), fatigue, heartburn and debilitating nausea. The nausea is constant but worse after eating; it is only partially controlled with oral cyclizine. He is a heavy smoker. He is cachexic and has a hard, red lump at his umbilicus and a lump palpable in his left supraclavicular fossa. He has routine bloods and is sent for a CT thorax, abdomen and pelvis.

What additional antiemetic should be given to this patient?

1. Amitriptyline
2. Domperidone
3. Levomepromazine
4. Metoclopramide
5. Ondansetron

Q204

A 30 year old man has 5 weeks of pain on defaecation associated with bleeding on wiping. He has a past medical history of constipation, and takes over-the-counter laxatives on occasion to help open his bowels. He is alert. His temperature is 37.1 °C, pulse 90 bpm, BP 134/72 mmHg, respiratory rate 16 breaths per minute, oxygen saturation 98% breathing air.

Given the most likely diagnosis, what is the most appropriate initial management?

1. Mebendazole
2. Oral antibiotics
3. Rubber band ligation
4. Surgical haemorrhoidectomy
5. Topical glyceryl trinitrate

Q205

A 78 year old woman hasn't opened her bowels for 4 days. She was admitted to the ward 6 days ago following a fall and would otherwise be medically fit for discharge. The issue has been intermittent for the last 6 months; she has to strain very hard to open her bowels – occasionally a mass exudes from her anus, which returns later. There is no abdominal pain or vomiting. Her observations are normal; her abdomen is soft and non-tender. There is evidence of a full-thickness rectal prolapse.

How would you manage this patient?

1. Commence a trial of laxatives and arrange colorectal surgical review
2. Give the patient an inpatient enema and ask the GP to follow her up
3. Manually attempt to reduce the prolapse
4. Order an urgent CT scan of her abdomen
5. Routine outpatient colorectal referral

Q206

A 28 year old man has recurrent abdominal pain, fatigue, and blood in his urine for the past 3 months. He has a recent history of travel to sub-Saharan Africa for a volunteer project. His temperature is 37.2 °C, pulse 95 bpm, BP 120/70 mmHg. He has a hepatosplenomegaly.

Investigations:

Elevated eosinophil count

Elevated liver enzymes

What is the most likely cause of his symptoms?

1. Amoebic abscess
2. Malaria
3. Schistosomiasis
4. Tuberculosis
5. Typhoid

7

General Duties

Q207

A 37 year old woman has a pruritic erythematous rash for 1 day. She complains that the itching is unbearable. She started a new medication for dysmenorrhea 3 days ago.

What is a requirement when reporting a suspected adverse drug reaction via the Yellow Card system?

1. The medication should be suspected as causing an adverse drug reaction
2. The medication should be under the black triangle monitoring scheme
3. The medication should have prescription-only status
4. The medication should have proven causality
5. The medication should not be a vaccine

Q208

A 53 year old woman receives a routine screening letter asking her to book a mammogram. She is uncertain about the benefits of the screening, worrying about the radiation exposure and the test's reliability.

In the context of a test with high sensitivity, which of the following is most accurate?

1. A negative result makes the condition less likely
2. A positive result makes the condition more likely
3. The test is prone to producing false negatives
4. The test is unlikely to produce false positives
5. The test has a high positive predictive value

Q209

A 52 year old woman has fatigue and right loin pain. Contrast-enhanced CT: a large right renal mass suggestive of tumour, and a likely metastatic mass within the liver.

What would be the most appropriate initial management for the patient?

1. Blood transfusion followed by referral to urology
2. Chemotherapy followed by surgery to remove liver mass
3. Chemotherapy followed by surgery to remove right kidney
4. Surgery to remove liver mass followed by adjuvant chemotherapy
5. Surgery to remove right kidney followed by adjuvant chemotherapy

Q210

A 28 year old woman has an ankle injury at work. She works as a builder. The ankle was openly reduced and internally fixed by an orthopaedic surgeon. She made an uneventful recovery on the ward. She has been deemed safe for discharge by the physiotherapist and the medical team. She has been told to be non-weight-bearing for 6 weeks, at which point the patient will be reviewed.

What is the most appropriate way of completing her fit note form?

1. Fit for work
2. May be fit for work with amended duties – no weight-bearing activities or lifting
3. May be fit for work with workplace adaptions – will need wheel-chair to get around site
4. Unfit for work for 2 weeks and GP to review
5. Unfit for work for 6 weeks

Q211

A 55 year old woman develops multi-organ dysfunction syndrome (MODS) involving respiratory and renal failure. She was admitted 3 days ago with pancreatitis, which developed into a systemic inflammatory response syndrome (SIRS).

What is the most likely reason for the progression from SIRS to MODS?

1. Delayed immune response
2. Genetic predisposition to organ failure
3. Inadequate fluid resuscitation
4. Infection spread to multiple organs
5. Persistent, uncontrolled systemic inflammation

Q212

A 65 year old man arrives in the emergency department confused. He has had 3 days of productive cough and pyrexia. He has no previous medical conditions. His temperature is 38.2 °C, pulse 110 bpm, BP 94/60 mmHg, respiratory rate 24 breaths per minute, oxygen saturation 87% breathing air.

What is the initial management?

1. Blood capillary glucose measurement
2. Commence intravenous fluid resuscitation
3. Estimate urine output
4. Oral antibiotics
5. Oxygen titrated to achieve an oxygen saturation 92–94%

Q213

A 22 year old man presents to the emergency department with 3 days of diarrhoea and vomiting. He is known to have type 1 diabetes mellitus. His blood gas shows a pH of 7.16, a pCO_2 of 3.0 kPa, lactate of 3.4 mmol/L, HCO_3 of 12 mEq/L and base excess of −8 mEq/L.

What abnormality does this blood gas show?

1. Metabolic acidosis with full respiratory compensation
2. Metabolic acidosis with partial respiratory compensation
3. Metabolic alkalosis with respiratory compensation
4. Respiratory acidosis with partial metabolic compensation
5. Respiratory alkalosis with no compensation

Q214

A 90 year old man has a gradual onset of shortness of breath, productive cough, fever and confusion. He has hypertension and benign prostatic hyperplasia.

His Glasgow Coma Score is 14/15. He is not orientated to time, place or person. He has normal heart sounds but decreased air entry at right lung base with crackles on auscultation.

Investigations:

Raised inflammatory markers

Chest X-ray shows consolidation on the right lung base

What assessment tool would you use to assess this patient for cognitive impairment?

1. CAM
2. CURB 65
3. Glasgow Blatchford score
4. HEART score
5. PESI score

Q215

A 26 year old man is brought to the emergency department with drowsiness. He has depression and a previous episode of deliberate self-harm. His heart rate is 115 bpm, BP 145/96 mmHg, respiratory rate 18 breaths per minute, oxygen saturation 96% on room air, temperature 37.5 °C. His capillary blood glucose is 6.4 mmol/L. On examination, he has a dry oral cavity, dilated pupils and a mildly tender suprapubic mass. His Glasgow Coma Score is 11 (E2, V4, M5).

An overdose of which drug could be causing his signs and symptoms?

1. Amitriptyline
2. Cocaine
3. Diazepam
4. Fentanyl
5. Paracetamol

Q216

A 53 year old woman attends the emergency department with severe breathlessness. She is centrally cyanosed. She has cardiomyopathy. She was turned down for heart transplant 3 years ago, and an implanted defibrillator (ICD) was turned off 2 weeks ago. Her Glasgow Coma Score is 8 (E2, M4, V2). She has pitting oedema to the lumbar region.

Investigations:

Potassium 8.1 mmol/L

Creatinine 2500 (< 140)

eGFR of 2 ml/min (baseline 85)

Her chest X-ray shows massive bilateral pleural effusions.

What is the next appropriate management?

1. Arrange bilateral chest drains
2. End of life care should be offered and promptly instituted
3. Give intravenous calcium chloride 20 ml of 10%, with 10 units of insulin and dextrose
4. Order an echocardiogram
5. Refer for dialysis

Q217

A 74 year old woman is confused on the ward and disturbing the other patients. She underwent surgical fixation of her neck of femur fracture 2 days ago and now appears confused. She has atrial fibrillation and type 2 diabetes mellitus. Her catheter bag urine looks cloudy. Her temperature is 38.2 °C, pulse 94 bpm, BP 84/60 mmHg, respiratory rate 18 breaths per minute, oxygen saturation 96% breathing air. Urine output 120 ml over the last 10 hours.

Her urine is sent for microscopy. Intravenous access is gained.

What would be the next course of action?

1. Arrange admission to ITU
2. Arrange full blood count
3. Arrange sedation
4. Request a senior review
5. Set up 0.9% saline solution

Q218

A 76 year old is brought into the emergency department by her son. She has rectal bleeding. She is haemodynamically stable but needs a colonoscopy. She has a history of moderate dementia. She can understand, weigh and retain the information you have presented to her about the procedure and she says that she would like to proceed. Her solicitor has lasting power of attorney.

What should you do next?

1. Consult an independent mental-capacity advocate

2. Continue with the procedure as consent is not required
3. Discuss the procedure with the patient's lasting power of attorney for health and welfare and ask them to consent
4. Discuss the procedure with the patient's son and ask him to consent
5. Invite the patient to sign a consent form

Q219

A 27 year old woman was diagnosed with epilepsy 9 months ago. Her last seizure was 6 months ago, just before starting medication. She has driven to her appointment today.

What is the most appropriate first course of action?
1. Confiscate the patient's car keys
2. Do nothing
3. Inform the DVLA
4. Inform the police
5. Remind the patient of their duty to inform the DVLA

Q220

A 92 year old woman is drowsy and unwell and unable to tell you the reason for her admission. The paramedic notes report concerns that she was febrile in the nursing home with a cough for the preceding 2 days. On examination, her fingernails are long and there is faecal matter underneath. She has a Grade 2 pressure sore on her sacrum.

What type of abuse might the patient have been experiencing?
1. Financial
2. Neglect
3. Physical
4. Psychological
5. Sexual

Q221

A 39 year old woman has had back pain for the last 10 years. She reports that the back pain has become progressively worse over the last 18 months and that her current analgesics are not working any more. She requests further analgesia to help her symptoms. She takes morphine sulphate (slow-release) 80 mg twice daily, naproxen

500 mg twice daily, paracetamol 1 g four times a day. She is referred to the pain clinic and physiotherapist.

What would be the most appropriate prescribing advice for the long-term management of her chronic pain?

1. Add in gabapentin
2. Add in pregabalin
3. Increase dose of morphine sulphate to 100 mg twice daily
4. Reduce the dose of morphine sulphate gradually
5. Use morphine sulphate liquid for breakthrough pain

Q222

A 45 year old man with advanced lung cancer has been admitted for treatment of a right-sided pneumonia, but deteriorated despite treatment. He is now held to be dying by the ward multidisciplinary team. At home, he had symptoms of pain and breathlessness for which he used 60 mg morphine sulphate modified release twice daily. He can no longer swallow.

How much morphine should he have in his subcutaneous driver over 24 hours?

1. 15 mg
2. 30 mg
3. 45 mg
4. 60 mg
5. 120 mg

Q223

An 80 year old woman has had recurrent falls in recent months. The falls often occur when walking or changing position, and she sometimes experiences dizziness during these episodes. She denies loss of consciousness, chest pain or palpitations. She has well-controlled hypertension, osteoarthritis and mild cognitive impairment. She lives independently at home with her husband and uses a cane for mobility. She takes losartan, ibuprofen and vitamin D supplements. Her BP is 130/70 mmHg.

What is the most likely cause of her falls?

1. Age-related gait disturbance
2. Cardiovascular syncope

3. Cognitive impairment
4. Drug-induced orthostatic hypotension
5. Osteoarthritis-related joint instability

Q224

An 86 year old man presents to the emergency department having been found on the floor by his neighbour. For the last 3 weeks he says his legs have – 'not been quite right'. He has macular degeneration, prostate cancer and type 2 diabetes. He lives independently. His BMI is 22 kg/m².

Which part of the history indicates the presence of a frailty syndrome?

1. Age of 86
2. BMI 22 kg/m²
3. History of macular degeneration
4. History of prostate cancer
5. Presenting with a fall

Q225

A 43 year old man presents to the emergency department with sudden-onset left loin pain that started 3 hours ago. The pain is intermittent, but very sharp, and radiates to his suprapubic region. It is the worst pain he has ever experienced, and it only settled with rectal diclofenac 100 mg. He is alert, his temperature is 37.3 °C, pulse 84 bpm, BP 134/73 mmHg, respiratory rate 22 breaths per minute, oxygen saturation 97% breathing air. He has a soft abdomen, with maximal tenderness in the left renal angle, and no pulsatile mass.

Given the likely diagnosis, what is the best imaging modality to diagnose this patient?

1. CT abdomen and pelvis with contrast
2. CT abdomen and pelvis without contrast
3. CT abdominal angiogram
4. CT kidney, ureter and bladder
5. US abdomen

Q226

A 77 year old man requires enteral feeding and medications due to an unsafe swallow after a stroke. A nasogastric tube was passed and secured at 60 cm. He could not swallow to help during tube insertion and coughed repeatedly during the procedure; 40 ml of green fluid was aspirated. pH testing on the sample reveals a pH of 5.8. He has a past history of reflux and hypertension. He takes omeprazole and losartan.

What is the most appropriate next step?

1. Document the tube is safe to use as the large volume of green fluid is clearly gastric
2. Flush 40 ml of air down the tube and listen for air flow over the stomach
3. Perform a chest X-ray
4. Remove the tube immediately as his coughing suggests placement in the respiratory tract
5. Remove the tube immediately as the pH suggests placement in the lung

Q227

A 23 year old woman is brought to the emergency department having taken an unknown amount of paracetamol 30 minutes ago. Her friends say that they found one empty paracetamol tablet packet in her room.

When should a blood sample be drawn, from the woman, to determine her plasma-paracetamol concentration?

1. 1 hour after paracetamol ingestion
2. 4 hours after paracetamol ingestion
3. 8 hours after paracetamol ingestion
4. 24 hours after paracetamol ingestion
5. As soon as possible

Q228

A 76 year old woman has been brought to the GP by her neighbour, who is concerned about her. She lives on her own and is generally independent. She admits she has been skipping meals and not taking her statin regularly. She has no past medical history other than hyperlipidaemia. Self-neglect is suspected. She is mildly pale and shows signs of poor personal hygiene.

What would constitute a holistic wellbeing check?

1. Drug and alcohol consumption review
2. Mental and physical health review
3. Mental health assessment
4. Mental, physical and social health assessment
5. Physical health assessment with general blood test

Q229

A 67 year old man is admitted for an elective right hemicolectomy for cancer; 6 days after his operation he becomes unwell, an anastomotic leak is identified and he is taken back to theatre for a further operation and is then admitted to the ICU for a week due to sepsis and post-operative instability.

What Clavien–Dindo grade of complication has the patient suffered?

1. Grade I
2. Grade II
3. Grade III
4. Grade IV
5. Grade V

Q230

An 89 year old woman has 2 days of a cough. She has type 2 diabetes and osteoarthritis, but lives independently on her own. She is mildly confused, her temperature is 38.1 °C, pulse 90 bpm, BP 140/72 mmHg. Right basal crepitations are noted on chest auscultation.

What is the most important factor when assessing her need for admission?

1. Chest X-ray
2. Collateral history from a family member
3. Her confusion precludes management at home
4. Sputum culture
5. Urea and electrolyte bloods

Q231

A 58 year old man is found to have a right renal mass on ultrasound which was arranged for his biliary colic. He is currently an inpatient in the surgical unit and waiting for discharge. The report suggests clinical correlation and further imaging with CT if indicated. He is clinically well and his symptoms have subsided, and home transport has arrived.

What is the most appropriate action?

1. Arrange urgent outpatient CT scan with clinic follow-up
2. Ask the patient to contact GP for the follow-up scan
3. Cancel the discharge and request a CT scan the next day
4. Cancel the discharge and send an inpatient referral to the urology team
5. Write in discharge summary for the GP to contact the patient

Q232

A 44 year old woman has pain all over her body for 2 years, which is constant and unremitting. She has had to give up work and her symptoms have disrupted family life. She now lives alone. She feels exhausted and is taking several medications including opiates. All investigations have been negative and physical examination reveals only apparent widespread tenderness on palpation and most movements. She walks with a crutch and wears dark glasses because she says that the light hurts her eyes.

What is the most appropriate management?

1. Advise her that it is all in her head and to get on with life
2. Agree that her pain is real, provide explanations and explore non-drug options
3. Arrange a whole-body scan to find the source of her pain
4. Refer to neurology
5. Suggest a step-wise increase in her analgesics

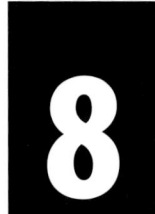

Haematology

8

Q233

A 34 year old woman feels tired. She eats an exclusively vegan diet.

Investigations:

Haemoglobin 104 g/L (115–165)

White cell count 6.8 x10⁹/L (4–11)

Platelets 382 x10⁹/L (150–400)

MCV 82fL (80–100)

MCH 26.4pg (28–32)

CRP 2 (< 6)

What is the most likely diagnosis?

1. Acute myeloid leukaemia
2. Anaemia of chronic disease
3. Iron deficiency anaemia
4. Paroxysmal nocturnal haemoglobinuria
5. Vitamin B12 deficiency

Q234

A 34 year old woman suddenly becomes short of breath on the acute medical ward. This is associated with agitation, nausea and stomach cramps; 30 minutes ago, she took her evening antibiotics. Her pulse is 120 bpm, BP 70/40 mmHg, respiratory rate 30 breaths per minute. She has a widespread wheeze.

What is the most appropriate initial management?

1. Chlorpheniramine 10 mg intravenously
2. Epinephrine 0.5 mg intramuscularly
3. Epinephrine 1 mg intravenously

4. Hydrocortisone 100 microgrammes intravenously

5. Salbutamol 5 mg nebulized

Q235

A 25 year old Black woman complains of recent onset of pallor, shortness of breath and tiredness. She has moderate conjunctival pallor, but is otherwise normal.

Investigations:

Haemoglobin 72 g/L (115–165)

White cell count 7.0 x 10^9/L (4.0–11.0)

Platelet count 350 x 10^9/L (150–400)

Reticulocytes 256 x 10^9/L (20–85)

Serum bilirubin 43 μmol/L (5–22)

Blood film: microspherocytes with severe polychromasia and occasional nucleated red blood cells

Direct antiglobulin (Coombs) test = Positive

What is the most likely diagnosis?

1. Autoimmune haemolytic anaemia

2. Glucose-6-phosphate dehydrogenase deficiency

3. Hereditary spherocytosis

4. Pyruvate kinase deficiency

5. Sickle cell anaemia

Q236

A 74 year old man has rectal bleeding and spontaneous bruising. He was admitted with a community-acquired pneumonia 4 days ago. He takes warfarin and bisoprolol for atrial fibrillation. He has been treated with intravenous antibiotics but his clinical condition is deteriorating.

Investigations:

Hb 100 g/L (120–160)

MCV 87fL (80–100)

WCC 18.6 x10^9/L (3.5–10.2)

Platelets 75 x 10^9/L (150–400)

Prothrombin time 30 sec (12–16)

APTT 79s (25–34)

Fibrinogen 1.3 g/L (1.5–4)

What is the most likely diagnosis?

1. Disseminated intravascular coagulation
2. Liver disease
3. Thrombocytopenia
4. Vitamin K deficiency
5. Warfarin overdose

Q237

A 23 year old woman of Cypriot origin is in her first pregnancy. Antenatal testing identifies her as being a carrier of beta thalassaemia minor with a β/β0 genotype. Partner testing finds that her partner has the same genotype (β/β0). What is the risk of the child developing beta thalassaemia major?

1. 0%
2. 25%
3. 50%
4. 75%
5. 100%

Q238

A 12 year old boy develops a swollen calf following a minor football injury. There is no family history of bleeding disorders. On examination, the calf is swollen, red and shows extensive bruising; a diagnosis of an intramuscular haemorrhage is made. Investigations:

White cells	8.9 x 10^9/L	(3.6–9.2)
Haemoglobin	189 g/L	(130–175)
Platelets	279 x 10^9/L	(140–400)
Prothrombin time	13.7 sec	(12.5–15.5)
Activated partial thromboplastin time	60.3 sec	(25.5–34)
Factor VIII	8 u/dL	(50–150)
Factor IX	80 u/dL	(50–150)
Von Willebrand antigen	99 u/dL	(50–150)
Von Willebrand activity	91 u/dL	(50–150)

What is the most likely diagnosis?

1. Acquired haemophilia A
2. Immune thrombocytopenia
3. Mild haemophilia A
4. Severe haemophilia B
5. Type 1 von Willebrand's disease

Q239

A 21 year old man has lost 10 kg weight in 4 months (previously 70 kg). This has been associated with drenching night sweats and a large left-sided neck lump. Biopsy of the neck lump confirms a diagnosis of Hodgkin lymphoma. PET–CT scan demonstrates multiple groups of involved nodes on both sides of the diaphragm but no extranodal sites.

What Ann Arbor stage is his lymphoma?

1. Stage IB
2. Stage IIA
3. Stage IIIB
4. Stage IVA
5. Stage IVB

Q240

A 52 year old man comes to the emergency department with excessive tiredness. He is pale, anxious and has bruises over his arms and legs. His temperature is 39 °C.

Investigations:

Haemoglobin 62 g/L (115–165)

WBC 100 x 10^9/L (4–11)

Platelets 40 x 109/L (150–400)

The lab confirms the existence of blasts on blood film.

What is the most likely diagnosis?

1. Acute lymphoblastic leukaemia
2. Acute myeloid leukaemia
3. Chronic lymphocytic leukaemia
4. Chronic myeloid leukaemia
5. Richter's syndrome

Q241

A 74 year old man has 1 week of abdominal and generalised bone pain. He has type 2 diabetes. He is a retired builder and a lifelong smoker.

Investigations:

Haemoglobin	109 g/L	(130–175)
White cells	6.2×10^9/L	(3.6–9.2)
Platelets	300×10^9/L	(140–400)
Neutrophils	4.4×10^9/L	(1.7–6.2)
Creatinine	194 µmol/L	(64–111)
Corrected calcium	3.10 mmol/L	(2.1–2.55)
Parathyroid hormone	1.0 pmol/L	(1.6–7.2)

Immunoglobulins

Ig   G 5.43 g/L   (5.4–18.2)

Ig   A 1.05 g/L   (1.01–6.45)

Ig   M < 0.05   (0.22–2.4)

Serum free light chains

Kappa   8.7 units   (3.3–19.4)

Lambda   8492 units   (5.7–26.3)

Serum immunofixation demonstrates a lambda light chain paraprotein of 2 g/L.

Urine immunofixation is positive for Bence–Jones proteins identified as lambda light chains.

What is the most likely diagnosis?

1. Bronchogenic carcinoma
2. Diabetic nephropathy
3. Monoclonal gammopathy of undetermined significance
4. Multiple myeloma
5. Primary hyperparathyroidism

Q242

A 19 year old man has 5 days of sore throat, fever and tender neck swelling. On examination, his fauces are indurated and there are multiple 1–2 cm lymph nodes palpable in the anterior triangle of the neck bilaterally. He has 1 finger-breadth of splenomegaly palpable in the abdomen.

What investigation is most likely to confirm the diagnosis?

1. CT scan of neck, thorax, abdomen and pelvis
2. EBV IgM serology
3. Full blood count
4. Lymph node biopsy
5. Ultrasound scan of neck

Q243

A 61 year old woman has a full blood count performed as part of a routine health check. Her platelet count was 789 x 10^9/L (150–400); the remainder of her bloods were normal. She is well with no symptoms; examination is unremarkable. Investigations:

Ferritin	121 ug/L	(10–204)
CRP	2 mg/L	(< 6)
JAK2 val617phe mutation	DETECTED	
CALR mutation	Not detected	
MPL mutation	Not detected	
BCR-ABL mutation	Not detected	

What is the most likely diagnosis?

1. Acute infection
2. Essential thrombocythaemia
3. Iron deficiency
4. Polycythaemia vera
5. Primary myelofibrosis

Q244

A 28 year old man has 3 weeks of worsening breathlessness on exertion and a sensation of 'the blood pounding in his ears'. He is pale, there is no splenomegaly and he has a purpuric rash over his ankles.

Investigations:

White cells	2.1 x 10^9/L	(3.6–9.2)
Haemoglobin	62 g/L	(130–175)
Platelets	12 x 10^9/L	(140–400)
Neutrophils	0.2 x 10^9/L	(1.7–6.2)

Blood film shows circulating blasts with minimal differentiation. There is pancytopenia with a leucoerythroblastic picture.

What is the most likely diagnosis?

1. Acute leukaemia
2. Chronic lymphocytic leukaemia
3. Folate deficiency
4. Metastatic malignancy
5. Myelofibrosis

Q245

A 62 year old man has chest pain diagnosed as acute coronary syndrome. A decision is made to treat with percutaneous coronary intervention. He is clinically stable and there is time to initiate oral therapy.

What is the recommended anti-platelet regimen in this scenario?

1. Aspirin 75 mg only
2. Aspirin and modified-release dipyridamole
3. Aspirin and ticagrelor or prasugrel
4. Clopidogrel 75 mg only
5. Ticagrelor or prasugrel

Q246

A 57 year old man has 2 years of gradual worsening shortness of breath. His exercise tolerance is limited to one flight of stairs before stopping to catch his breath. He has hypertension and takes bend-roflumethiazide 2.5 mg daily. He smokes 20 cigarettes a day with a 40 pack year history. He is plethoric with a reduced chest expansion and expiratory wheeze throughout all lung fields. His oxygen saturation is 91% breathing air.

Investigations:

Haemoglobin	182 g/L	(130–175)
White cells	12.1 x 10^9/L	(3.6–9.2)
Platelets	398 x 10^9/L	(140–400)
Haematocrit	0.61	(0.4–0.5)
Neutrophils	8.8 x 10^9/L	(1.7–6.2)
JAK2 val617phe mutation	Not detected	

What is the most likely cause of his polycythaemia?

1. Chronic obstructive pulmonary disease
2. EPO-secreting tumour
3. Gaisbock's syndrome
4. Polycythaemia vera
5. Relative polycythaemia

Q247

A 24 year old woman has recently had genetic tests because her father has haemophilia A. Her results were normal (she is not a carrier).

What is the most likely reason for her genetic results?

1. Cross-over at meiosis
2. Cross-over at mitosis
3. Non-maternity
4. Non-paternity
5. She has an XY karyotype

Q248

A 70 year old woman is admitted from the emergency department with epistaxis. She has a mechanical heart valve, atrial fibrillation (AF) and moderately impaired cardiac function. She takes amiodarone, bisoprolol, digoxin, diltiazem, flecanide and warfarin.

Investigations:

INR 8.4 (target 3.0)

What medication may have led to her being over anti-coagulated?

1. Amiodarone
2. Bisoprolol
3. Digoxin
4. Diltiazem
5. Flecanide

Q249

A 3 year old boy has a sudden-onset severe abdominal pain. He has sickle cell anaemia and has been taking prophylactic penicillin. His temperature is 37.7 °C, pulse 165 bpm, respiratory rate of 44 breaths per minute, capillary refill time 3.5 seconds. He has conjunctival pallor and a large, tender mass left upper quadrant. His bloods show a haemoglobin of 67 g/L with reticulosis.

What is the most likely diagnosis?

1. Acute chest syndrome
2. Acute cholecystitis
3. Mesenteric adenitis
4. Parvovirus B19 infection
5. Splenic sequestration crisis

Q250

A 64 year old man started a red blood cell transfusion approximately 10 minutes ago and now appears to be having a **moderate** transfusion reaction.

What is the **first** thing you should do before any further assessment?

1. Check the patient's temperature
2. Continue the transfusion at a slower rate
3. Inform the blood bank that the patient is having a transfusion reaction
4. Set up a saline infusion to run alongside the transfusion
5. Stop the transfusion

Q251

A 56 year old woman bleeds excessively during a routine cholecystectomy. She has had heavy periods, almost from menarche, and easy bruising as a child. She had a significant postpartum haemorrhage following the birth of her son 30 years ago and required a blood transfusion. Her mother also had heavy periods. Her clotting screen, FBC, renal and liver function are all normal.

What is the most likely diagnosis?

1. Disseminated intravascular coagulation
2. Immune thrombocytopenia
3. Haemophilia A
4. Haemophilia B
5. von Willebrand's disease

Q252

A 22 year old woman has a growing tender midline neck swelling. She has had some neck swelling since childhood. She has no changes to her voice or difficulty breathing. She feels tired. On examination, she has a 3 x 2 cm midline lump which moves cranially when she sticks out her tongue.

What is the underlying aetiology?

1. Fascial weakness between the cricopharyngeus and thyropharyngeus muscle
2. Incomplete embryonic epithelial growth at lines of fusion
3. Persistent thyroglossal duct
4. Proliferation of a clone of malignant B cells
5. Second branchial cleft which has failed to obliterate

Q253

A 35 year old woman becomes short of breath over a period of 3 minutes, following an intravenous injection of amoxicillin. Her heart rate is 110 bpm, BP 72/44 mmHg (previously 116/72).

What is the next step in management?

1. Administer 0.5 mg intramuscular adrenaline (1:1000)
2. Administer 10 mg intramuscular chlorphenamine
3. Administer 200 mg intravenous hydrocortisone
4. Fast-bleep the on-call allergy/immunology team
5. Take further collateral history

Infectious Disease

9

Q254

A 10 year old girl has difficulty swallowing. She has recently had braces fitted. She has creamy white plaques on the surface of her tongue extending down the back of the throat. It is possible to gently scrape away this plaque to reveal underlying inflamed tissue.

What is the most likely causative agent?

1. Candida albicans
2. Corynebacterium diphtheriae
3. Epstein–Barr virus
4. Porphyromonas gingivalis
5. Streptococcus mitis

Q255

A 26 year old man has an increasing number of painful lumps on his penis, progressing over the last 24 hours. He has never had these lesions before. Examination confirms a cluster of ten small vesicles, filled with clear fluid. There is no significant crusting or swelling.

What treatment would be most appropriate in this case?

1. No treatment required
2. Oral aciclovir
3. Oral doxycycline
4. Topical aciclovir
5. Topical fucidin cream

Q256

A 70 year old man suddenly becomes unwell with fever, tachycardia, hypotension, diarrhoea and new confusion. He was admitted to hospital 1 week ago following a fall where he sustained a fractured neck of femur. He underwent a hemi-arthroplasty 6 days ago and is currently on day 3 of ciprofloxacin. He is isolated; his wound is reviewed; a stool sample is taken for Clostridium difficile; a urine dip and MC&S are performed. His ciprofloxacin is stopped.

What is the most appropriate additional action?

1. Abdominal CT scan
2. Blood cultures x 2
3. Lumbar puncture
4. Prepare for theatre for exploration of wound
5. Sputum sample

Q257

A 78 year old man presents to the emergency department with 24 hours of fever and delirium. He is cared for in a residential home and is normally alert and orientated. He has type 2 diabetes mellitus (metformin only) and benign prostatic hypertrophy with a long-term urethral catheter *in situ*. He has had six attendances in the last year with similar symptoms; the last time he had a traumatic catheter change which required input by the urology team.

His temperature is 39.1 °C, pulse 87 bpm, BP 136/74 mmHg, respiratory rate 13 breaths per minute, oxygen saturation 96% breathing air, capillary refill 2 seconds. He is tender in the suprapubic region. There is no blood in the catheter bag, but the urine is concentrated and still draining well. His bedside glucose is 12 mmol/L. Urine is sent for MC&S. Intravenous fluids are commenced.

What is the most appropriate management?

1. Change the urethral catheter and send the tip to the laboratory for culture
2. Commence empirical intravenous antibiotics based on the hospital antibiotic guidance
3. Defer antibiotic administration until cultures return
4. Give antipyretics such as intravenous paracetamol and seek to optimise his blood glucose
5. Review the patient's previous microbiology results and discuss with the microbiologist

Q258

A 29 year old man presents to the emergency department with 2 days of fever, cough and shortness of breath, particularly on exertion. He is known to be HIV positive for the past 5 years but has not been compliant with antiretroviral medication due to side effects. He has been started on oxygen, given fluids and paracetamol, and referred to the medical team. He is Covid negative.

Investigations:

CD4 count 50 per mm^3

Viral load of 250,000 per ml

Chest X-ray: perihilar pulmonary infiltrates with sparing of the peripheral lung fields

What is the next management step?

1. High-dose trimethoprim/sulfamethoxazole
2. Immediately start Truvada plus dolutegravir
3. Intravenous co-amoxiclav and clarithromycin
4. Meropenem and gentamicin
5. Oral aciclovir

Q259

A 33 year old man has been feeling feverish and achy for the last 3 weeks, now with a painful swollen right knee joint; 2 weeks ago, he had an erythematous rash on his right leg. He has some soreness and redness in both eyes. He works as a tree forester.

His temperature is 37.8 °C, pulse 76 bpm, BP 124/82 mmHg, respiratory rate 14 breaths per minute, oxygen saturation 98% breathing air. Both knees are warm and swollen, with a mildly reduced range of movement. His eyes demonstrate mild erythema with no significant photophobia. Skin examination is now normal. A possible diagnosis of Lyme disease is made. Blood is sent away for microbiological confirmation.

What is the next step in management?

1. Admit for intravenous antibiotics
2. Reassure and review if symptoms get worse
3. Start oral antibiotics immediately
4. Start oral steroids
5. Wait for the microbiology report and treat accordingly

Q260

A 34 year old man has 10 kg unintentional weight loss in the last 3 months. This has been associated with night sweats and a low-grade fever. He has also had a productive cough for the last 6 months. He moved to this country from South East Asia, 2 months ago. He lives alone and works from home.

What is the most appropriate initial management?

1. Arrange a TB Gold QuantiFERON test
2. Check Vitamin D level
3. Collect three early morning sputum samples and refer to a respiratory physician urgently
4. Give 1-week course of amoxicillin and follow-up on completion of treatment
5. Refer to the emergency department for urgent chest X-ray

Q261

A 64 year old man has 2 days of intermittent fever and chills. He reports having severe myalgia, headaches and malaise. He recently returned from a business trip to Nigeria. He did not take any chemo-prophylaxis against malaria. You suspect he may have malaria.

Which investigation would most likely lead to confirmation of the diagnosis?

1. Blood cultures
2. CT thorax, abdomen, pelvis
3. Full blood count
4. Microscopy of thick and thin smears
5. Throat swab

Q262

A 5 year old boy has been unwell for 3 days with a low-grade fever. He has been off food but still drinking, and less interested in playing. He developed a bilateral parotid swelling this morning, suggesting mumps. His temperature is 38.1 °C. His other observations are normal. He has no rash.

What course of action should be taken in terms of notifying the local public health team of this patient?

1. Admit to paediatrics and expect them to notify if appropriate

2. Do nothing unless a second case presents
3. No action is needed, mumps is not a notifiable disease
4. Report the case the same day
5. Undertake testing for mumps and report it if the results come back as positive

Q263

A 57 year old man is pyrexial and has an increasingly painful wound 24 hours post-operatively from a left hemicolectomy for bowel cancer. He has opened his bowels post-operatively and is not vomiting.

He is alert, his temperature is 38.4 °C, pulse 104 bpm, BP 136/86 mmHg, oxygen saturation 98% breathing room air. His abdomen is slightly distended, and he is tender around the surgical wound site with some erythema. On palpation, moderate amounts of purulent exudate can be expressed. The surgical clips appear to be holding well and are not under significant amounts of strain.

What are your next steps in management?

1. Ask nursing team to change wound dressing and monitor the observations
2. Commence immediate intravenous fluid resuscitation and discuss transfer to theatres for emergency laparotomy with senior members of the team
3. Draw around the area of erythema and ask the nursing team to contact you if he continues to deteriorate
4. Order an urgent CT scan and await the results
5. Swab the exudate, mark the area, change the dressing, commence antibiotics according to local protocol and discuss imaging with senior members of the team

Q264

A 67 year old woman has pyrexia and general malaise. She hit her right leg on a stool 4 days ago, since when the leg has become swollen with a large area of erythema anteriorly, which has spread rapidly over the last 24 hours.

What is the most appropriate management plan?

1. Cryotherapy
2. Fluid resuscitation

3. Intravenous antibiotics
4. Oral antibiotics
5. Surgical debridement and intravenous antibiotics

Q265

A 20 year old woman presents to the emergency department with 3 days of fever, myalgia, diarrhoea, rash, general malaise and syncopal symptoms. She is disorientated and confused, her temperature is 39.4 °C, pulse 122 bpm, BP 86/50 mmHg, respiratory rate 24 breaths per minute, oxygen saturation 99% breathing air.

Which dermatological condition is most associated with a diagnosis of toxic shock syndrome?

1. Desquamation of palms and soles
2. Dry gangrene
3. Erythema multiforme
4. Erythema toxicum
5. Erythroderma

Q266

A 21 year old man attends a travel clinic appointment asking about how to reduce his risk of catching malaria when he goes to Kenya in 2 months' time. You discuss bite prevention strategies with him.

What does the ABCD guide to preventing malaria stand for?

1. Assessment, Bite avoidance, Chemoprophylaxis, Diagnosis
2. Assessment, Bite prevention, Covering up, Drugs
3. Avoidance, Bite prevention, Covering up, Drugs
4. Awareness, Bite avoidance, Chemoprophylaxis, Deterrence
5. Awareness, Bite prevention, Chemoprophylaxis, Diagnosis

Q267

A 24 year old man has 3 weeks of productive cough, night sweats and 6 kg weight loss. His observations are normal and chest X-ray shows right upper lobe cavitating lesions. Sputum is smear positive for acid-fast bacilli. He was started on standard four-drug anti-TB therapy and is currently in isolation.

When can he start going out in public again?

1. Immediately, if he is wearing a face mask

2. When he has a normal chest X-ray
3. When he has been taking his medication for 3 weeks
4. When he has completed 6 months of anti-TB therapy
5. When his symptoms have improved and he is no longer coughing

Q268

A 2 year old boy has 24 hours of fever, a vesicular rash on his torso associated with itching, and general malaise, suggestive of chickenpox.

What is the most suitable laboratory investigation to undertake?

1. Full blood count
2. IgG antibodies to varicella zoster virus
3. IgM antibodies to varicella zoster virus
4. No test required
5. Polymerase chain reaction for varicella zoster virus

Q269

A 55 year old man presents to the emergency department with 3 days of cough and worsening shortness of breath. He denies any purulent sputum. He is overweight and has type 2 diabetes mellitus. His temperature is 39 °C, respiratory rate 24 breaths per minute, oxygen saturation 94% breathing 15 L oxygen. He is clammy and lethargic. Chest auscultation reveals poor air entry on both sides.

Investigations:

Creatinine 100 μmol/L (60–90)

CRP 65 mg/L (< 6)

SARS-CoV-2 PCR result is pending

Chest X-ray shows bilateral diffuse opacities.

What are the next best steps in management?

1. Admit to hospital and give O_2, intravenous fluids, antibiotics, dexamethasone and remdesivir
2. Admit to hospital for observations only
3. Consider contacting ITU as a matter of urgency
4. Give the patient the Covid vaccine
5. Give reassurance and advice, discharge home for 10 days of isolation

Mental Health

Q270

A 28 year old woman has experienced a 2 week worsening in her mental state. She has become increasingly withdrawn in the past month, and her partner reported that she has been restricting her diet. She is underweight, with scratches on her knuckles and a swollen neck. Her BMI is 14 kg/m², and her ECG shows QT prolongation and U waves. Blood is taken for urea and electrolytes, glucose, LH, FSH and GH.

What is the most likely laboratory finding on her blood test?

1. High blood sugar
2. High LH and FSH
3. Hypernatremia
4. Hypokalaemia
5. Low growth hormone

Q271

A 29 year old woman feels anxious and 'on edge' most of the time, since the birth of her baby 8 weeks ago. This is associated with guilt and shame. She had a prolonged and frightening labour and birth, requiring an emergency caesarean section after signs of fetal distress. She explains that she keeps 'going back' and re-experiencing her labour. While having these episodes, she feels extremely frightened, out of control and worried for the safety of her baby and herself. She describes feeling numbed and is having difficulty bonding with her baby.

What is the most accurate diagnosis?

1. Acute stress disorder
2. Agoraphobia

3. Generalised anxiety disorder
4. Post-traumatic stress disorder
5. Severe depressive disorder

Q272

A 22 year old woman has a year's history of intensive and distressing intrusive thoughts pertaining to locking and cleaning. She explained to the general practitioner that her lateness was due to her checking five times that all the electrical sockets and equipment around the house were switched off. She explained that she has to follow these rituals every time she leaves her house, which has been causing her trouble at work. She has also been in conflict with her family as she spends a significant time obsessively cleaning and tidying. She has little tolerance of any perceived mess, and this leads to big arguments. On observation, she is fidgety, she looks anxious, and she has dermatitis on both hands.

What would be the most suitable initial management?

1. Diazepam
2. Intensive CBT combined with SSRI
3. Low-level CBT with Exposure and response prevention
4. Propranolol
5. Watch and wait approach

Q273

A 25 year old woman has severe anxiety and depression for the last 3 weeks. She takes lithium 1000 mg at night for bipolar affective disorder. She was admitted last year with a manic episode.

The local formulary has the following medications for severe anxiety and depression in bipolar disease: aripiprazole, diazepam, lamotrigine, quetiapine and sodium valproate.

Which one of the formulary medications is contraindicated in this situation?

1. Aripiprazole
2. Diazepam
3. Lamotrigine
4. Quetiapine
5. Sodium valproate

Q274

A 32 year old man has 2 months of low mood, associated with lethargy, low self-esteem and impaired concentration. He has no suicidal ideation. He has never spoken with a professional about his mental health before. He has stable employment, a supportive partner and cannot recall any recent psychosocial stressors.

Which of the following is the most appropriate first management step?

1. Commence an SSRI
2. Individual guided self-help based on cognitive behavioural therapy (CBT)
3. Psychodynamic psychotherapy
4. Reassurance
5. Referral to secondary care services

Q275

A 64 year old man believes that his bowel has stopped working and faeces are now leaking out and travelling around his body. He is low in energy, appears tired, doesn't show any emotional reactivity and has poor eye contact. He hasn't eaten anything for the last week and has a minimal fluid intake. He wakes very early in the morning and believes it would be better off if he were dead. He has no past psychiatric history.

What is the likely diagnosis?

1. Bipolar disorder
2. Delusional disorder
3. Schizoaffective disorder
4. Schizophrenia
5. Severe depression with psychosis

Q276

A 25 year old woman presents to the emergency department with palpitations. She reports feeling very cold, despite it being a warm day. She is exhausted and frequently faints. She has been at university doing a PhD but has become increasingly stressed due to pending deadlines. Her food intake has reduced over recent months; she currently eats 800 calories a day as a means of managing her anxiety. Her pulse is 42 bpm, lying BP 96/54 mmHg. Her BMI is 13.2 kg/m².

What is the next step of management?

1. Admit to the medical wards for monitoring and weight restoration
2. Discharge with Eating Disorders Service follow-up
3. Discharge with GP follow-up
4. Refer to acute psychiatry team for admission to eating disorder unit
5. Refer to self-help services

Q277

A 55 year old woman is depressed and considering harming herself. Three years ago, she took an overdose of paracetamol thinking this would be fatal. She drinks 2 glasses of wine each evening. She is menopausal, married, with two grown-up children.

Which factor in her history has most influence on her suicide risk?

1. Being menopausal
2. Female gender
3. Her alcohol intake
4. Married status
5. Previous impulsive suicide attempt

Q278

A 23 year old man presents to the emergency department with suicidal ideation. He is very tearful and quick to get angry. He split with his partner 2 weeks ago. Since then, he has been binge drinking and having unprotected sex with several partners whilst intoxicated. He has impulsively punched walls in frustration and cut himself several times with a razor blade when feeling distressed. He has a plan to take an overdose of paracetamol but is amenable to working with the liaison psychiatry team.

Which of the following is most appropriate as a treatment for this patient?

1. Dialectal behaviour therapy
2. Diazepam 10 mg twice daily for 3 weeks

3. Intensive community support for crisis management
4. Quetiapine as a mood stabiliser
5. Voluntary inpatient psychiatric admission

Q279

A 27 year old man is brought into the emergency department by his partner. She is concerned as he has been behaving out of character. He has not slept for 3 days, has been uncontactable for much of the time, and she is worried he has been spending lots of money on clothing, gambling and a car. This has never happened before; he has no previous physical or mental health conditions and takes no medication. The triage nurse tells you he has been overfamiliar with her, asking to swap phone numbers. The observations are normal apart from a heart rate of 105/min.

What is the next step?

1. Arrange Mental Health Act assessment
2. Bloods and a urine dip and drug screen
3. Call security as he has spoken inappropriately to a member of staff
4. Contact the psychiatric liaison team
5. CT scan head

Q280

A 42 year old man experiences auditory hallucinations and holds delusional beliefs that he is part of a 'national elite crime squadron'. He was diagnosed with schizophrenia 12 years ago and has had three hospital admissions under the Mental Health Act. He is under the care of the community mental health team, with daily support from carers.

He has previously been treated with aripiprazole and olanzapine and is currently taking haloperidol 5 mg twice daily, although he admitted to non-adherence with medication. He has recently become more concerned about his neighbours, believing they are not following instructions from 'high command'. He has approached them about this on multiple occasions.

He does not use drugs or alcohol.

What is the most appropriate management?

1. Admit to hospital under the Mental Health Act
2. Consider a trial of clozapine

3. Increase the frequency of visits from the Community Psychiatric Nurse
4. Request a blister pack for his medication
5. Switch haloperidol to a depot formulation

Q281

A 35 year old woman has been experiencing a wide array of physical symptoms across multiple organ systems for the past several years. She frequently visits various healthcare providers seeking relief from her symptoms but fails to find any medical explanation for her complaints. She reports experiencing pain, gastrointestinal disturbances, neurological symptoms, and other bodily sensations that vary in intensity and location. Her symptoms cause significant distress and impairment in her daily functioning. On mental status examination, she appears preoccupied with her physical health and expresses frustration about not receiving a definitive medical diagnosis.

What is the most likely diagnosis?

1. Factitious disorder
2. Functional neurological symptom disorder
3. Generalised anxiety disorder
4. Illness anxiety disorder
5. Somatic symptom disorder

Q282

A 30 year old woman is found unconscious and clammy. Her temperature is 36.8 °C, pulse 60 bpm, BP 110/70 mmHg, respiratory rate 6 breaths per minute, oxygen saturation 85% breathing air. She has miosis. High-flow oxygen has been applied via a non-rebreathe mask.

What is the most appropriate initial management step?

1. Artificial ventilation
2. Bolus of intravenous fluids
3. Intravenous infusion of adrenaline (epinephrine)
4. Intravenous lorazepam
5. Therapeutic trial of intravenous naloxone

Q283

A 16 year old woman attends the emergency department after being found by her mother, having taken a large overdose of paracetamol 6 hours ago. She has a severe personality disorder. Her serum paracetamol level is above the cut-off range, indicating that she needs treatment with N-acetylcysteine. During the assessment process, she indicates she wishes to leave, indicating no regrets about the overdose. She is frustrated at having been brought to hospital and is at risk of death from the overdose.

What would be the most appropriate next step?

1. Conduct a mental capacity assessment
2. Discharge the patient as requested
3. Refer for Mental Health Act assessment
4. Treat her against her wishes as she could die from the overdose
5. Watch and wait to see whether she stays in hospital and changes her mind

Q284

A 32 year old woman is brought to the emergency department by paramedics with an acute confusion. She is very tearful, dazed, agitated – picking her skin and hitting herself in the face, requiring restraint by police officers. She is unable to take in any information from those around her. She was robbed at knife point by an assailant 1 hour ago. She was not physically harmed during the assault.

What is the most appropriate next step?

1. CT head scan
2. Mental Health Act assessment
3. Nurse 1:1 in a quiet area
4. Oral lorazepam
5. Take MSU and bloods for delirium markers

Q285

A 34 year old man presents to the emergency department with 6 hours of increasing anxiety. He usually drinks 30 units of alcohol a day and last drank alcohol 20 hours ago. His pulse is 105 bpm. He is clammy and has a tremor. On mental state examination, he is

dishevelled, irritable, and complains of low mood. He wants something to make these symptoms better.

What would be the most appropriate next management step?

1. Admit him to a medical ward for a reducing regimen of
   benzodiazepines
2. Advise him to self-refer to the local substance misuse service and
   to keep drinking alcohol in the meantime
3. Phone the community drug worker to arrange an inpatient detox
4. Prescribe him acamprosate and advise follow-up by his GP
5. Provide a prescription for a reducing regimen of chlordiazepoxide
   with GP follow-up

Q286

A 70 year old woman has 3 weeks of agitation and confusion. She hasn't
eaten or drunk anything in the last 24 hours as she believes the water is
poisoned. She is unable to follow conversations. She saw her general
practitioner last month, who changed some of her medications. She has
no past psychiatric history but she does have hypertension, heart failure
and diabetes. There is no illicit substance or alcohol use.

The patient appears distressed and is reporting that there are
insects on her bed. She does not wish to stay in hospital, and although
you were able to take her blood earlier, she is declining any further
investigations or treatment.

What would be the next step?

1. Allow her to self-discharge
2. Investigate which medications have been changed
3. Refer to the psychiatry liaison team
4. Restrain the patient to administer medications and fluids as
   indicated
5. Undertake a full Mental Health Act assessment

Q287

An 18 year old man has been brought to his GP surgery by his
mother, due to concerns about his mental health. He says that, for
the last 4 months, he has been followed by the police who have been
trying to find a reason to arrest him. He reports that they have put
cameras in his house and have been following him in public and

recording his movements. He has also noticed members of the public giving him odd looks and looking at their phones.

He has not heard anyone talking about him or heard any strange noises. He did not find any cameras in his house when he looked. He becomes angry with his general practitioner when she suggests that he might be misunderstanding things. He has become increasingly withdrawn and lost interest in many of his hobbies and friendships.

His mother reports that she has searched the house and could not find any hidden cameras. She has also not noticed any odd behaviours from members of the public when she has been with her son. When she has spoken to him about this, he has become angry and shouted at her.

What is the most likely diagnosis to give at this stage?

1. Bipolar disorder
2. Mania
3. Panic disorder
4. Psychosis
5. Severe depression with psychosis

Q288

A 19 year old woman requests a genetic test to prove her royal status. For the last 2 weeks, she has been spending lots of time in pubs talking to strangers, asking them inappropriate personal questions. She has told people that she is related to the royal family, a cousin of Prince Harry.

Her flatmate says that this is not characteristic for her: she is normally shy and retiring. He is not aware of any connections with the royal family.

There is no medical or psychiatric history; she is on no medication and her observations are normal.

She is appropriately dressed and has pressure of speech.

What is the most appropriate diagnosis to give at this stage?

1. Bipolar disorder
2. Delusional disorder
3. Mania
4. Personality disorder
5. Schizophrenia

Q289

A 30 year old man arrives in the emergency department saying he wishes to kill the chief executive of the hospital, and asks where her office is. He says he has started to make a plan, but will not give further details in case it jeopardises his mission. On further questioning, he discusses a government plot against him.

He has had depression over the past 2 years, treated with sertraline 200 mg. He stopped working a year ago. He smokes cannabis daily. You suspect this is a first episode of psychosis. When attempting to discuss this with him, he becomes irate at the suggestion of him being mentally unwell.

What would be the most appropriate next step?

1. Admit under medics
2. Complete a mental capacity assessment
3. Discharge into the community with psychiatric follow-up
4. Physical health screening
5. Refer for Mental Health Act assessment

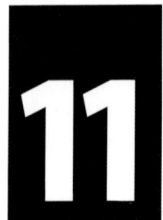

Neurology

Q290

A 58 year old man has 2 days of worsening headaches, later associated with reduced consciousness, seizures and left-sided weakness. He has a background of diabetes and is an intravenous drug user. His MRI head confirmed a large right-sided abscess. He underwent a craniotomy for excision of the abscess, with a pus sample sent to the lab for microbiological assessment.

What is the most likely causative organism?

1. Escherichia coli
2. Herpes simplex virus
3. Mycobacterium tuberculosis
4. SARS-CoV-2
5. Staphylococcus aureus

Q291

A 75 year old man has headaches, unintentional weight loss, haemoptysis, nausea, vomiting and unsteadiness. He drinks 20 units of alcohol per week and has a 50 year pack history. An MRI shows a mass lesion measuring 3 cm in diameter in the vermis of the cerebellum.

What is the most likely diagnosis?

1. Meningioma
2. Primary brain tumour
3. Primary central nervous system lymphoma
4. Prostatic metastasis
5. Small cell lung metastasis

Q292

A 74 year old man is admitted to hospital with pneumonia. Admission bloods suggest an acute kidney injury which resolves following fluids and antibiotics. He has severe osteoarthritis. He takes gabapentin and has a morphine patch for analgesia. During admission he is noted to have brief, shock-like jerks of the whole body. The jerks settle over a few days.

What is the most likely cause for the abnormal movements?

1. Drug-induced myoclonus
2. Drug-induced tremor
3. Epileptic seizures
4. Functional movement disorder
5. Hemiballismus

Q293

A 46 year old woman has 12 months of post-exertional extreme tiredness associated with non-refreshing sleep, headaches and poor concentration. She was referred to a rheumatology clinic with pain in multiple joints and muscles without signs of inflammation. Her pain is widespread but particularly over the right neck and right shoulder. FBC, urea and electrolytes, TSH, HbA1c, cancer markers and rheumatology markers are all within normal limits. The ultrasound scan of the hands does not reveal any inflammation and an MRI of the whole spine shows minor degenerative changes.

What would be the best rational approach to manage her pain?

1. Initiate opiate medication
2. Oral steroids for 3 weeks
3. Pain clinic referral
4. Regular anti-inflammatory medication
5. Steroid injection into trigger points

Q294

A 61 year old man has a slow development of restlessness and a short temper with regular outbursts of anger. Family members noticed that he often talked to objects and people who were not present. He could no longer concentrate on television programmes. Over the past 2 years he developed smaller handwriting than usual and his walking has become 'shuffling'. There is no family history. On examination, he walked slowly with reduced arm swing on the left. An MRI show age-related atrophy in the frontal and parietal lobes, with an intact hippocampus and temporal lobe. No scarring was detected.

What is the most likely diagnosis?

1. Alzheimer's disease
2. Creutzfeldt–Jakob disease
3. Dementia with Lewy bodies
4. Frontotemporal dementia
5. Vascular dementia

Q295

A 48 year old man has 2 days of lethargy, headache and confusion. On arrival at the emergency department, his Glasgow Coma Score is 14 and he scores 1 in the Abbreviated Mental Test 4. His temperature is 38.4 °C.

There is no meningism or photosensitivity. He goes on to have a witnessed 30 second seizure in the emergency department. A CT head is normal. A lumbar puncture is performed, revealing 670 lymphocytes, 3 polymorphs, protein of 0.76 g/L and glucose of 3.5 mmol/L (serum 4.6 mmol/L).

What is the most appropriate initial management?

1. Aciclovir
2. Benzylpenicillin
3. Ceftriaxone
4. Dexamethasone
5. Phenytoin

Q296

A 17 year old woman is referred to the neurology clinic after a second event in 1 month in which she fell to the ground and was seen to rhythmically shake for 90 seconds. She bit her tongue and took around 30 minutes to fully wake up. She has infrequent arm jerks in the mornings and occasional blank spells at school. Her neurological examination is normal and an MRI head scan shows no abnormalities. The neurologist suspects generalised epilepsy and discusses starting antiseizure medications. They also arrange a standard EEG.

What benefit might the EEG add to this patient's management?

1. It can confirm a diagnosis of epilepsy
2. It can demonstrate that the collapse was actually a syncope
3. It can determine whether she is allowed to drive
4. It can help define an epilepsy syndrome
5. It can rule out epilepsy as a cause of her collapses

Q297

A 21 year old man is brought to the emergency department after his friends witnessed him collapse. His arms were seen to stiffen and then shake for 1 minute. Following this, he was sleepy and took about 45 minutes to recognise his friends and respond to their questions. He now feels fully recovered, his neurological examination is normal and his temperature is 36.5 °C.

Which of the following is the most important investigation?

1. CT head
2. ECG
3. Lumbar puncture
4. MRI head
5. Serum prolactin

Q298

An 83 year old woman has tremors in both of her hands for the last 3 years. The tremors are worse when she is under stress or trying to perform precise movements. She has a bilateral action tremor that affects her hands and forearms.

What is the most appropriate initial management of this patient's tremor?

1. Initiate deep brain stimulation
2. Primidone
3. Propranolol
4. Recommend lifestyle modifications
5. Refer to physiotherapy

Q299

A 19 year old man was involved in a road traffic accident 1 day ago. After a brief period of loss of consciousness, he was able to extricate himself from the vehicle and walk home. He attended the emergency department as he had some ongoing headaches. He is otherwise fit and well. On assessment, he is mildly confused and has a wound on the side of his head but is otherwise well. He is given analgesia and the wound is glued and dressed.

What would the most appropriate next step in management be?

1. Admit for neuro-observation and review again in 4 hours
2. Arrange an urgent CT head
3. Call the neurosurgeons immediately to review him for theatre
4. Chest X-ray, ECG and routine bloods
5. Discharge home with head injury advice

Q300

A 50 year old man has recurrent, disabling headaches that prevent him from doing his job. This often comes on following exercise. The headache is preceded by visual disturbance. It has a pulsating quality, and is associated with nausea and occasionally vomiting. The duration of the last one was 5 days. A diagnosis of migraine is made.

Which part of the history is unusual for migraine?

1. Always preceded by visual disturbance
2. Headache is aggravated by routine physical activity
3. Headaches last 5 days at a time
4. Presence of nausea/vomiting during the headache
5. Pulsating quality

Q301

A 67 year old man has 6 months of fasciculation, muscle atrophy and weakness. This initially started in the right hand but has since progressed to involve both upper limbs and his left lower limb. On examination, the patient has brisk reflexes in all affected limbs, with generalised atrophy and reduced power. The neurologist suspects motor neurone disease.

Which is the most likely form of motor neurone disease?

1. Amyotrophic lateral sclerosis
2. Kennedy disease
3. Primary lateral sclerosis
4. Progressive muscular atrophy
5. Spinal muscular atrophy

Q302

A 78 year old man becomes confused 2 days after a left hip hemi-arthroplasty. He becomes irritable, having visual hallucinations and being disorientated in time and place. He has a history of atrial fibrillation, hypertension and diabetes mellitus.

What is the most appropriate next action?

1. Call family members to ask about the patient's baseline cognitive function
2. Organise a chest X-ray, a set of confusion screen blood and urine tests
3. Organise CT head scan
4. Perform a set of observations and assess the patient clinically
5. Prescribe lorazepam

Q303

A 37 year old man has progressive unsteadiness of gait, numbness and weakness of the lower limbs. His symptoms started 14 months ago. He has spasticity of the lower limbs, with brisk reflexes, bilateral upgoing plantars, and a sensory level at the level of the umbilicus. His imaging shows two spinal cord T2 hyperintense lesions (at C5 and at T10). His brain imaging was normal. His blood tests including antibody testing (including for neuromyelitis optic spectrum disorder) are negative, and his chest X-ray is normal. His lumbar puncture showed oligoclonal bands not matched in blood.

What is the most likely diagnosis?

1. Clinically isolated syndrome (albeit with two lesions)
2. It is not possible to make a diagnosis at this stage
3. Primary progressive multiple sclerosis
4. Relapsing multiple sclerosis
5. Secondary progressive multiple sclerosis

Q304

A 3 year old boy started walking 6 months ago and has frequent trips and falls. He is able to use a few words to describe objects. There is no family history of muscle weakness. His gait is unsteady and he walks on his toes as he enters the room.

What would be the most appropriate next investigation?

1. Creatine kinase
2. Genetic test for Duchenne muscular dystrophy
3. Karyotype analysis
4. Muscle biopsy
5. Ultrasound scan of muscle

Q305

A 56 year old man has 6 months of 'slowing down'. He now finds it difficult to use a knife and fork. His family state that, having been a very 'jolly' man, he now rarely smiles. He has been constipated and lost his sense of smell some years ago. He has a reduced arm swing on his right. There was a paucity of facial expression. The amplitude of right-hand finger tapping reduced progressively. Slight rigidity of the right wrist was detected when he tapped his left hand on his lap. A right-hand tremor was present when his hand was on his lap, which temporarily resolved, then restarted when he held his arms outstretched.

What is the most likely diagnosis?

1. Alzheimer's disease
2. Essential tremor
3. Motor neurone disease
4. Multiple sclerosis
5. Parkinson's disease

Q306

A 40 year old woman has 2 weeks' left foot drop associated with numbness and tingling over the dorsum of her foot. She has a recent history of trauma to the knee and fracture of the fibula on the affected side. She has a history of hypertension and type 2 diabetes.

What is the most likely diagnosis?

1. Diabetic neuropathy
2. Injury to the lateral cutaneous nerve of the thigh
3. Prolapsed intervertebral disc
4. Traumatic common peroneal nerve injury
5. Traumatic sural nerve injury

Q307

A 22 year old man is brought to the emergency department with reduced consciousness. He is not opening his eyes to pain, is groaning and is not obeying commands. Collateral history reveals he hit his head whilst playing football and had a brief period of unconsciousness followed by a lucid interval. His CT head shows a left biconvex lens-shaped bleed.

What is the most likely diagnosis?

1. Acute subdural haematoma
2. Chronic subdural haematoma
3. Extradural haematoma
4. Intracerebral haemorrhage
5. Traumatic subarachnoid haemorrhage

Q308

A 49 year old woman has low back pain and severe left-sided sciatica. She has hesitancy when passing urine and sensory loss on both buttocks and down the back of both legs.

She has a reduced straight leg raising on the left, normal power (in the context of assessment difficulties caused by pain), bilateral saddle numbness, and numbness in the S1 and S2 dermatomes. Her ankle reflexes were also both absent.

In addition to prescription of pain relief, what is the most appropriate management?

1. Arrange an emergency whole spine MRI
2. Mobilisation as tolerated
3. Refer to neurosurgery for urgent assessment
4. Refer urgently to physiotherapy
5. Undertake a urine microscopy and culture, commence antibiotics and review in 48 hours

Q309

A 62 year old man is brought into the emergency department with reduced consciousness and a fixed and dilated pupil. His observations and blood sugar are normal.

What is the most appropriate next investigation?

1. CT head scan
2. Fundal photography
3. Lumbar puncture
4. MRI
5. Transcranial doppler

Q310

A 55 year old man is admitted to hospital following a fall from a bicycle. No other vehicles were involved. He has signs of an incomplete spinal cord injury at the T8 level.

Which of the following options should be undertaken within 24 hours of the injury?

1. Administration of hypertonic saline
2. Administration of methylprednisolone
3. Referral to the Regional Spinal Cord Injury Centre
4. Spinal angiography
5. Ventilation to avoid hypoxia

Q311

An 81 year old woman presents to the emergency department, having fallen down 12 stairs. She reports severe thoracolumbar spinal pain. She is mildly confused (Glasgow Coma Score 14) and has normal lower limb neurology.

What is the most appropriate initial investigation to perform?

1. Bone scan
2. Lumbar puncture
3. Pan-CT
4. Whole body MRI
5. X-ray of the spine

Q312

A 68 year old man has had three falls in the last 12 months. He says he is otherwise well. On examination, he has postural hypotension along with unilateral resting tremor, bradykinesia and rigidity.

What is the most likely diagnosis?

1. Autonomic neuropathy
2. Essential tremor
3. Hereditary spastic paraparesis
4. Idiopathic Parkinson's disease
5. Paraneoplastic cerebellar degeneration

Q313

An 84 year old woman suddenly becomes unresponsive. She has been treated for an acute ischaemic stroke. The Glasgow Coma Score is 9 (E2, V3, M4). Her temperature is 36.7 °C, pulse 105 bpm, BP 160/70 mmHg, oxygen saturation 92% breathing air. While you are conducting your initial assessment, she begins to have a seizure.

What is the most likely complication?

1. Allergic reaction to alteplase
2. Aspiration pneumonia
3. Concomitant myocardial infarction
4. Haemorrhagic transformation
5. Venous thromboembolism

Q314

A 55 year old woman collapses at home. Her husband tells you she clutched her head before collapsing and shouted out. Her Glasgow Coma Score is 9 (E2, V3, M4). Her temperature is 37.2 °C, pulse 110 bpm, BP 168/72 mmHg, oxygen saturation 94% breathing air. Her blood sugar is normal.

Which test is most appropriate to confirm the suspected diagnosis?

1 CT angiogram
2 CT scan of the head
3 Full blood count
4 Lumbar puncture
5 MRI of the head

Q315

A 36 year old woman has recurrent episodes of headaches that last for 4 days at a time. They occur 5 times per month and are dull, aching and band-like. There is no associated photophobia, phonophobia, nausea or vomiting. She uses paracetamol only when she feels she must, 5 days per month.

Which is the most appropriate preventive management?

1. Amitriptyline 10 mg once nightly
2. Oramorph as required for acute episodes
3. Regular aspirin 600-1200 mg four times daily
4. Regular paracetamol 1 g four times daily
5. Triptans as required for acute attacks

Q316

A 72 year old man has a 15 minute episode of right facial droop and right arm heaviness, along with some slurring of his speech. His urological examination is normal. His ECG shows normal sinus rhythm. His MRI head shows cerebral microvascular disease.

What is the most appropriate immediate treatment for this patient?

1. Alteplase
2. Aspirin
3. Atorvastatin
4. Dabigatran
5. Warfarin loading dose

Q317

A 75 year old man presents in the emergency department with 1 day of confusion, visual hallucinations and unsteadiness. He has ischaemic heart disease, diabetes, atrial fibrillation, depression and a recent diagnosis of tremor-predominant Parkinson's disease. His observations are within normal limits and he is afebrile. He is agitated and not cooperative, and is severely ataxic in all limbs, with bilateral visual field defects. Routine bloods are unremarkable. There are no recent medication changes.

What is the next step in management?

1. Electroencephalogram (EEG)
2. Lumbar puncture
3. MRI brain
4. Psychiatry review
5. Referral to Parkinson's team

Q318

A 65 year old man has 1 week of excruciating electric shock-like pain on the left side of his face, radiating between his mouth and cheek. The pain lasts between 30 seconds and 2 minutes. He describes the pain intensity by sharply clapping his hands. He has 5 or 6 episodes of pain each day.

The pain is triggered when he smiles, eat, laughs, and sometimes when he talks.

Clinical examination is normal, although he is fearful of the examination triggering an attack of pain.

What is the most likely cause of his pain?

1. Brainstem glioma
2. Dental abscess
3. Maxillary sinusitis
4. Subarachnoid haemorrhage
5. Trigeminal neuralgia

Q319

A 42 year old man is found wandering confused and unsteady. He is homeless and has a past history of alcohol excess, type 2 diabetes, COPD and AIDS. There is no evidence of head injury or trauma. He is apyrexial and has a Glasgow Coma Scale (Glasgow Coma Score) of 14/15. He is disorientated, and mentally slow. Blood sugar is normal. Wernicke's encephalopathy is suspected clinically.

Other than alcohol excess, which feature in the history also increases this patient's risk of Wernicke's encephalopathy?

1. Age
2. AIDS
3. COPD
4. Normal temperature
5. Type 2 diabetes

Q320

An 80 year old man has a gradual decline in mobility over the last week, and 2 days of increased confusion and dragging his right leg. He has recurrent falls and a previous stroke. He is mildly confused. His temperature is 36.8 °C, pulse rate 96 bpm regular, BP 150/70 mmHg, oxygen saturation 98% breathing air. Neurological examination reveals slight reduction in right lower limb power.

What is the most likely diagnosis?

1. Acute subdural haematoma
2. Chronic subdural haematoma
3. Extradural haematoma
4. Intracerebral haematoma
5. Ischaemic stroke

Q321

A 35 year old man has symmetrical numbness and weakness in his arms and legs. It started distally and has been progressing proximally for the last 10 days. He also has 'shooting' pain in his back that radiated round to his abdomen. Three weeks prior to this presentation, he had fever and bloody diarrhoea.

Which of the following is the most likely diagnosis?

1. Amyotrophic lateral sclerosis
2. Guillain–Barre syndrome
3. Multiple sclerosis
4. Myasthenia gravis
5. Parkinson's disease

Q322

A 75 year old man has the sensation of hearing loud noises. He has no past medical history of note. His neighbours inform him there is no noise. He has marked hearing loss bilaterally and no disorders of thoughts or mood.

What is the most likely cause for this man's symptoms?

1. Epilepsy
2. Head injury
3. Hearing loss
4. Parkinson's disease
5. Schizophrenia

Q323

An 85 year old woman has several episodes of brief loss of consciousness after standing up from her chair. She recovers fully and feels well in between episodes. She has no history of chest pain or shortness of breath. Her examination is normal.

What is the most appropriate next management?

1. Arrange an MRI head
2. Arrange for routine blood test
3. Perform lying and standing BP
4. Refer immediately to emergency department for full work-up
5. Start anti-epileptic medication

Q324

A 68 year old man has a sudden onset of double vision. He has had no headache and no loss of function or sensation in his limbs. He has hypertension and type 2 diabetes. He takes atorvastatin, ramipril and amlodipine. His pulse rate is 74 bpm, BP 158/92 mm Hg. His external eye movements show diplopia on looking in most directions, but when looking to his right and down there is no diplopia. The right pupil measures 4 mm and has direct and consensual reflexes. The left pupil measures 3 mm and is reactive.

What is the most likely pathology to account for this problem?

1. Abscess
2. Demyelination
3. Haemorrhage
4. Infarction
5. Malignancy

Q325

A 65 year old woman has a sudden onset of left-sided facial weakness. She is a smoker with a 40 pack year history. She has muscle weakness on the left side of her face, incomplete closure of the left eye, inability to puff her cheek. Her left arm and leg has slightly reduced power.

What is the most appropriate next step in management?

1. Anti-viral therapy
2. Chest X-ray
3. High-dose corticosteroid
4. MRI brain
5. Urgent CT head

Q326

A 45 year old woman has paroxysms of shooting pain in the right cheek, over the last year. The symptoms are worse at mealtimes and in winter, when she has to cover her face with a scarf.

What is the most appropriate first-line medication to commence?

1. Amitriptyline
2. Carbamazepine
3. Duloxetine
4. Lidocaine patch
5. Pregabalin

Q327

A 55 year old woman has a left facial droop. She woke this morning and noticed a unilateral facial paralysis on the left side, which was not present the previous night. She also reports hyperacusis in her left ear and says food tastes different. She has type 2 diabetes, hypertension and hyperlipidemia. There is a left facial droop and she is unable to close her left eye or wrinkle the left side of her forehead. The rest of the examination is normal.

What is the most likely diagnosis?

1. Bell's palsy
2. Lyme disease
3. Multiple sclerosis
4. Pontine stroke
5. Right MCA territory stroke

Q328

A 63 year old woman has suspected myasthenia. Her symptoms have come on over a few months, and are worse at the end of the day. She is otherwise fit and well, and on no regular medication.

What is the usual first symptom of myasthenia gravis?

1. Confusion
2. Double vision
3. Foot drop
4. Headache
5. Hip girdle stiffness

Q329

A 50 year old man is concerned regarding muscle twitches he is having in his legs, particularly in his calves after running. He is a keen runner and has been having these twitches intermittently for the last 5 years, always in the back of his legs. They have not changed over this time, and he has not noticed any pain or weakness. He has asthma but is otherwise fit and well. Neurological examination reveals no abnormal findings.

What is the most likely cause of his fasciculation?

1. Amyotrophic lateral sclerosis
2. Benign fasciculation syndrome
3. Chronic inflammatory demyelinating polyneuropathy
4. L5/S1 nerve root lesion
5. Multifocal motor neuropathy

Q330

A 45 year old woman presents to the emergency department with an occipital headache that began 5 days previously. It had a rapid onset, reaching maximum severity within 5 minutes. A neurological examination reveals no focal abnormalities, and no abnormalities on fundoscopy.

Which of the following is the most appropriate initial management?

1. Lumbar puncture
2. Preventive migraine treatment
3. Reassurance and discharge
4. Referral to neurology outpatients
5. Urgent CT head scan

Q331

A 62 year old man with a history of poorly controlled insulin dependent diabetes presents to his GP surgery with an infected ulcer on the base of his foot. Neurofilament testing reveals that he has no sensation below his knees. Investigations:

HbA1c 96 mmol/mol (< 46)

Which of the following is the most appropriate management to prevent progression of his diabetic neuropathy?

1. Amitriptyline
2. Duloxetine
3. Gabapentin
4. Improved glycaemic control
5. Midodrine

Q332

A 60 year old man presents to the emergency department with sudden-onset right leg weakness with slurred speech and urinary incontinence. He is known to have hypertension and paroxysmal atrial fibrillation. What is the most likely diagnosis?

1. Guillain–Barre syndrome
2. Left anterior cerebral artery stroke
3. Myasthenia gravis
4. Normal-pressure hydrocephalus
5. Todd's paresis

Q333

A 72 year old man has 3 months of progressive right leg weakness, pain and numbness. This started with buttock pain, progressing to severe pain radiating down the leg and causing a right foot drop. He has been losing weight during this period. He has significant weakness in the right lower limb (3/5 in multiple muscle groups), absent ankle reflex, and sensory deficits over the lateral foot and calf. MRI of the lumbosacral spine is normal, and nerve conduction studies have been requested.

What is the most appropriate next investigation?

1. HbA1c and bloods, including a vasculitis panel, hepatitis, Lyme and syphilis screen

2. Lumbar puncture, antibody panel +/− nerve biopsy
3. MRI brain and whole spine
4. MRI lumbosacral plexus
5. Ultrasound of the course of the sciatic, tibial and peroneal nerves

Q334

An 86 year old man has 12 months of worsening memory and now finds it difficult to manage his financial affairs and medication. He has no family history. He smokes 15 cigarettes a day (having a 65 pack year history).

He is obese, his pulse rate is 96 bpm and irregular, BP 160/70 mmHg. His neurological examination is grossly normal. His gait is normal but is limited by claudication in his calves bilaterally.

What is the most likely cause of his memory loss?

1. Alzheimer's disease
2. Delirium
3. Dementia with Lewy bodies
4. Pick's disease (frontotemporal dementia)
5. Vascular dementia

Q335

A 65 year old woman has a severe headache, high fever and neck stiffness. This was preceded by general malaise for the past 2 days. Her temperature is 38.6 °C, pulse 105 bpm, BP 95/60 mmHg. A lumbar puncture reveals elevated white blood cells, decreased glucose, and increased protein in the cerebrospinal fluid.

What is the most likely causative organism?

1. Escherichia coli
2. Haemophilus influenzae
3. Listeria monocytogenes
4. Neisseria meningitidis
5. Streptococcus pneumoniae

Q336

A 64 year old woman has 3 months of swallowing difficulties. In the last 3 weeks, she has developed right eyelid ptosis and bilateral proximal upper limb weakness, with no associated myalgia. Her symptoms are usually worse in the evening and after activity.

Investigations:

Creatinine kinase normal

Anti-acetylcholine receptor antibodies positive

What is the most likely diagnosis in this patient?

1. Congenital myopathy
2. Inflammatory myopathy
3. Motor neurone disease
4. Myasthenia gravis
5. Peripheral neuropathy

Q337

A 58 year old man arrives in the emergency department, having fallen from scaffolding. Resuscitation is immediately started.

Which of the following clinical signs is consistent with spinal cord compression?

1. Absent tendon reflexes
2. Downgoing plantar
3. Hypotonia
4. Muscle fasciculation
5. Sustained clonus

Q338

A 78 year old woman has 3 days of diplopia. She is otherwise well. She has a partial left ptosis with the left eye depressed and abducted. Her visual acuity is 6/6 in each eye and her pupils are normal. Her BP is 146/92 mmHg.

What is the nerve affected?

1. Abducens
2. Facial
3. Oculomotor
4. Optic
5. Trochlear

Q339

A 51 year old woman has 2 months of excessive daytime sleepiness and fatigue. She usually completes her work shifts in the daytime only, and her partner complains that she snores very loudly at night. She has smoked 20 cigarettes daily for the past 30 years and her past medical history includes type 2 diabetes mellitus and COPD. On examination, she appears sleepy during the consultation and her BMI is 41.3 kg/m^2.

What is the most likely diagnosis?

1. Circadian rhythm sleep–wake disorder
2. Insomnia
3. Narcolepsy
4. Obstructive sleep apnoea
5. Restless leg syndrome

Q340

A 62 year old man has 6 weeks of falling to the right and clumsiness in his right hand. He has had headaches at night and has vomited before breakfast over the last 3 days. He has normal visual acuity and visual fields. He has an intention tremor on the right, fundoscopy reveals bilateral swollen optic discs, and he has unsteadiness on walking.

What is the most likely site of pathology?

1. Cervical spine
2. Foramen magnum
3. Left internal capsule
4. Pituitary fossa
5. Right cerebellar hemisphere

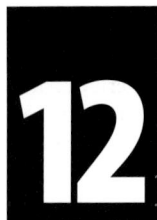

Obstetrics, Gynaecology and Breast

Q341

A 34 year old woman attends late for her cervical smear. Her last smear 8 years ago tested positive for human papillomavirus with no abnormal cytology. Examination shows a lesion suggestive of cervical cancer extending from her cervix to the upper third of her vagina.

Which stage of cervical cancer is this?

1. Stage 0
2. Stage 1
3. Stage 2
4. Stage 3
5. Stage 4

Q342

A 59 year old woman has a constant burning sensation in perineum for 2 years. It is associated with back pain, dysuria and dyspareunia. She has five children, all vaginal births, with no complications reported. There is no evidence of abnormal bleeding or vaginal discharge or lesions at present. On examination, erythema and dryness are noted externally and inside vaginal canal with poor skin turgor.

What is the most likely diagnosis?

1. Atrophic vaginitis
2. Bacterial vaginitis
3. Endometrial cancer
4. Pelvic inflammatory disease
5. Uterine prolapse

Q343

A 32 year old woman has 6 days of clear, fishy smelling, vaginal discharge. This started 3 days after her last menstrual period. She is otherwise well. She has never been pregnant and she has had the same sexual partner for the last 4 years. She has had two previous episodes but is not sure how it was treated.

What would be the most appropriate management?

1. Aciclovir
2. Azithromycin
3. Metronidazole
4. No treatment now but await swab findings
5. Refer to the sexual health clinic

Q344

A 46 year old woman has requested a smear test. She has three children. She has a period once a month which is intermittently heavy. Her last smear was 4 years ago – reported as human papilloma virus (HPV) not detected. Speculum examination reveals a dry but otherwise healthy-looking vagina and cervix with no worrying features.

What is the most appropriate next step?

1. As she is HPV negative, she no longer needs smear tests
2. Perform a smear test as she is a year overdue
3. Reassure her that her next test is not due for another year
4. Stop and rearrange smear after 2 weeks of topical oestrogen therapy
5. Urgent referral to gynaecology as her periods are intermittently heavy

Q345

A 27 year old woman is 31 weeks pregnant and has been admitted to the antenatal ward with ruptured membranes with a breech presentation. She calls the midwife because she can feel something between her legs. The midwife diagnoses cord prolapse. What is the next management step?

1. Bleep the anaesthetist
2. Check the woman's observations

3. Insert a cannula
4. Pull the emergency buzzer
5. Start cardiotocography

Q346

A 29 year old woman contacts primary care for the result of her cervical smear.

The result is: human papilloma virus positive. No abnormal cells detected.

What is the most appropriate management?

1. Immunisation with human papilloma virus vaccine
2. No additional action necessary
3. Referral to the colposcopy clinic
4. Repeat smear in 12 months
5. Treatment with antivirals

Q347

A 21 year old woman who is currently 28 weeks pregnant has been diagnosed with gestational diabetes on an oral glucose tolerance test (OGTT). The results were: fasting blood sugar 6.0 mmol/L, 2-hour blood sugar 8.0 mmol/L. Her BMI was 39 kg/m² at booking. Her growth scan shows a normal size for dates boy with normal amniotic fluid measurement.

What is the most appropriate management?

1. Advise weight loss due to her BMI
2. Commence insulin only
3. Commence metformin and insulin
4. Give advice regarding diet and exercise changes and review again in 1–2 weeks
5. Repeat the OGTT to confirm the result

Q348

A 24 year old woman has a right lower quadrant pain for 1 day. This is associated with light vaginal bleeding. Her last period was approximately 2 months ago. Her temperature is 36.8 °C, pulse rate 110 bpm, BP 110/70 mmHg. She is guarding in the left lower quadrant of her abdomen. Her urine pregnancy test is positive.

What is the most likely diagnosis?

1. Appendicitis
2. Ectopic pregnancy
3. Normal menses
4. Ovarian cyst
5. Urinary tract infection

Q349

A 32 year old woman has cyclical abdominal pain. This is associated with pain on sexual intercourse, especially on deeper penetration. She also has pain and bleeding when defaecating during menstruation. She has been trying to conceive for the last 2 years and therefore has not used any contraception. An ultrasound scan suggests that her pelvic organs have limited mobility.

What would be the most appropriate management?

1. Diagnostic laparoscopy +/- excision of endometriosis
2. GnRH agonists
3. Hysterosalpingogram
4. MRI
5. Referral to the fertility team for IVF

Q350

A 35 year old woman has mild stress incontinence and urinary urgency. She has regular but very heavy menstrual bleeding. She has no bowel symptoms. She has two children. Her BMI is 19 kg/m²; pelvic examination reveals a slightly bulky uterus. FBC shows that she is mildly anaemic.

What is the most likely diagnosis?

1. Cervical cancer
2. Ovarian cancer
3. Overactive bladder
4. Pregnancy
5. Uterine fibroids

Q351

A 26 year old woman has severe, worsening nausea and vomiting at 11 weeks gestation in her second pregnancy. Her first pregnancy was normal. Her temperature is 36.9 °C, pulse 82 bpm, BP 160/110 mmHg (110/65 at booking, 6 weeks ago). The fundus is not palpable above the symphysis pubis.

What is the most likely explanation for this presentation?

1. Anxiety
2. Hyperemesis gravidarum
3. Molar pregnancy
4. Multiple pregnancy
5. Pre-eclampsia

Q352

A 26 year old woman attends for fitting of an IUD 6 months after the birth of her first child. She denies any unusual vaginal bleeding or discharge. She has had previous genital warts, successfully treated with cryotherapy. She was pregnant at the time of her call for her first smear and did not attend. She is breastfeeding. She is a non-smoker, with normal BMI and she is in a monogamous relationship for the last 5 years.

Speculum examination reveals a cervix with small ectropion.

Vaginal swabs taken 5 days ago show no infection. Her pregnancy test is negative.

In addition to your fitting of a coil, what further action should be undertaken?

1. Full set of bloods including CA125
2. Perform a smear test
3. Prescribe antibiotics
4. Refer to sexual health clinic
5. Urgent referral to colposcopy

Q353

A 29 year old woman is diagnosed with gestational diabetes in her first pregnancy. She has a BMI of 35 kg/m².

What is the likely mechanism for her development of gestational diabetes?

1. Increased excretion of insulin
2. Increased metabolism of insulin
3. Insulin resistance

4. Lack of production of insulin
5. Overproduction of insulin

Q354

A 48 year old woman has had regular hot flushes for the past 6 months. She has regular monthly periods, the last one 2 weeks ago. After discussion of her options, she requests hormone replacement therapy (HRT).

Which is the most suitable type of HRT to start her on?

1. Continuous combined HRT
2. Oestrogen only HRT – oral tablets
3. Oestrogen only HRT – patches or gel
4. Sequential combined HRT
5. Tibolone

Q355

A 59 year old woman has 4 months of bloating, a feeling of indigestion and frequent urination. Her urine dipstick is negative.

What is the first investigation that should be arranged?

1. Bloods (FBC, urea and electrolytes, liver function tests, CA125)
2. CT CAP
3. Referral for colonoscopy
4. Referral for gastroscopy
5. Transabdominal and transvaginal ultrasound scan

Q356

A 34 year old woman has bleeding at 26 weeks gestation in her first pregnancy. The bleeding is similar to her period. The bleeding has now stopped, and she can feel fetal movements. She is clinically stable, her temperature is 36.4 °C, pulse rate 80 bpm, BP 125/70 mmHg. Her latest scan was normal.

Which is the next step in management?

1. Admit to the maternity department for assessment and ongoing management
2. Perform a manual vaginal examination

3. Reassure the patient and discharge them
4. Request an ultrasound
5. Start intravenous fluids

Q357

A 32 year old woman had a vaginal delivery for her first baby 60 minutes ago. Her labour was induced because of pre-eclampsia, with intravenous syntocinon. She received a syntocinon bolus for the third stage of labour, but the placenta remains *in situ* and she has bled over 700 ml so far. Her temperature is 36.9 °C, pulse rate 105 bpm, BP 136/82 mmHg, respiratory rate 18 breaths per minute, oxygen saturation 100% breathing air. Bloods are taken.

What is the definitive management?

1. A compression balloon
2. Blood transfusion
3. Ergometrine
4. Theatre for an examination under anaesthesia and removal of placenta
5. Tranexamic acid

Q358

A 36 year old nulliparous woman attends maternity triage with a frontal headache and reduced fetal movements. She is at 34 weeks gestation. She is otherwise fit and well and has no past medical history and no allergies. She takes aspirin 150 mg once daily.
Her BP is 181/113 mmHg.

Which anti-hypertensive would be most appropriate to prescribe?

1. Atenolol
2. Enalapril
3. Labetolol
4. Methyldopa
5. Nifedipine

Q359

A 29 year old woman has a tender, painful lump near the vaginal opening. Her temperature is 36.9 °C, pulse 82 bpm, BP 120/75 mmHg. There is exquisitely tender, fluctuant labial mass at junction of upper 2/3rd and lower 1/3rd, with surrounding erythema and oedema.

What is the most appropriate management?

1. Antibiotics
2. Cystectomy
3. Incision and drainage
4. Marsupialisation
5. Refer to sexual health clinic

Q360

A 32 year old woman has a small, fresh antepartum haemorrhage. She is 36 weeks into her first pregnancy. Her last ultrasound scan at 20 weeks gestation was normal.

She reports no pain and no fetal movements.

The maternal observations are within normal limits and the uterus is soft and non-tender. There is fresh blood on speculum examination mixed with liquor. The CTG (cardiotocograph) has shown a sinusoidal pattern for the last 30 minutes.

Which of the following is the most appropriate management?

1. Category 1 (Immediate) caesarean section
2. Category 2 (Urgent) caesarean section
3. Discharge home with the plan for outpatient monitoring
4. Induction of labour with prostaglandin pessary
5. Induction of labour with syntocinon

Q361

A 24 year old woman presents to the emergency department with a sudden-onset shortness of breath and chest pain. She is 32 weeks into her first pregnancy, has a BMI of 39 kg/m² and has been recently diagnosed with gestational diabetes. She has no other clinical history of note. She is haemodynamically stable and examination is unremarkable. ECG and chest X-ray are normal. She is started on low molecular weight heparin.

What is the next step in management?

1. Check her D-dimer and calculate her Wells score
2. Discussion with the woman concerning a ventilation/perfusion scan or CT pulmonary angiogram

3. Repeat chest X-ray in 4 hours
4. Request bilateral compression duplex ultrasound
5. Start thrombolysis

Q362

A 42 year old woman has hot flushes, irritability and has not had a period for 12 months. Her periods in the year prior to that were very irregular. She does not know when her mother's or older sister's periods stopped. She is not depressed.

Her BMI is 24 kg/m². Her abdominal examination is normal (she does not consent to vaginal examination).

Her pregnancy test is negative. Routine bloods are requested including FSH.

What would be the most appropriate next step in her management?

1. Ask her to make an appointment at the sexual health clinic
2. Refer for transvaginal ultrasound
3. Routine referral to endocrinology
4. Start treatment for hormone replacement therapy
5. Urgent referral to a gynaecologist

Q363

A 23 year old woman has a sudden onset of severe abdominal pain and vaginal bleeding that she describes as spotting. She is pregnant but has not attended antenatal clinic and does not know her expected due date. She admits to recent cocaine use. Her BP is 162/104 mmHg; symphysis–fundal height is 31 cm; her uterus feels tense.

What is the most likely diagnosis?

1. Placental abruption
2. Placental praevia
3. Preterm premature rupture of membranes
4. Uterine rupture
5. Vasa praevia

Q364

A 65 year old woman has heavy vaginal bleeding for the last 2 weeks. She has type 2 diabetes for which she takes metformin. She has had three children and went through the menopause 15 years ago. She has no history of past gynaecological problems. Her BMI is 35 kg/m².

Which factor is protective against endometrial cancer?

1. Age 65
2. Multiparity
3. Obesity
4. Time elapsed since menopause
5. Type 2 diabetes

Q365

A 32 year old woman has persistent vaginal blood loss and feels lightheaded just after giving birth, at 38 weeks gestation. On examination, the fundus of the uterus is at the level of the umbilicus.

What is the commonest cause of this presentation?

1. Abnormal coagulation
2. Normal postpartum discharge
3. Retained placenta
4. Trauma to the birth canal
5. Uterine atony

Q366

A 38 year old woman is undergoing induction of labour (at term for her fourth pregnancy) and had a single dose of vaginal prostaglandin E2, 6 hours ago. She is admitted to the delivery suite for artificial rupture of the membranes at 3 cm cervical dilatation. The procedure is performed in the lithotomy position and within 3 minutes she becomes acutely breathless with audible wheeze, followed 1 minute later by circulatory collapse. She has a history of asthma, is a heavy smoker and has a BMI of 34 kg/m².

What is the most likely diagnosis?

1. Amniotic fluid embolism
2. Anaphylaxis
3. Asthma attack with tension pneumothorax
4. Myocardial infarction
5. Pulmonary embolism

Q367

A 25 year old woman presents to her general practitioner with regular cramping pelvic and abdominal pains. She has a history of irregular menstrual cycles and is unsure of date of her last period. On examination, she appears to be in active labour, her cervix is 8 cm dilated. On phoning for an ambulance, the emergency control room ask whether she has entered the second stage of labour.

What defines the start and end points of the second stage of labour?

1. Cervical dilatation to 4 cm and delivery of the placenta
2. Cervical dilatation to 4 cm to delivery of the fetal head
3. Cervical dilatation to 10 cm and delivery of the placenta
4. Cervical dilatation to 10 cm to delivery of the fetal head
5. Uterine contractions occurring regularly for 1 hour or more

Q368

A 47 year old woman has 5 months of debilitating hot flushes, night sweats and mood swings. She is still having periods although these have become less frequent. She does not have any urogenital symptoms, nor is she sexually active. She has a history of deep vein thrombosis during her last pregnancy but otherwise no significant past medical history. Her BP is 119/67 mmHg. She is asking for hormone replacement therapy (HRT).

Which would be the best choice of HRT for this patient?

1. None, HRT is contraindicated
2. Oral oestrogen alone
3. Oral oestrogen with progesterone
4. Transdermal oestrogen with progesterone
5. Vaginal oestrogen

Q369

A 28 year old woman in her first pregnancy is attending her booking appointment. She smokes ten roll-up cigarettes a day, with variable tobacco in each.

Which of the following tests is used to assess risk to the pregnancy from smoking?

1. Carbon monoxide breath test
2. Nicotine level testing
3. Oxygen saturations
4. Peak expiratory flow rate
5. Serum tar level

Q370

A 21 year old woman presents to general practice with heavy, painful periods. Her cycle is regular, with 5 days of bleeding and 21 days in between. She denies she has ever been pregnant, but is sexually active. She has a progesterone implant and does not wish to conceive in the near future. She has no personal or family history of deep vein thrombosis or pulmonary embolism. She suffers from migraines with aura. She has tried simple analgesia with no effect. Her BMI is 19 kg/m².

What is your first management step?

1. Provide a prescription for codeine for the pain
2. Reassure her that this is normal and needs no medical intervention
3. Refer for endometrial ablation
4. Start the combined oral contraceptive pill
5. Trial of tranexamic acid

Q371

A 24 year old woman has missed two periods. She has poorly controlled epilepsy, hypertension and bipolar disorder. She takes amlodipine, escitalopram, lamotrigine, quetiapine and sodium valproate.
Urine HCG confirms pregnancy.

Which of her medications is contraindicated during pregnancy?

1. Amlodipine
2. Escitalopram
3. Lamotrigine
4. Quetiapine
5. Sodium valproate

Q372

A 65 year old woman has 3 weeks of abdominal bloating. She has a family history of breast cancer. She is otherwise well and has no change in bowel habit. Abdominal and pelvic examinations are unremarkable.

What is the next appropriate investigation?

1. Colonoscopy
2. CT scan of thorax, abdomen and pelvis
3. Serum CA125
4. Serum CEA
5. Ultrasound scan of pelvis

Q373

A 35 year old woman is currently 11 weeks into her first pregnancy. She had her height and weight measured at her booking appointment, with a calculated BMI of 48 kg/m².

What should be the next step in her management?

1. Advise her to increase her exercise to at least 1 hour every day of the week
2. Advise her to lose weight to reduce her BMI towards the normal range
3. Continue with routine low-risk care
4. Discuss her increased risk of back pain in pregnancy
5. Refer to a consultant obstetrician for an individualised management plan

Q374

A 26 year old woman has 24 hours of intense, sharp pain in the right lower quadrant of her abdomen. The pain came on suddenly. It is not associated with nausea or vomiting. She had pelvic inflammatory disease 12 months ago, which was treated. She has been trying to conceive for 1 year with no success. She normally has a 29-day menstrual cycle and her last menstrual period was 6 weeks ago, but she thinks that she has started her menstrual period yesterday because she has had some vaginal bleeding. Her temperature is 37.2 °C, pulse rate 114 bpm, BP 98/63 mmHg. Her urinary hCG test is positive.

What is the most likely diagnosis?

1. Endometriosis
2. Ovarian torsion
3. Recurrent pelvic inflammatory disease
4. Ruptured ectopic pregnancy
5. Tubo-ovarian abscess

Q375

A 42 year old woman delivers a stillborn son at 42 weeks. Fetal monitoring in labour had been by intermittent auscultation. The last recorded fetal heart rate was 165 bpm, 15 minutes before delivery. The boy weighs 2.8 kg and has no obvious dysmorphic features. Investigation of the mother after delivery shows a normal glucose tolerance test. Serology (mother): Toxoplasmosis IgM negative, Toxoplasmosis IgG positive, and Cytomegalovirus IgM and IgG both negative.

What is the most likely cause for stillbirth?

1. Chromosomal abnormality
2. Congenital infection
3. Intrapartum asphyxia
4. Maternal autoimmune disease
5. Placental abruption

Q376

A 36 year old woman presents to general practice at 29 weeks into her first pregnancy. She complains that the fetus has not yet developed a pattern of movements, and she will have days when she cannot feel the fetus move.

Which of the following is the next course of action?

1. Arrange ultrasound scan
2. Ask patient to go home and concentrate on their movements for an hour before coming in
3. Reassure her that this is normal
4. Refer for review by the maternity department via their triage service
5. Send to the emergency department for review

Q377

A 30 year old woman has decreased fetal movements. She is in the 34th week of her first pregnancy. She is a smoker at ten cigarettes a day. The fetal heart is normal. The symphysis–fundal height is 37 cm (above the 95th centile).

What is the next step in management?

1. Arrange caesarean section at 36 weeks because of the risk of shoulder dystocia
2. Arrange glucose tolerance test
3. No action is required
4. Request a senior clinician to repeat the examination
5. Ultrasound scan to check the fetal size

Q378

A 36 year old woman has constant lower abdominal pain following a horse-riding accident. She is 37 weeks pregnant. Her temperature is 37.1 °C, pulse 115 bpm, BP 96/64 mmHg, fetal pulse rate is 160 bpm, her abdomen is hard with size consistent with 37-week pregnancy. She is cannulated and fluid is started. Ultrasound reveals a concealed haemorrhage around a partially detached placenta. There is no other sign of injury.

What is the most appropriate management?

1. Category 1 caesarean section
2. Category 2 caesarean section
3. Induction of vaginal delivery with oxytocin
4. Intravenous tocolytics
5. Strict bed rest and review in 4 hours

Q379

A 44 year old woman has a sensation of a mass 'coming down her vagina'. She feels that she needs to apply digital pressure on the posterior vaginal wall to empty her rectum. She has stress incontinence of urine but not faeces. She has seven children, all by normal vaginal deliveries. Her periods are normal.

What is the likely next stage of management?

1. Oestrogen pessary
2. Radical hysterectomy
3. Ring pessary
4. Vaginal hysterectomy and repair
5. Vaginal mesh

Q380

A 45 year old woman has a vulval lump and itching. This has not been relieved with over-the-counter medications and causes slight pain on intercourse. She is a heavy smoker and has a history of two LLETZ procedures to her cervix. She is currently in a new sexual relationship but not using condoms. There is a 5 mm slightly raised papule; there is no ulceration or bleeding. Areas of the surrounding vulval skin appear red or white.

What is the most likely diagnosis?

1. Allergic reaction
2. Lichen sclerosis
3. Sexually transmitted infection
4. Vulval cancer
5. Vulval intraepithelial neoplasia

Q381

A 36 year old woman has a lump in her right breast. She delivered a healthy baby girl, at term, 3 months ago. She is breastfeeding. She takes carbamazepine for epilepsy. Her temperature is 36.9 °C, pulse 82 bpm, BP 120/60 mmHg, there is a 1 x 1.5 x 1.5 cm firm lump in her right breast.

What is the most appropriate management?

1. Advise her to stop the carbamazepine and review in 1 month
2. Prescribe antibiotics and review
3. Reassure and review in 1 month
4. Refer to breastfeeding advisory nurse
5. Request an urgent (2-week-wait) appointment

Q382

A 28 year old woman has a very painful red area on her left breast for the last 2 days. She is now 2 weeks after a normal vaginal delivery. She has been exclusively breastfeeding her baby since birth. Her temperature is 36.4 °C, pulse 78 bpm, BP 110/70 mmHg. There is a tender, hard, wedge-shaped area of redness on the inferior aspect of the left breast.

What is the most appropriate advice?

1. Continue to feed from both breasts
2. Only feed from the affected breast
3. Only feed from the non-affected breast
4. Stop breastfeeding for 24 hours
5. Stop breastfeeding until symptoms resolve

Q383

A 42 year old woman has a breast lump, which has been present for the last 2 months. This has remained the same size. There is no nipple discharge, nipple inversion or any breast skin changes. She does not have fever or weight loss. There is 2 x 2 cm lump situated in the right upper quadrant of the right breast. The lump is mobile, fluctuant, non-tender and there is no erythema over the lump.

What is the most appropriate next investigation?

1. Biopsy of lump
2. BRCA-1 genetic profiling
3. Breast ultrasound
4. CT chest, abdomen and pelvis
5. FBC

Q384

A 22 year old woman has had a palpable pea-sized lump in her right breast for the last month. She is nulliparous and not pregnant.

What is the most likely cause of this lump?

1. Breast cancer
2. Breast cyst
3. Fibroadenoma

4. Intraductal papilloma
5. Lipoma

Q385

A 46 year old woman noticed a mass 3 weeks ago in the right upper portion of her left breast. She has no family history; the mass is not painful and there is no visible 'dimpling' or change in shape of the breast. She attends the breast clinic and, following palpation and a visual examination, she is sent for a mammogram, an ultrasound and a core biopsy.

Which of the following is most likely to indicate that the mass is malignant?

1. Adipose tissue
2. An infiltrative border
3. Fluid-filled cysts
4. Micro-calcifications
5. Oedema

Q386

A 32 year old woman has a 3 x 3 cm tender warm left-sided breast lump at 4 weeks postpartum. Her temperature is 37.9 °C, pulse 98 bpm, BP 100/60 mmHg. She is prescribed flucloxacillin 500 mg qds and advised regarding paracetamol.

What is the recommended advice regarding continuation of breastfeeding?

1. Continue to breastfeed or express both sides
2. Continue to breastfeed or express on the affected side, letting the normal side rest
3. Continue to breastfeed or express only on the normal side, letting the affected side rest
4. Stop breastfeeding altogether
5. Stop breastfeeding while taking antibiotics, then try to restart

Q387

A 34 year old woman has pain in her left breast for which she takes simple analgesics. She regularly self-examines and has not noticed any lumps. She is not pregnant. Her last pregnancy was 12 years ago.

Her temperature is 36.4 °C, pulse 86 bpm, BP 140/80 mmHg; her breasts and axillae are normal.

What is the best course of action?

1. No further action needed
2. Prescribe the combined oral contraceptive
3. Request a mammogram
4. Routine outpatient appointment
5. Urgent (2-week-wait) outpatient appointment

Q388

A 40 year old woman is consulting over the phone; she has a 4-week history of white nipple discharge associated with early morning headaches. She has also had acne and irregular periods. She has had four pregnancies in the past with no complications. When asked, she mentions that she has also been experiencing changes in her vision, especially the peripheries.

What is the most appropriate next step?

1. Arrange an MRI head
2. Complete a breast and ophthalmic examination
3. Prescribe cabergoline/bromocriptine
4. Reassure
5. Refer to the 2-week-wait breast clinic

Ophthalmology

13

Q389

A 65 year old white man has 6 months of a raised lesion on the inner corner of the right upper eye lid. This has recently become larger and has bled twice while wiping his eyes at work. He works as a farmer. The lesion looks rough and slightly dark compared to the adjacent area. He gives a past history of a lump removed from his forehead.

What would be the next step in management?

1. Crush the lesion with forceps and apply cryopexy
2. Excision biopsy
3. Prescribe topical antibiotic cream
4. Reassurance and review in 6 months
5. Take a scraping from the surface looking for fungal hyphae

Q390

A 72 year old man has 6 months of crusting of his lashes, with early morning discharge and redness of his eyes. He was prescribed chloramphenicol eye drops by his general practitioner, which gave some improvement, but his symptoms persist. After examination, he is prescribed a course of doxycycline for chronic blepharitis.

Which gland is associated with blepharitis?

1. Accessory lacrimal gland of Krause
2. Glands of Moll
3. Lacrimal gland
4. Meibomian gland
5. Parotid gland

Q391

A 65 year old man has 2 days of double vision on looking to his left; this he can overcome by closing one eye. It is associated with headache and watering in both eyes while attempting to read. He has poorly controlled type 2 diabetes mellitus and has had laser treatment for diabetic maculopathy. There is no evidence of papilloedema on examination.

What is the most appropriate immediate management?

1. Ask optician to review prescription for glasses
2. Hess screening to measure the deviation
3. Patch one eye
4. Referral to GP for improving diabetic control
5. Urgent MR scan of head

Q392

A 56 year old man is seen in the eye clinic with 5 months of gradual dimming of his vision. He denies trauma to the eye. He is not on any regular medication but has used steroid skin cream for atopic dermatitis for the last 10 years. His best corrected visual acuity is 6/18 in both eyes. He has cataracts in both eyes with a very poor view of the retina. He needs to drive for his living.

What is the next management step?

1. Advise surgery as soon as possible for the cataracts
2. Advise that he takes vitamins A and E
3. Prescribe regular aspirin
4. Review in 6 months' time to check cataract maturity
5. Stop the steroid cream

Q393

A 72 year old man has 4 hours of sudden-onset, painless loss of vision in the right eye. He has ischaemic heart disease and takes aspirin and atorvastatin. Fundoscopy of his right eye reveals a cholesterol embolus in the branch retinal artery.

What is the next step in management of this patient?

1. High-dose intravenous corticosteroids
2. Immediate CT head

3. No treatment needed for this patient
4. Ocular massage to the right eye
5. Urgent temporal artery biopsy

Q394

A 24 year old man has a painless loss of vision in his left eye 1 day ago. He describes first noticing a dark cobweb effect and says that the vision then became globally blurred. There were no visual symptoms prior to this. He has type 1 diabetes mellitus and takes insulin and oral hypoglycaemics. His latest HbA1c is 104 mmol/mol (< 48). He has not attended his most recent retinal screening appointments.

What is the most likely cause of his sudden vision loss?

1. Cataract
2. Diabetic macular oedema
3. Open angle glaucoma
4. Optic neuritis
5. Vitreous haemorrhage

Q395

An 18 year old man has unilateral redness of his right eye. He was treated with chloramphenicol eye drops 2 weeks ago with some response, but the redness has returned.

Investigations:

Chlamydia PCR positive

What is the appropriate treatment strategy for this patient?

1. Topical beta-blocker eye drops
2. Topical chloramphenicol eye drops with oral doxycycline
3. Topical fusidic sodium eye ointment
4. Topical prednisolone eye drops with oral penicillin
5. Topical quinolone antibiotic drops

Q396

A 48 year old man attends eye casualty with a right-sided painful eye, blurred vision and photophobia. He wears monthly contact lenses which he has been cleaning with tap water. In addition, he occasionally forgets to remove them at night. He denies any discharge.

His visual acuity is 6/36 in the right eye, and 6/4 in the left eye. His right eye is red and there is a 3.5 mm circular epithelial defect that stains with fluorescein. The defect is surrounded by a whitish infiltrate in the stroma; however, there is mild anterior chamber inflammation.

What would be your first step in the management?

1. Prescribe topical tear supplements
2. Start broad-spectrum topical antibiotics
3. Start oral antibiotics
4. Start topical steroids
5. Take corneal scrape for gram stain and bacterial culture sensitivity

Q397

A 42 year old man with a history of sore throat and a runny nose presents to the emergency eye department with pain in his eyeball. He had a thorough ocular examination.

What feature suggests preseptal cellulitis rather than orbital cellulitis?

1. Diplopia
2. Normal eye movements
3. Pain on eye movements
4. Proptosis
5. Reduced vision

Q398

A 24 year old man presents to the eye department with 5 days of a red and sore right eye with associated photophobia. He has some pain which is mostly relieved by paracetamol, but this wakes him up at night. There is no discharge from his eyes. He had a previous history of red eye but this resolved within a few days. He has had low back pain for the last couple of years and is currently being investigated for ankylosing spondylitis.

What is the most likely ocular diagnosis?

1. Bacterial keratitis
2. Endophthalmitis
3. Iritis

4. Ocular migraine

5. Viral conjunctivitis

Q399

A 65 year old man is referred to the eye hospital with a diagnosis of suspected primary open angle glaucoma. His visual acuity is 6/9 in the right and 6/7.5 in the left eye. His intraocular pressure by Goldman applanation tonometer is 34 mmHg in the right eye and 36 mmHg in the left. Visual field examination shows early arcuate scotoma in both eyes.

Which is the most appropriate treatment option?

1. Cyclocryopexy

2. Drainage tube

3. Goniotomy

4. Latanoprost eye drops

5. Peripheral iridotomy

Q400

A 79 year old woman has 2 days of central vision loss with distortion of images. She complains of inability to do her crossword puzzles, and narrowly missed falling over the kerb the previous evening. She is an ex-smoker and was diagnosed with dry age-related macular degeneration (AMD) 3 years ago.

What is the most likely type of macular degeneration?

1. Disciform scar

2. Early AMD

3. Late and dry AMD

4. Late and wet active AMD

5. Late and wet inactive AMD

Q401

A 22 year old woman presents to the emergency department with ocular discomfort and blurred vision. She was diagnosed with multiple sclerosis 2 years ago. She is in good health otherwise.

What should be the next step?

1. Arrange an urgent CT scan of the brain
2. Immediate lumbar puncture to look for CSF proteins
3. Establish diagnosis by examining the affected eye
4. Reassure patient and order next-day electrodiagnostic test
5. Treat urgently with bolus of intravenous methylprednisolone

Q402

A 65 year old man has a sudden onset of loss of vision. He is diagnosed with an acute retinal detachment involving the upper retina, but not yet involving the fovea.

When should retinal detachment repair surgery be carried out?

1. Within 24 hours
2. After 24 hours, up to 1 week
3. After 1 week but within 3 months
4. After 3 months
5. Timing is irrelevant

Q403

A 54 year old woman presents to the emergency department with 3 days of a severely painful right eye. This has woken her at night. Paracetamol does not give her full relief. She has been undergoing investigation by her physician for a suspected autoimmune disorder. On examination, there is localised redness in the temporal part of the sclera and the intraocular pressure reading is 24 mmHg.

What is the most likely diagnosis?

1. Acute angle closure glaucoma
2. Diffuse scleritis
3. Orbital pseudotumour
4. Superior limbic keratoconjunctivitis
5. Typical migraine

Q404

A 21 year male has 2 hours of pain in his right eye. He has been using a metal trimmer while gardening without protective goggles. His visual acuity is reduced to counting fingers in the right eye and 6/9 unaided in the other eye. There is a perforation in the limbal area of the right eye measuring 2 by 3 mm. The intraocular pressure is 5 mmHg. There is hyphaema, making the view to the eye beyond the cornea difficult.

What is the next appropriate radiological investigation?

1. Bedside rapid assessment by ultrasound of the globe and orbit
2. CT scan orbits
3. MRI of orbits
4. PET scan of the orbit
5. X-rays of the globe in two positions of gaze

Q405

A 26 year old woman has double vision; a sore, blurry right eye; and a prominent eyeball, as noticed by her family. She is not on any medication, but lately, she mentioned having palpitation and weight loss.

What would be the first line of management?

1. Broad-spectrum antibiotics
2. Detailed ocular assessment to rule out compression of the optic nerve
3. Referral to the cardiologist
4. Routine blood tests
5. Topical lubricants and reassurance

Q406

A 36 year old man has unilateral ocular pain, photophobia and redness for the last 2 weeks. His vision is slightly hazy, and there is no discharge. He admits to ongoing back pain that he has previously managed with NSAIDs.

What is the most likely diagnosis?

1. Anterior uveitis
2. Conjunctivitis
3. Episcleritis
4. Intermediate uveitis
5. Posterior uveitis

Q407

An 82 year old woman presents to the emergency department with 2 days of visual impairment in the right eye. She has loss of weight and appetite, and pain while eating her food and combing her hair. Examination reveals best corrected visual acuity of 6/36 in the right eye and 6/9 in the left eye. Her optic disc in the right eye shows oedema in the inferior half with indistinct margin in the superior half.

What would be the next step in the management?

1. Carotid duplex scan
2. Reassure and review in outpatients in 2 weeks
3. Reassure her and request routine blood test
4. Refer to the optician for corrective lenses
5. Urgent blood test consisting of CRP, FBC and plasma viscosity

Q408

A 68 year old man presents to the emergency department with 3 days of swelling of his right eye associated with the sensation of tightness behind the eye. He feels unwell. His temperature is 38.4 °C. He has an axial proptosis with painful and restricted eye movements.

What is the next step in the management?

1. Blood sample to exclude immunodeficiency
2. CT scan of brain and orbits
3. ENT review
4. Intravenous antibiotics
5. Intravenous steroids

Q409

A 25 year old man presents to the emergency department with 2 hours of severe pain, photophobia and tearing in his right eye, which he cannot open He had been gardening a few hours before and not using protective goggles. He has no past ocular history of significance.

What is the most likely diagnosis?

1. Acute mucopurulent conjunctivitis
2. Necrotising scleritis

3. Ruptured hordeolum externum
4. Traumatic carotico-cavernous fistula
5. Traumatic corneal abrasion

Q410

A 40 year old woman presents to the urgent eye care department after a splash by caustic soda into her eye 1 hour ago. She complains of tearing, severe burning sensation and blurred vision. Her visual acuity on presentation was counting fingers in the affected eye.

What is the immediate and critical management step?

1. Exploration of the eyeball in theatre to rule out a globe rupture
2. Immediate, intense topical steroids to counter the inflammation
3. Intramuscular analgesia and discharge her with topical lubricants
4. Irrigate her eyes with saline checking the pH of the conjunctival sac periodically
5. Urgent CT scan

Q411

A 59 year old man presents with 2 days of flashes and floaters in his right eye. The flashes are like lightning and occur every few hours, especially in dim light. He has a history of myopia and migraines, and his visual acuities are normal.

What is the most appropriate management?

1. Immediate laser photocoagulation
2. Start oral steroids
3. Perform tonometry to check intraocular pressure
4. Refer for urgent MRI of the brain
5. Urgent ophthalmology referral

Q412

A 10 year old boy has difficulty seeing, associated with tiredness of his eyes with watering in the evening. He squints his eyes and sits very close to watch the television. His teacher has moved him to the front row of the class and this has improved his performance. His visual acuity is 6/36 in both eyes, improving to 6/9 with pin hole. His eye examination was otherwise normal.

What is the next step towards assessing his visual status?

1. Advise pencil push-ups
2. Arrange urgent MRI/CT
3. Optometrist assessment
4. Tear supplements
5. Urgent ophthalmological review

Q413

A 10 year old boy is seen in eye clinic with a greyish-white pupillary reflex in his right eye. He has had worsening blurred vision since he had trauma to his right eye while playing rugby at school 3 days ago. He has been wearing glasses for myopia since the age of 6. His father has Stickler syndrome (a connective tissue disease). He has an obvious bruise above the right eye.

What is the next step in management?

1. Arrange an urgent geneticist appointment
2. Arrange an urgent MR scan
3. Dilated eye examination with ultrasound
4. Reassure and discharge
5. Topical steroids and antibiotics

Q414

A 65 year old man has a unilateral painful red eye, nausea and vomiting. His past ocular history was unremarkable except for wearing glasses for hypermetropia since the age of 6. He has conjunctival injection, corneal oedema, and shallow anterior chamber with an intraocular pressure of 60 mmHg (< 20) by Goldmann applanation tonometer.

What is the initial management?

1. Arrange an urgent CT scan to rule out intracranial lesion
2. Arrange an urgent laser peripheral iridotomy
3. Refer the patient to a physician for his vomiting
4. Treat with intravenous acetazolamide 500 mg
5. Treat with topical beta-blocker (timolol 0.5%) eye drops

Q415

A 19 year old woman has 1 day of increasing pain, redness and photophobia in her right eye. She accidentally slept with her contact lens *in situ* the previous night.

Her best corrected visual acuity is 6/9 in her right eye and 6/6 in her left eye. The right eye has diffuse conjunctival injection in all four quadrants. There is some watery discharge. There is a small well-circumscribed white opacity on the cornea. Some anterior chamber cells are visible. The left eye is normal.

What is the most appropriate initial empirical treatment?

1. Ganciclovir gel
2. Hypromellose 0.3%
3. Levofloxacin
4. Natamycin 5%
5. Prednisolone eye drops

Q416

A 65 year old woman has a vague headache of 2 months' duration, associated with a shadow in the inferior field of vision. A few months before this presentation, she was diagnosed with early cataract in her left eye. She has systemic hypertension and is on medication for the same. An automated visual field test showed a right homonymous inferior quadrantic visual field defect.

Where is the most likely lesion?

1. Lens of the eye
2. Occipital cortex
3. Optic chiasma
4. Parietal lobe
5. Retina

Orthopaedics and Trauma

14

Q417

An 80 year old woman was found on the floor in her nursing home. She has hypertension, ischaemic heart disease and dementia. She normally walks unaided indoors.

Clinical examination reveals a short and externally rotated right leg.

An X-ray reveals a displaced intracapsular neck of femur fracture.

What is the appropriate operative management plan?

1. Cannulated screws
2. Dynamic hip screw
3. Hemiarthroplasty
4. Intramedullary nail
5. Total hip arthroplasty

Q418

A 38 year old man presents to the emergency department after being pushed through a window. He has a shard of glass 1 x 0.3 cm penetrating 20 cm directly inferior to the anterior superior iliac spine. There is a 10 x 8 x 3 cm swelling on the lateral aspect of the thigh.

Which structure lies immediately deep to the glass entry site?

1. Femoral artery
2. Femoral nerve
3. Femoral vein
4. Vastus lateralis
5. Vastus medialis

Q419

A 60 year old man has 2 days of severe back pain and weakness in both legs. He has ischaemic heart disease, diabetes and prostate cancer. Examination reveals a sensory level at T10, and 3/5 weakness of the proximal hip muscles. X-ray of the spine shows collapse of the T9 vertebra. The patient is placed on flat bed rest and given analgesia by the nursing staff. A bladder scan shows 280 ml of urine in the bladder.

What is the most appropriate next step in management?

1. CT-guided biopsy of the T9 vertebra
2. MRI of the whole spine
3. Occupational therapist assessment
4. Referral to the spinal surgery team for spinal stabilisation
5. Urinary catheter

Q420

An 11 year old girl has pain in the left elbow following a fall from monkey bars. A supracondylar fracture of the distal humerus is suspected, and she is unable to make an 'OK sign'.

Injury to which nerve is likely to have caused this?

1. Anterior interosseous branch of median nerve
2. Axillary nerve
3. Dorsal branch of the ulnar nerve
4. Lateral cutaneous nerve of the forearm
5. Posterior interosseous branch of radial nerve

Q421

An 80 year old woman was brought to the emergency department by her son, who has subsequently left. He stated that she has become more immobile and isolated over the past 3 weeks, not coming out of her house and sleeping in her living room chair rather than her bed.

On superficial examination, she is unkempt and confused (abbreviated mental test score 5/10). She has several bruises of various ages around her body.

What is the next appropriate management step?

1. Contact the police
2. Obtain corroborative history followed by a detailed clinical examination
3. Occupational therapy assessment
4. Refer to the dietitians
5. Routine blood investigations – full blood count, renal function

Q422

A 25 year old man has a chronically discharging sinus in his distal right lower leg; 3 years ago, he had an open fracture of his right tibia requiring intermedullary nailing. He feels systemically well but complains of pain on walking, partially relieved by using crutches. He is given appropriate antibiotics.

What should the initial stage of his treatment comprise of?

1. Above-knee amputation
2. Long-term antibiotics only
3. Surgical debridement, removal of the intermedullary nail
4. Surgical debridement of discharging tract
5. Symptom control with analgesia and physiotherapy

Q423

A 56 year old woman has right knee pain for the last 2 days, with associated joint effusion. She has hypertension. Her temperature is 37.6 °C, pulse 86 bpm, BP 130/70 mmHg. The joint is hot to the touch. Her inflammatory markers are raised.

What is the appropriate next management?

1. Joint aspiration
2. Reassure and review in 2 weeks
3. Routine referral to rheumatology
4. Start on intravenous antibiotics
5. Take to theatre for debridement of joint

Q424

A 67 year old woman has pain in both of her hands. It is worse in the morning and the pain is mostly in the metacarpophalangeal and proximal interphalangeal joints in her hands. On examination of her hands and wrists, there are subcutaneous nodules and an ulnar deviation of her metacarpophalangeal joints.

What is the most likely diagnosis?

1. Ankylosing spondylitis
2. Gout
3. Osteoarthritis
4. Psoriatic arthritis
5. Rheumatoid arthritis

Q425

A 26 year old man has increasingly severe pain in his right leg. He had a closed right transverse tibial fracture following trauma and was placed into a plaster cast 3 days ago. His leg is elevated on a pillow and the cast is split. His pain is increasing despite having been given analgesia.

What is the most appropriate next step?

1. Assess the neurovascular status of his leg
2. CT scan of his leg
3. Elevate his limb more to relieve dependent oedema
4. Ice application to whole area
5. Venous ultrasound of the leg to exclude a venous thrombosis

Q426

A 76 year old woman has pain in her right thigh, particularly when mobilising. She has osteoporosis and a past breast cancer. She has pain on palpation and gentle mobilisation of her right thigh. Chest and breast examination are normal.

Blood tests are unremarkable. Radiograph shows a lucent area with ill-defined margins in the middle third of her femur. X-ray of the pelvis, femur and knee are normal.

What is the next best step in her management?

1. Commence bisphosphonates
2. Femoral MRI and a CT chest, abdomen and pelvis
3. Primary excision of the lesion and referral to oncology
4. Primary stabilisation with an intramedullary nail
5. Radiotherapy followed by excision of the lesion

Q427

A 25 year old man is brought to the emergency department with an incised wound on the right wrist, sustained while at work. He has complete loss of sensation on the palmar surface of his right little finger and half of his ring finger, but dorsal sensation is intact.

Which movement is most likely to be compromised?

1. Abduction of the fingers
2. Extension of the little finger
3. Flexion of the distal interphalangeal joint of the little finger
4. Flexion of the interphalangeal joint of the thumb
5. Palmar abduction of the thumb

Q428

A 57 year old man attends the emergency department with a laceration to the base of his left thumb. The wound occurred less than 1 hour ago and was made with a clean knife. He is haemodynamically stable, the base of the wound is slowly oozing blood and the patient cannot adduct their thumb.

What is the most appropriate initial management?

1. Admit for elevation and intravenous antibiotics
2. Close the wound with interrupted sutures and refer for outpatient follow-up
3. Close with wound closure strips and cover with non-adherent dressings
4. Control any bleeding with topical dressings and refer for immediate specialist assessment
5. X-ray the thumb

Q429

A 23 year old man is brought into the emergency department following a road traffic accident.

His pulse is 136 bpm, BP 85/49 mmHg, respiratory rate 22 breaths per minute, oxygen saturation 94% breathing air. He has a lot of blood around his face and mouth and is gurgling.

His left pupil is 8 mm and non-reactive. His right pupil is 3 mm and reactive. He has bruising over his right upper quadrant and a large scrotal haematoma. He has an absent radial pulse and a weak femoral one. He has an obviously deformed, open fracture of his ankle.

His airway is secured and he is started on oxygen.

What are the priorities for managing this patient?

1. Antibiotics, reduction and splintage of his fracture
2. Cervical spine X-rays
3. Large-bore intravenous access and 1 L of Hartmann's solution
4. Pelvic binder application
5. Urgent neurosurgical opinion

Q430

A 40 year old man has a swelling on his left arm. It appeared when, while carrying a heavy sofa up a flight of stairs 3 days ago, he slipped and injured himself. He has no significant past medical history but smokes 10 cigarettes a day. He is neurovascularly intact but has bruising around the elbow and the proximal forearm. He has a 3 × 3 cm swelling over the anterior aspect of the left upper arm and is tender in the medial antecubital fossa. He has a full range of flexion and extension at the elbow but this is sore.

What is the most likely diagnosis?

1. Distal biceps tendon rupture
2. Elbow dislocation
3. Lateral epicondylitis
4. Proximal biceps tendon rupture
5. Teres minor tear

Q431

A 34 year old man is involved in a head-on collision with a car while riding his horse. He has multiple limb fractures. On arrival in the emergency department, his temperature is 36.4 °C, pulse 135 bpm, BP 90/60 mmHg, respiratory rate 32 breaths per minute, oxygen saturation 93% breathing air, capillary refill 3 seconds. Class III haemorrhagic shock is suspected.

What is the primary intervention for this patient, according to the ATLS classification?

1. Administer crystalloid solutions to stabilise the patient
2. Initiate the Massive Haemorrhage Protocol and call for a blood transfusion
3. Order a CT angiogram to identify the source of bleeding
4. Perform early definitive airway management with an endo-tracheal tube
5. Splint and align long bone fractures promptly

Q432

A 14 year old boy has a 10-day history of lumbar back pain. This occurred the day after trampolining. He has no red flags. He takes regular ibuprofen and paracetamol; however, this does not settle the pain completely.

What is the most appropriate management option?

1. Active rehabilitation
2. Add opiate pain relief
3. Blood test for FBC and PSA
4. Lumbar spine X-ray
5. MRI lumbar spine

Renal and Urology

15

Q433

An 18 year old woman has dysuria and lower abdominal and flank pain for the past 48 hours. Her temperature is 38.5 °C. She has a negative pregnancy test.

Urine dipstick is as follows:

Specific gravity – high

pH – 8.5

Blood – trace

Protein – negative

Glucose – negative

Ketones – 1+

Bilirubin – negative

Nitrites – 2+

Leukocytes – 2+

What is the most likely diagnosis?

1. Diabetic ketoacidosis
2. Ectopic pregnancy
3. Glomerulonephritis
4. Lower urinary tract infection
5. Pyelonephritis

Q434

A 65 year old woman presents to the emergency department with abdominal pain, nausea and vomiting. She passed very little urine 2 days ago, and none in the last 24 hours. She has poorly controlled diabetes mellitus and hypertension. She takes ramipril and amlodipine. Her temperature is 39.2 °C, pulse 110 bpm, BP 105/60 mmHg.

Investigations:

Haemoglobin	165 g/L (120–150)
PCV	0.56% (0.37–0.47)
Sodium	147 mmol/L (135–145)
Potassium	6.0 mmol/L (3.5–5.0)
Serum urea	28 mmol/L (2.5–6.7)
Serum creatinine	375 μmol/L (54–145)
eGFR	42 mL/min/1.73 m2
Bicarbonate	19 mmol/L (22–30)
Albumin	46 g/L (32–45)
Calcium	2.3 mmol/L (2.1–2.6)
Phosphate	1.85 mmol/L (0.8–1.5)

What is the next step in the management of this patient?

1. 1 L of 0.9% saline
2. 40 mg intravenous furosemide
3. Infusion of calcium gluconate, rehydration
4. Intermittent haemodialysis
5. Parenteral nutrition

Q435

A 75 year old man has 2 months of difficulty initiating his urinary flow, incomplete emptying of his bladder and terminal dribbling. It is significantly impacting his quality of life. He has type 2 diabetes, hypercholesterolaemia and postural hypotension secondary to diabetic neuropathy. His medications include atorvastatin 20 mg daily, metformin 500 mg twice daily and fludrocortisone 100 micrograms daily. On digital rectal examination, he has a large smooth prostate with no masses and soft stool in the rectum.

Given the likely diagnosis, what is the most appropriate initial management plan?

1. Doxazosin
2. Finasteride
3. Stop fludrocortisone
4. Tamsulosin
5. Transurethral resection of the prostate

Q436

A 74 year old man has progressive renal impairment. He has type 2 diabetes and hypertension; 4 months ago, his eGFR was 30 ml/min/1.73m^2. He takes amlodipine 5 mg once daily and atorvastatin 20 mg once daily.

Investigations:

BP 156/78 mmHg

Blood glucose 6.5 mmol/l

Serum creatinine 197 μmol/L (60–110)

Serum albumin 36 g/L (37–49)

eGFR 28 ml/min/1.73m^2 (> 60)

HbA1c 45 mmol/mol

Urinalysis protein 2+, blood negative

Urinary protein:creatinine ratio 255 mg/mmol (< 15)

What is the most appropriate next step in the management?

1. Add indapamide 2.5 mg once daily
2. Add metformin 1 g twice daily
3. Add ramipril 2.5 mg once daily
4. Increase amlodipine to 10 mg once daily
5. Prepare for dialysis

Q437

A 26 year old woman has uncontrolled voiding of urine when she laughs or sneezes. The urge to urinate does not occur frequently or with urgency. She is nulliparous. Her BMI is 46 kg/m^2, her abdomen is soft with no palpable bladder mass.

What would be the most suitable first-line treatment for this patient?

1. Bladder training
2. Oestradiol ring
3. Pelvic floor exercises
4. Topical oestrogen gel
5. Weight loss

Q438

A 65 year old man has a diabetes review. He has had type 2 diabetes mellitus for 10 years and had a myocardial infarction 13 years ago. He takes aspirin, atorvastatin and the maximum tolerated dose of ramipril and metformin. His glycaemic control is satisfactory. His BP is 135/85 mmHg, eGFR > 90 ml/min, ACR of 25 mg/mmol (< 2.5).

What is the next appropriate class of medication he should be started on?

1. Beta-blocker
2. Calcium channel blocker
3. Dipeptidyl peptidase intravenous (DPP IV) inhibitor
4. Sodium-glucose cotransporter-2 (SGLT2) inhibitor
5. Sulphonylurea

Q439

A 65 year old man has 72 hours of testicular pain. This started gradually and has been getting worse. He now has swelling of his left testis and redness of the overlying scrotal skin. An ultrasound scan confirms an epidydimo-orchitis.

What is the most likely infecting organism?

1. Chlamydia trachomatis
2. Escherichia coli
3. Group B streptococcus
4. Neisseria gonorrhoeae
5. Staphylococcus aureus

Q440

A 67 year old man has nocturia and hesitancy, getting progressively worse over 6 months. His abdomen is soft and he has a hard, irregular prostate. His serum PSA test is 35. Prostate cancer is suspected.

Which lobe is most commonly affected first in prostate cancer?

1. Anterior
2. Left Lateral
3. Median
4. Posterior
5. Right lateral

Q441

A 25 year old man has a pea-sized, painless swelling on his left testis. He is normally fit and well and has had no previous surgeries. His temperature is 36.8 °C, pulse 78 bpm, respiratory rate 12 breaths per minute. He has a small hard lump on the left testicle that does not transilluminate and was non-tender. Right testicular examination was unremarkable.

What is the most likely diagnosis?

1. Epididymo-orchitis
2. Hydrocele
3. Inguino-scrotal hernia
4. Testicular cancer
5. Testicular torsion

Q442

A 28 year old woman has 1 day of severe left flank pain that comes in waves and radiates to her groin. She passes urine more frequently, occasionally with some blood in it. She returned from holiday, in Spain, 2 days ago. Urine pregnancy test is negative.

What would be the most appropriate next investigation?

1. Bloods for kidney function
2. Contrast CT kidney, ureters and bladder
3. Non-contrast CT kidney, ureters and bladder
4. Ultrasound scan abdomen
5. Urine dipstick

Q443

A 27 year old woman has increased urinary frequency and dysuria. There is no visible blood in her urine. She has no fevers, chills, flank pain or vaginal discharge. She is sexually active with her long-term partner and takes the combined oral contraceptive pill. Her temperature is 36.8 °C, pulse 86 bpm, BP 110/ 68 mmHg. She has a soft, non-distended abdomen with normal bowel sounds. She has moderate discomfort in her suprapubic region but no other tenderness. A pelvic examination is normal with no evidence of abnormal vaginal or cervical discharge or inflammation.

What is the most likely diagnosis?

1. Acute kidney injury
2. Cystitis
3. Pyelonephritis
4. Renal calculi
5. Sexually transmitted disease

Q444

A 38 year old woman has 6 weeks of intermittent left flank pain and bloody urine. She has felt fatigued over the last few months and recently saw her general practitioner because she was worried her ankles were swollen. She has hypertension and systemic lupus erythematosus. She takes valsartan.

Her abdomen is soft with mild left flank tenderness. There is no palpable hepatosplenomegaly. She has pitting oedema to the knee. Urinalysis shows 3+ of protein and 1+ RBCs.

Investigations:

Hb	119 g/L	(115–160 g/L)
WBC	9.2 x 10^9/L	(4.0–11.0 x 10^9/L)
Platelets	423 x 10^9/L	(150–400 10^9/L)
Na+	135 mmol/L	(135–145)
K+	4.5 mmol/L	(3.5–5.0)
Urea	13.4 mmol/L	(2.0–7)
Creatinine	325 μmol/L	(55–120)
ALT	38 iu/L	(3–40)
Bilirubin	16 μmol/L	(3–17)
Alkaline phosphatase	80 μmol/L	(30–100)
Albumin	21 g/L	(35–50)
CRP	12 mg/L	(< 10)

What is the most likely diagnosis?

1. Acute interstitial nephritis secondary to valsartan
2. AKI secondary to pyelonephritis
3. Portal vein thrombosis secondary to nephrotic syndrome
4. Renal colic
5. Renal vein thrombosis secondary to nephrotic syndrome

Q445

A 48 year old man presents to his general practitioner after noticing that his urine has been intermittently bloodstained over the last 2 weeks. He is otherwise well. His urine looks clear, urine dip is negative for protein, leukocytes and nitrites, 1+ positive for blood.

What is the most appropriate management?

1. Immediate 2-week-wait referral to urology
2. Make a follow-up appointment following mid-stream urine analysis
3. Make a non-urgent referral to urology
4. Prescribe antibiotics for presumed urinary tract infection
5. Reassure the patient that the symptoms should resolve spontaneously without further treatment

Q446

A 77 year old man has 6 hours of hypotension and vomiting associated with a constant thirst. He has essential hypertension and mild asthma, taking ramipril and using a salbutamol inhaler. One day ago, he had a laparotomy and bowel resection for acute perforation.

His temperature is 36.8 °C, pulse 108 bpm, BP 93/56 mmHg, respiratory rate 20 breaths per minute, oxygen saturation 96% breathing air, capillary refill 5 seconds. His chest is clear bilaterally; heart sounds S1 + S2 + 0; his skin feels cold to touch and he has dry mucosae; abdomen is soft but mildly tender around the wound site and urine bag has 200 ml of dark, concentrated urine since surgery finished.

What is the most likely diagnosis?

1. Asthma exacerbation
2. Oliguria due to hypovolaemia
3. Perioperative fluid overload
4. Postoperative opioid overdose
5. Septic shock

Q447

A 70 year old man has a single episode of painless visible haematuria. He is otherwise well and has no lower urinary tract symptoms. He has COPD and had a myocardial infarction 2 years ago. He is a current smoker. He takes aspirin, amlodipine and inhalers.

Observations were in the normal range. Abdominal examination was also unremarkable.

What is the best next immediate investigation?

1. Check his prostate specific antigen levels (PSA)
2. Full blood count
3. Perform bedside urinalysis
4. Refer for 2-week-wait urology referral
5. Refer for CT urogram

Q448

A 35 year old man has a painless, progressive swelling in the right hemiscrotum, which he first noticed 1 year ago. He has no past history. His temperature is 36.8 °C, pulse 78 bpm, respiratory rate 12 breaths per minute. There is a large, cystic swelling in the right hemiscrotum that is transilluminant. Left testicular examination was unremarkable.

What is the most likely diagnosis?

1. Epididymal cyst
2. Hydrocele
3. Inguinal hernia
4. Testicular tumour
5. Varicocele

Q449

A 63 year old man has 6 months of a worsening weak stream when urinating. This is associated with straining to empty his bladder. He has no new back pain; he denies any blood in his urine. He does not get any bed-wetting at night-time. He has type 2 diabetes for which he takes metformin. His BMI is 34 kg/m²; abdominal examination is otherwise normal. He has an enlarged, benign-feeling, non-tender prostate on digital rectal examination. You offer him lifestyle advice.

What is the most appropriate next management step?

1. 5-alpha reductase inhibitor
2. Anticholinergic medication
3. Ask him to complete a symptom score
4. Bladder outlet surgery
5. Urgent bladder scan

Q450

A 22 year old man presents to the emergency department with 2 hours of severe left-sided testicular pain. On examination, he has a tender, high-riding left testis with absent cremasteric reflex.

What is the most appropriate next management?

1. CT scan of the abdomen and pelvis
2. Discharge with analgesia and antibiotics and review in the STI clinic
3. Intravenous antibiotics and review by the urology team
4. Refer to the on-call urologist for operation imminently
5. Ultrasound scan of his scrotum

Respiratory

16

Q451

A 62 year old man presents to the emergency department with 3 days of worsening shortness of breath. He has a cough productive of green sputum. He has a 40 pack year history of smoking. His pulse is 110 bpm, BP 96/61 mmHg, respiratory rate 20 breaths per minute, oxygen saturation 84% breathing air. He appears anxious and is using his accessory muscles, and has an audible expiratory wheeze.

Arterial blood gas taken on room air:

  pH 7.26
  pCO_2 7.9 kPa
  pO_2 7.2 kPa
  Lactate 2.4 mmol/L
  Bicarbonate 34 nmol/L

What is the most appropriate initial management of this patient?

1. Apply oxygen to target SpO_2 of 88–92%
2. Contact the critical care registrar on call
3. Give an intravenous antibiotic
4. Give an intravenous fluid bolus of 250 ml Hartmann's solution
5. Start non-invasive ventilation

Q452

A 45 year old man is found quiet, unconscious and cyanosed on the ward; 3 hours before, he was admitted from the emergency department after a sudden collapse while shopping at the supermarket. He was complaining of headache, neck pain and nausea. On admission, he was given 15 mg morphine and 4 mg ondansetron.

What is the most appropriate next step?

1. Administer 400 mcg naloxone intravenously
2. Begin bag-mask ventilation with a self-inflating bag
3. Call for help and begin CPR
4. Open the airway and assess for breathing and a pulse
5. Perform a primary survey to rule out any trauma

Q453

A 78 year old man has progressive breathlessness over 6 months, with more recent onset of worsening right-sided chest pain that disturbs his sleep. He describes lethargy and 11 kg weight loss. He is an ex-smoker of 8 cigarettes per day for 35 years, and is a retired dockyard worker. His BMI is 19 kg/m^2. He has quiet breath sounds on the right posteriorly with dullness to percussion. There is no digital clubbing. Chest X-ray: large right pleural effusion but clear lung fields otherwise.

What is the most likely diagnosis?

1. Asbestosis
2. Benign asbestos-related effusion
3. Mesothelioma
4. Pleural plaques
5. Pneumonia

Q454

A 75 year old man has 6 months of progressively worsening shortness of breath. He is breathless on climbing a flight of stairs and has a dry cough present throughout the day. He last smoked 20 years ago with a 30 pack year history. His occupation prior to retirement was as a painter and decorator. He has no hobbies involving birds. His past medical history is hypertension and osteoarthritis. Clinical examination demonstrates loss of the nail-fold angle and bi-basal 'velcro-like' crackles on auscultation of his chest. His chest X-ray demonstrates peripheral and basal reticular shadowing.

What is the most likely diagnosis?

1. Asthma
2. Bronchiectasis

3. Chronic obstructive pulmonary disease

4. Lung cancer

5. Pulmonary fibrosis

Q455

A 24 year old man has signs and symptoms consistent with influenza. PCR testing confirms influenza A with Covid absent. There are no signs of end-organ involvement, and the patient has someone at home to look after him. The illness occurs during an influenza epidemic.

What is the most appropriate management?

1. Admit to a side-room on a general ward for observation, requesting echo to rule out myocarditis

2. Direct patient to self-care with support of friends and family and with appropriate safety netting

3. Discharge to isolate at home with no personal contact allowed

4. Give oseltamivir 75 mg PO twice daily for 5 days

5. Keep in side-room in the emergency department, inform ICU

Q456

An 18 year old man has 1 hour of shortness of breath and lightheadedness. He developed right-sided chest pain which was exacerbated by inspiration. He is 195 cm tall with a slim build; his pulse is 160 bpm, BP 85/30 mmHg, oxygen saturation 90% breathing air. There is reduced air entry on the right hemithorax and his apex beat is in the 5th intercostal space in the anterior axillary line.

What is the most likely diagnosis?

1. Acute myocardial infarction

2. Asthma exacerbation

3. Pneumonia

4. Pulmonary embolism

5. Tension pneumothorax

Q457

A 72 year old woman has 2 days of fever, green sputum and dyspnoea. Her temperature is 38.4 °C, pulse 122 bpm, BP 110/40 mmHg, respiratory rate 22 breaths per minute, oxygen saturation 88% breathing air. She is oriented. Investigations:

Urea 8.2 mmol/L

What is their CURB 65 score?

1. CURB 65 = 1
2. CURB 65 = 2
3. CURB 65 = 3
4. CURB 65 = 4
5. CURB 65 = 5

Q458

A 33 year old man has 3 days of right-sided chest pain. He has hay fever and he is a current smoker. His temperature is 36.5 °C, pulse 75 bpm, BP 110/85 mmHg, oxygen saturation 98% on room air, and a chest X-ray shows a small apical right-sided pneumothorax. His repeat chest X-ray after 4 hours shows no change in the size of the pneumothorax. He is discharged home with outpatient respiratory clinic follow-up.

What advice should be given about flying?

1. As long as he stops smoking to reduce his risk of a recurrent pneumothorax, he can fly at any time
2. Flying is not recommended until 1 week after a chest X-ray demonstrating complete resolution
3. He can fly 6 weeks after symptom resolution
4. He can fly but should arrange supplemental oxygen for his next flight
5. Unless a surgical pleurectomy is completed, the patient should never fly again

Q459

A 74 year old man has had 3 months of intermittent haemoptysis, characterised by spitting out a small amount of blood-stained saliva first thing most mornings when he cleans his teeth.

He has a history of diabetes, hypertension, previous stroke and atrial fibrillation. He is an ex-smoker of 5 pack years and used to work as a postman. He has not travelled outside the UK. He has no breathlessness, chest pain, wheeze or rash. He has no constitutional symptoms. Chest X-ray was normal.

What is the most likely cause of his haemoptysis?

1. Abnormal clotting
2. Bronchiectasis
3. Pulmonary embolus
4. Tuberculosis
5. Vasculitis

Q460

A 44 year old man has had a cough for 10 days. His cough is productive of purulent sputum. He is feeling tired but not breathless. He has asthma and cystic fibrosis. His temperature is 37.9 °C; there are audible crackles in both lungs. He has had two negative PCR tests for SARS-Cov-2.

What part of his history most indicates the need to prescribe antibiotics?

1. A history of asthma
2. A history of cystic fibrosis
3. Crackles audible on both lungs
4. Repeat SARS-Cov-2 PCR test remains negative after a week
5. Sputum remaining purulent for more than 1 week

Q461

A 45 year old man has had 9 months of chronic cough associated with shortness of breath and occasional wheeze. Following investigations, he has been diagnosed with asthma COPD overlap syndrome.

What is the most appropriate first line of treatment?

1. Adequate controller therapy, including inhaled corticosteroid but not a long-acting beta-agonist, nor long-acting muscarinic antagonists
2. Inhaled corticosteroid and short-acting beta-agonist when required
3. Specialist referral before starting any treatment
4. Start treatment for COPD until further investigations have been performed
5. Treatment including corticosteroid with add-on long-acting beta-agonist

Q462

A 55 year old woman has 4 months of slowly worsening shortness of breath. She has rheumatoid arthritis. She has no history of inhaled noxious agents. Her spirometry shows airflow obstruction but no variability.

What is the most likely diagnosis?

1. Bronchiolitis
2. Fibrotic lung disease
3. Pneumonia
4. Pulmonary embolism
5. Upper respiratory tract infection

Q463

A 63 year old woman has several years of worsening breathlessness. She also has a cough producing less than a teaspoon of grey sputum most days. She is an ex-smoker of 34 pack years, works as a solicitor, has hypertension, and has a pet dog. She is slower than the rest of her walking group now, so has had to give it up. Her heart sounds and chest sounds are normal. Spirometry: FEV1 2.3 litres (73% predicted), FVC 3.8 litres (90% predicted). Chest X-ray is clear.

Which of the following is the most appropriate intervention?

1. Arrange a CT scan of the chest
2. Prescribe a salbutamol nebuliser for use as required
3. Refer for pulmonary rehabilitation
4. Send sputum for culture
5. Start a combined long-acting beta-agonist and inhaled steroid inhaler

Q464

A 75 year old man has a general decline, being confused and increasingly constipated. He is undergoing investigation for a new diagnosis of lung cancer. Investigations:

Corrected calcium 3.22 mmol/L (2.2–2.6)

CT head is normal

What type of lung cancer is hypercalcaemia most associated with?

1. Atypical carcinoid

2. Non-small cell lung cancer – adenocarcinoma
3. Non-small cell lung cancer – squamous cell carcinoma
4. Small cell lung cancer
5. Typical carcinoid

Q465

A 67 year old man has 6 months of breathlessness on exertion. He previously worked as a carpenter in a shipyard. He has fine crackles at the lung bases but otherwise examination is normal. Chest X-ray looks clear.

What is the most appropriate next test?

1. CT chest
2. Echocardiogram
3. Rheumatoid factor
4. Serial peak flow monitoring
5. Spirometry

Q466

A 56 year old woman arrives in the emergency department with 2 days of dyspnoea. She is a construction worker and broke her left femur 8 weeks ago and spent 6 weeks in a cast. She collapses in the waiting room and is rushed to the resus area. Her pulse is 115 bpm, BP 74/42 mmHg, oxygen saturation 90% on room air.

What is the next most appropriate investigation?

1. Bedside echo
2. CT pulmonary angiogram
3. D-dimer
4. ECG
5. V/Q scan

Q467

A 54 year old woman collapsed whilst shopping in the supermarket. She has had worsening breathlessness and fatigue for several months. She has type 2 diabetes, hypertension and high cholesterol. She has a 10 pack year smoking history and she works as a barmaid. Her observations are normal; she has a loud second heart sound, parasternal heave and peripheral pitting oedema to the knees. ECG shows a rightward axis deviation and P-pulmonale. Chest X-ray is normal.

What is the most appropriate next investigation?

1. 24-hour ECG recording
2. Coronary angiography
3. Echocardiogram
4. High-resolution CT chest
5. Right heart catheterisation

Q468

A 60 year old man has had a dry cough for the last 8 months. The cough is worse at night-time and also triggered by bending forwards. There are no associated red flag symptoms and no prior history of respiratory disease.

Chest X-ray and spirometry are normal.
What is the most appropriate therapy?

1. Amlodipine orally
2. Lpratropium bromide nasal spray
3. Omeprazole orally
4. Prednisolone orally
5. Salbutamol inhaler

Q469

A 35 year old woman has 3 days of cough, fevers and bloodstained sputum. She is a smoker with a 12 pack year history.

Her temperature is 38.6 °C, pulse 95 bpm, respiratory rate 24 breaths per minute, oxygen saturation 84% breathing air. She has central and peripheral cyanosis.

What is the most likely diagnosis?

1. Acute severe asthma
2. Lung cancer
3. Pneumonia
4. Pneumothorax
5. Pulmonary embolism

Q470

A 22 year old man has a sudden-onset right-sided pleuritic chest pain. He reports this came on suddenly after lifting heavy boxes and was associated with breathlessness. He smokes cannabis. His father had Marfan's disease.

Which of the following investigations is most likely to lead to the diagnosis?

1. Arterial blood gas
2. Chest X-ray
3. D-dimer
4. ECG
5. Troponin

Q471

A 27 year old man has 4 weeks of increasing shortness of breath, occasional cough, ankle swelling and occasional frothy urine.

His pulse is 92 bpm, respiratory rate 22 breaths per minute, oxygen saturation 96% breathing air. His chest expansion is reduced on the left; trachea is deviated to the right; absent breath sounds on the left base and dull to percussion.

His urinalysis shows 3+ protein, chest X-ray reveals a large left pleural effusion.

What is the most likely cause of this presentation?

1. Carcinoid syndrome
2. Mesothelioma
3. Nephrotic syndrome
4. Pancreatitis
5. Pulmonary tuberculosis

Q472

A 24 year old woman presents to the emergency department with dyspnoea and chest tightness; she has a history of asthma but ran out of her inhalers a few weeks ago. Her temperature is 36.7 °C, pulse 105 bpm, BP 120/70 mmHg, respiratory rate 33 breaths per minute, oxygen saturation 94% breathing 35% oxygen; her chest is quiet on auscultation.

Investigations:

Arterial blood gas:

pH 7.32

PaO$_2$ 12.1 kPa

PaCO$_2$ 7.0 kPa

What is the next management step?

1. Call for immediate review from the intensive care team
2. Give a salbutamol and ipratropium nebuliser and review in 1 hour
3. Give her nebulised magnesium and intravenous hydrocortisone
4. Reduce oxygen saturation target to 88–92% and repeat ABG in 1 hour
5. Start her on non-invasive ventilation and inform the medical registrar

Q473

A 44 year old man has intermittent frontal headache, nasal congestion, sneezing and rhinorrhoea (pale green mucus) which has been present for 5 days. It is interfering with his ability to concentrate at work. He has no fever, no sweats, no difficulty swallowing, and no change in hearing. He is allergic to penicillin and takes bendroflumethiazide for hypertension. He has never smoked. Examination is normal apart from nasal inflammation with pale green mucus and erythema of the oropharynx.

You give him advice about the probable duration and which symptoms would require reassessment.

What is the next step?

1. Advise over-the-counter antihistamines
2. Arrange a CT scan of the head and sinuses
3. No treatment
4. Prescribe a 5-day course of doxycycline
5. Take a nasal swab for culture

Q474

A 26 year old man presents to the emergency department with an acute wheeze. He has no history of respiratory illness, no rash and no swelling in the neck.

On examination, his pulse is 95 bpm, respiratory rate 24 breaths per minute, oxygen saturation 92% breathing air. He has widespread wheezing through both lungs.

What is the most important immediate management step?

1. Arterial blood gas
2. Chest X-ray
3. Intramuscular adrenaline
4. Nebulised salbutamol
5. Oxygen therapy

Q475

A 30 year old woman has a persistent cough for the last 14 years, productive of a tablespoon of yellow sputum per day. Approximately three times a year, she experiences worse symptoms, characterised by the sputum becoming thick and dark, a feeling of chest tightness, and lethargy. Antibiotics help, but she often needs two courses before the problem resolves. There is no past or family history of atopy; she has been prescribed an inhaled steroid with no benefit. She smoked 5 cigarettes a day for 8 years but stopped last year. Her BMI is 18 kg/m². She has clubbing and there are bi-basal crackles on auscultation. Sputum culture is negative.

What is the most likely diagnosis?

1. Asthma
2. Bronchiectasis
3. COPD
4. Chronic bronchitis
5. Foreign body inhalation

Q476

A 59 year old man is being treated on the medical admissions unit (MAU) for community-acquired pneumonia. He has no recent travel, no pets, and no past medical history. He has never smoked. His blood cultures have grown Streptococcus pneumoniae, but despite 48 hours of intravenous antibiotics he remains febrile and tachycardic, though respiratory rate is normal and oxygen saturation 94% on air.

What is the most likely diagnosis?

1. Acute respiratory distress syndrome
2. Atrial fibrillation
3. Delirium
4. Empyema
5. Pleurisy

Rheumatology

17

Q477

A 43 year old woman has 12 months of insidious onset of fatigue, recurrent mouth ulcers, arthralgias and Raynaud's phenomenon. Last summer, she had a sun-sensitive facial rash; 5 years ago, she was investigated for a pulmonary embolus but no evidence of one was found, and she describes not receiving anti-coagulation. Her mother had recurrent miscarriages.

Which is the most likely diagnosis?

1. Giant cell arteritis
2. Reactive arthritis
3. Rheumatoid arthritis
4. Sarcoidosis
5. Systemic lupus erythematosus

Q478

A 25 year old man has 6 months of lower back pain, occasionally radiating to the posterior thigh. It is relieved by staying active, exacerbated by rest. In recent weeks, the symptoms have woken him at 4 a.m. He takes no regular oral medication. His father had lower lumbar decompression surgery for an L4/5 root impingement when 45 years old.

His observations are stable, he has a scaly rash on his scalp, and he has global reduction of lumbar spinal movements in all directions. Flexing his hips produces pain in the posterior thigh bilaterally. Cervical spinal and upper and lower limb appearance and movements are otherwise unremarkable.

What is the most likely diagnosis?

1. Axial spondyloarthritis
2. Cauda equina syndrome

3. Lumbar L4/L5 root impingement
4. Lumbar spinal malignancy
5. Psoriatic arthritis

Q479

A 45 year old man has 8 weeks of lateral and anterior shoulder pain. He is a kitchen fitter and the pain is particularly associated with fitting wall-hung kitchen units and lifting other objects. There is no preceding trauma. He has taken ibuprofen regularly and has tried self-directed shoulder exercises from the NHS website. His shoulder movements are decreased because of pain, including elevation, internal rotation, and abduction, especially beyond 70 degrees of abduction. A diagnosis of subacromial bursitis is made.

What is the next management step?

1. Intra-articular injection of glucocorticoid
2. Oral glucocorticoid course for 1 week
3. Partial immobilisation with a simple sling
4. Radiograph of shoulder
5. Referral to physiotherapy

Q480

A 35 year old woman has 6 months of widespread non-specific pain and post-exertional fatigue affecting most joints. This has been associated with non-refreshing sleep and increased sensitivity to light, sound and smell. She is diagnosed with fibromyalgia.

Which of the following is advised in her management?

1. 2 weeks of complete bed rest
2. 3 trigger point injections with steroids, 1 month apart
3. A short course of prednisolone
4. Regular oxycodone, gradually increasing as needed
5. Regular slow rhythmic exercise

Q481

A 73 year old woman has 1 week of progressive, proximal muscle pain. She has had no skin rashes, infective symptoms or trauma. She had an ischaemic stroke 4 months ago and takes clopidogrel, atorvastatin and amlodipine. She drinks a glass of wine twice a week and does not smoke. Physical examination is unremarkable.

Investigations:

Normal full blood count, liver function tests and renal function

Creatine kinase 1050 IU/L (25–200)

What is the most likely cause of her myalgia?

1. Amlodipine
2. Atorvastatin
3. Duchenne dystrophy
4. Inflammatory autoimmune myositis
5. Myasthenia gravis

Q482

A 73 year old woman has 6 months of aching in her left groin moving down her thigh into her left knee. This is worse when walking and sometimes she has to stop because of the pain. The pain occasionally disturbs her sleep and is only partly relieved by paracetamol. She is otherwise fit and healthy.

What is the most appropriate imaging?

1. Hip arthrogram
2. Lumbar spine X-ray
3. Plain X-ray of the left knee
4. Plain X-ray of the pelvis
5. Ultrasound of the pelvis

Q483

A 60 year old man has 3 months of unsteadiness, falls and widespread diffuse limb pain. He relocated to the United Kingdom from North Africa 3 years ago. He mainly works indoors. After investigation, a diagnosis of osteomalacia due to insufficient vitamin D is made.

What investigation results would confirm the diagnosis?

1. High serum phosphate and high serum calcium
2. High serum phosphate and low serum calcium
3. Low bone alkaline phosphatase
4. Low serum phosphate or low serum calcium
5. Suppressed parathyroid hormone

Q484

A 70 year old man has a month of bilateral shoulder and pelvic girdle pain which is worse in the mornings. He has previously had a right-sided frozen shoulder, but this episode feels different. He has had problems turning in bed and getting off the toilet. Examination demonstrates restriction in shoulder abduction, no muscle weakness, no visible peripheral joint swelling.

Investigations:

CRP 18 mg/dL (< 6)

Thyroid function tests are normal

What is the most likely diagnosis?

1. Infective arthritis
2. Parkinson's disease
3. Polymyalgia rheumatica
4. Polymyositis
5. Rheumatoid arthritis

Q485

A 45 year old man is seen in the respiratory clinic with 4 months of recurrent, painful nodules over his shins. These resolve over several weeks, leaving a bruise-like appearance. He also has tender, swollen ankles. His weight and appetite are stable. He has no change in bowel habit. He is a non-smoker. Lung function is normal with a preserved transfer factor. A chest X-ray confirms symmetrical, bilateral hilar lymphadenopathy.

What would be the most appropriate management?

1. Endobronchial ultrasound and biopsy of hilar lymph nodes
2. Fractional exhaled nitric oxide test
3. High-resolution computed tomography
4. Review in clinic with repeat chest X-ray in 3 months
5. Serum ACE blood

Q486

A 30 year old woman has 3 days of a red painful eye and left knee pain; 2 weeks ago, she returned from a 3-week holiday abroad. She reports having unprotected sex whilst on holiday. She takes the oral contraceptive pill. Her mother and maternal aunt both have rheumatoid arthritis.

Her temperature is 36.2 °C; she has a right conjunctivitis. Her left knee is swollen, warm and globally tender. There is no specific tibial tuberosity tenderness.

What is the most likely diagnosis?

1. Osgood–Schlatter disease
2. Patellar tendonitis
3. Reactive arthritis
4. Rheumatoid arthritis
5. Septic arthritis

Q487

A 65 year old man presents to the emergency department with 1 day of hot, swollen and painful right knee. He has rheumatoid arthritis, takes 20 mg methotrexate once weekly, and leflunomide 10 mg daily. His temperature is 37.8 °C. His other observations are normal.

What is the correct immediate action?

1. Aspirate the affected joint and send for urgent microscopy and culture
2. Check a serum uric acid
3. Discharge home with advice to see his GP if things don't improve
4. Immediately commence broad-spectrum intravenous antibiotics
5. Start the patient on a reducing course of prednisolone

Q488

A 5 year old girl presents to her general practitioner with her mother. Over the past 4 weeks, she has been reluctant to play or to sit on the floor of the classroom. She is well otherwise.

Her observations are normal. She has a limp, with a mildly swollen right knee and elbow. She is started on regular NSAIDs and referred to the paediatric rheumatology service.

What is the most likely diagnosis?

1. Juvenile idiopathic arthritis (oligoarticular subtype)
2. Juvenile idiopathic arthritis (polyarticular subtype)
3. Juvenile idiopathic arthritis (systemic subtype)
4. Septic arthritis
5. Transient synovitis

Q489

A 72 year old woman has pain in her right (dominant) wrist, preventing her from washing. She has been in hospital for the last 6 days following a non-ST elevation myocardial infarction. She does not drink alcohol or smoke tobacco.

Her temperature is 37.3 °C; her other observations are normal. She has no tophi and she is systemically well. Her right wrist is red, warm, swollen, and there is some global limitation to movements. There is no skin rash, and she has evidence of osteoarthritis in her fingers and left knee.

Investigations:

CRP 18 (< 6)

Renal function normal

Wrist X-ray: chondrocalcinosis

What is the most likely diagnosis for her right wrist?

1. Calcium pyrophosphate dihydrate arthritis
2. Gout
3. Haemarthrosis
4. Rheumatoid arthritis
5. Septic arthritis

Q490

A 65 year old man has an acutely painful swelling of his left knee. He has a metallic mitral valve, hypertension, osteoarthritis, and received 5 days of clarithromycin recently for a community-acquired pneumonia. He usually takes amlodipine, paracetamol, and has had a stable dose of warfarin for the past 6 months. He drinks minimal alcohol and does not smoke. On examination, the knee is hot, swollen, exquisitely tender, and with very limited flexion. His temperature is 37 °C and he is systemically well. Blood tests in the past year show renal and liver function, and serum urate, in the normal ranges.

What is the most appropriate initial treatment?

1. Allopurinol and non-steroidal anti-inflammatories
2. Analgesics and non-steroidal anti-inflammatories
3. Colchicine and analgesics
4. Reversal of anti-coagulation
5. Temporary immobilisation and analgesics

Q491

A 52 year old woman has 12 months of pain in her hands, knees and hips. The pain is always present, worsening after activity. It intermittently flares for 1–2 weeks when individual joints swell; when that happens, the joints are warm and very tender. She has early morning stiffness of 20 minutes, and finds it difficult to open jars. Topical painkillers and ibuprofen worked initially but no longer help.

On examination, she is comfortable. There are hard, fixed, non-fluctuant swellings in her distal interphalangeal, proximal, and index and middle metacarpal phalangeal joints in both hands. She has left thumb carpometacarpal joint tenderness.

What is the most likely diagnosis?

1. Fibromyalgia
2. Gout
3. Osteoarthritis
4. Psoriatic arthritis
5. Rheumatoid arthritis

Q492

A 65 year old man has 2 weeks of neck pain and paraesthesia in his right fingertips. He is otherwise well and on no regular medication. Examination of all four limbs shows normal tone, power and reflexes. There is altered sensation in his right C6/C7 dermatome. A clinical diagnosis of degenerative cervical radiculopathy is made due to a C6/C7 disc prolapse. He is given appropriate analgesia.

Which is the most appropriate initial management?

1. Computer tomography scan
2. Magnetic resonance imaging
3. Nerve conduction studies
4. Neurosurgical opinion
5. Physiotherapy

Q493

A 76 year old woman has lost 8 cm in the last 18 months and has occasional mid back pain. Her menopause was at 42 years of age. She is otherwise healthy with no other past medical history. She takes calcium and vitamin D supplements. She currently smokes, she has a 35 pack year history. Her BMI is 19 kg/m^2. She has a slight kyphosis. Her bloods including urea and electrolytes, liver function tests, calcium, phosphate and parathyroid hormone are all normal.

Which is the most likely diagnosis?

1. Bronchial carcinoma
2. Growth hormone deficiency
3. Osteoporosis
4. Rickets
5. Tuberculosis

Sexual Health

18

Q494

A 23 year old man has a yellow penile discharge and intermittent dysuria for 2 weeks. He travelled to South East Asia 6 weeks ago and paid for sex; he did not use a condom. He has no allergies. Urine culture was negative 1 week ago in primary care. Urethral microscopy in clinic then demonstrates gram-negative intracellular diplococci.

Which antibiotic is likely to be the best choice for this infection?

1. Azithromycin 1 g PO stat
2. Ceftriaxone 1 g intramuscular stat
3. Ciprofloxacin 500 mg twice daily for 7 days
4. Metronidazole 400 mg three times daily for 7 days
5. Trimethoprim 200 mg twice daily for 7 days

Q495

A 22 year old man has a non-itchy rash which covers his whole body, including his palms and the soles of his feet. He has had unprotected anal sex with four men in the last 6 months. He had a full sexual health screen 9 months ago and he tested negative for chlamydia, gonorrhoea, HIV, syphilis, hepatitis B (surface antigen) and hepatitis C (antibody). He has no past medical history and takes no medications. His syphilis serology is now positive.

What is the most likely stage of his syphilis infection?

1. Early latent
2. Late latent
3. Primary
4. Secondary
5. Tertiary

Q496

A 26 year old woman requests advice about trying to conceive following a month of unprotected sex. She has normal but irregular periods. Her partner is a fit and well non-smoker with a normal BMI and works as a fitness instructor. She has a history of acne and concerns over excessive hair growth. She is a non-smoker. Her BMI is 32 kg/m^2, BP is 115/75. You discuss potential diagnosis of polycystic ovarian syndrome.

What is the next step in management?

1. Clomiphene ovulation induction
2. Intra-cytoplasmic sperm injection
3. Metformin
4. Semenalysis from partner
5. Supported weight reduction, and sexual intercourse every 2–3 days

Q497

A 42 year old woman has a 6 day history of scanty, yellow, frothy, vaginal discharge. This is associated with slight dysuria. She is otherwise well. She is not pregnant, and she has had three different sexual partners in the last 4 weeks. Trichomoniasis is suspected.

What would be the most appropriate area to swab to confirm your diagnosis?

1. Cervical
2. Low vagina
3. Mid vagina
4. Posterior fornix
5. Urethra

Q498

A 25 year old woman has vaginal bleeding after sex and yellow vaginal discharge for 1 month. She is sexually active and is currently with a long-term partner. She has taken the combined oral contraceptive pill (COCP) for 2 years. She has never had a smear test. Urinary pregnancy test is negative.

What is the most likely diagnosis?

1. Cervical cancer
2. Chlamydia infection

3. COCP adverse effect
4. Endometrial cancer
5. Endometriosis

Q499

A 36 year old woman is in a new sexual relationship and requests advice regarding which contraceptive to use. She has heavy painful periods; she does not suffer from migraines. She has no family history of note. She smokes 20 cigarettes per day and has an 18 pack year smoking history. Her BMI is 25 kg/m². Her BP is 115/75 mmHg.

Which method of contraception should you advise her to avoid?

1. Combined hormonal contraception (pill, patch or ring)
2. Hormonal intrauterine device
3. Injectable hormonal contraception (subcutaneous or intramuscular)
4. Progesterone only pill
5. Subdermal implant

Q500

A 52 year old man presents to his GP requesting tadalafil. His ability to maintain an erection has been diminishing for the past 9 months. Now he can't sustain it long enough to reach orgasm, which he finds frustrating. He blames a deterioration in the relationship between him and his partner for his erectile dysfunction, stating that there is no longer any foreplay. He does not have morning erections. He has hypertension and hypercholesterolaemia. He takes ramipril and atorvastatin. He is a smoker with a 26 pack year history. His BMI is 29 kg/m². He has tried sildenafil 50 mg, which did not work fully.

What is the most likely reason for the sildenafil not working?

1. He is not receiving sufficient sexual stimulation with his current relationship difficulties
2. He needs to lose weight and smoke less
3. He should have been prescribed tadalafil as requested
4. The statins he has started taking are interacting with the sildenafil
5. There is another organic cause of his erectile dysfunction

Q501

A 25 year old woman has 1 week of worsening right-sided lower abdominal pain, and irregular vaginal bleeding. She has recently broken up with her boyfriend, whom she suspected of having other sexual partners. She was using the progesterone only pill for contraception but was not always consistent with taking it. Pelvic inflammatory disease is suspected.

What is the most important differential diagnosis to rule out before starting treatment?

1. Appendicitis
2. Chlamydia
3. Diverticulitis
4. Ectopic pregnancy
5. Endometriosis

Q502

A 62 year old woman has vaginal dryness and pain on intercourse. She has had 2 years of reduced interest in sex. She reports no bleeding after intercourse and has no medical history of note. Examination reveals vaginal atrophy.

Which of the following options would be the most appropriate initial investigations/management?

1. Check blood hormone status (LH, FSH)
2. Mental health review
3. Oral oestrogen therapy
4. Topical testosterone therapy
5. Vaginal oestrogen

Q503

A 34 year old woman has 1 week of lower abdominal pain, mild dysuria and an increase in yellow vaginal discharge. She also has pain during sexual intercourse – she denies personally engaging in any sexual activity outside of her current relationship but is unsure about her partner.
She has had a copper coil for several years. Her observations are normal.

What is the most useful diagnostic investigation?

1. Abdominal CT

2. Abdominal ultrasound
3. High vaginal swab
4. NAAT (vulvo-vaginal) swab
5. Urinary pregnancy test

Q504
Q504(a)

A 19 year old woman has painful genital ulcers for the last 3 days which she has never had before. They started as blisters which then ulcerated. She also has pain on passing urine. She had a new sexual partner 3 weeks ago. The ulcers are widespread across the vulva and extend towards the anus. The local skin is swollen but is normal in colour with no spreading erythema.

What is the most likely diagnosis?

1. Aphthous ulceration
2. Cellulitis
3. Primary herpes simplex infection
4. Secondary herpes simplex infection
5. Syphilis

Q504(b)

A 45 year old woman has a new genital lump, which has bled and is itchy and sore. She has had cervical intra-epithelial neoplasia treated by LLETZ. She has never been vaccinated against human papilloma virus The lesion is large extending from the labia minora onto the posterior fourchette, and is pigmented in nature.

What is the safest management plan in this scenario?

1. Take a biopsy and treat accordingly
2. Treat with cryotherapy
3. Treat with imiquimod
4. Treat with podophyllotoxin
5. Treat with surgical excision

Q504(c)

A 65 year old man has a urethral discharge, and pain on passing urine. He has no testicular pain. He has a new male sexual partner who has no symptoms. The discharge is clear and only visible on opening the urethral meatus. He attends the sexual health clinic where a urethral swab is taken and a diagnosis of urethritis is confirmed.

What would be the best first-line antibiotic treatment?

1. Azithromycin 1 gm stat followed by 500 mg po daily for a further 48 hours
2. Azithromycin 1 gm stat followed by 500 mg daily for a further 48 hours with additional metronidazole 400 mg three times a day for 7 days
3. Ceftriaxone 1 gm intramuscular stat
4. Doxycycline 100 mg twice daily for 7 days
5. Nitrofurantoin MR 500 mg twice daily for 3 days

Q505

A 32 year old woman requests a termination for an unwanted pregnancy. She has four children, and is recently separated from her partner. She is certain that she is 5 weeks pregnant, and requests home treatment as she does not want to attend clinic due to family commitments. She has a thorough telephone appointment with the sexual health nurse.

What gestational age is the cut off for home medical terminations?

1. 6 weeks
2. 10 weeks
3. 14 weeks
4. 18 weeks
5. 24 weeks

Q506

A 21 year old woman has a week of offensive vaginal discharge. She reports it to be yellow in colour. She has had a recent change in sexual partner. She is using the combined oral contraceptive pill for contraception. There is a yellow/green discharge coming from the cervix. Investigation

Cervical swab for culture: gram-negative intracellular diplococci

What is the most likely causative organism?

1. Chlamydia trachomatis
2. Lactobacilli
3. Neisseria gonorrhoea
4. Staphlycoccus aureus
5. Trichomonas vaginalis

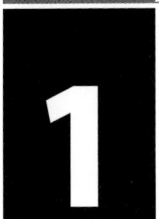

Answers

Cardiovascular

Q1 Acute Coronary Syndromes

Answer 1 – **Aspirin.** The patient's presentation (central chest pain, breathlessness, clammy and pale appearance, with ST elevation in leads II and III on the ECG) is highly suggestive of an ST-elevation myocardial infarction (STEMI). Immediate therapy should be aimed at reducing clot formation and improving perfusion. Aspirin (300 mg) should be administered immediately to inhibit platelet aggregation. **Atorvastatin:** while statins are important for long-term secondary prevention of cardiovascular events, they are not part of the immediate acute management. **Bisoprolol:** beta-blockers are used cautiously in STEMI and typically after renal and urohaemodynamic stabilisation. They are not given immediately in the community setting. **Inhaled oxygen:** oxygen is only recommended if the patient's oxygen saturation is < 94%. This patient has an oxygen saturation of 96%, so oxygen is not indicated. **Ramipril:** ACE inhibitors are important for long-term management post-STEMI but are not part of immediate therapy.

Q2 Aortic Aneurysm

Answer 1 – **CT angiogram**. CT angiogram is almost universally available – it gives detailed, accurate, speedy diagnosis as well as an assessment of surrounding structures. **Ultrasound** is useful for screening but gives less detail, as does **non-contrast CT** scanning. **MRA** is detailed, but takes longer and is not always available. **PET scan** is not used for diagnosing aneurysms.

Q3 Arterial Thrombosis

Answer 1 – **Acute mesenteric ischaemia**. In a 78 year old man, the most common cause would be aortic dissection. But there are pointers in the question away from this towards mesenteric ischaemia – notably, the recent myocardial infarction and going into atrial fibrillation, which makes thromboembolism much more likely. It is more likely than the other distractors to cause generalised peritonism. **Aortic dissection** typically occurs in the chest and back and often with a tearing sensation. **Colitis** usually presents more gradually. **Duodenal ulceration** is usually localised to the epigastrium. **Pancreatitis** is usually more epigastric and associated with nausea and vomiting.

Q4 Aortic Valve Disease

Answer 1 – **Aortic regurgitation**. The findings – exertional breathlessness, widened pulse pressure, and an early diastolic murmur – point to aortic regurgitation as the most likely diagnosis. **Hypertrophic obstructive cardiomyopathy** (HOCM) is typically associated with a systolic ejection murmur, dynamic outflow obstruction and sometimes mitral regurgitation. There is no widened pulse pressure or diastolic murmur in HOCM. **Mitral stenosis** presents with a mid-diastolic rumble at the apex and is often associated with pulmonary congestion. The absence of pulmonary symptoms and a normal JVP make mitral stenosis less likely. **Pulmonary regurgitation** causes a diastolic murmur, but this is best heard in the pulmonary area and is often associated with pulmonary hypertension. There is no evidence of pulmonary hypertension here. **Tricuspid stenosis** causes a diastolic murmur but is typically accompanied by systemic venous congestion, such as elevated JVP and peripheral oedema, which are not present in this case.

Q5 Arterial Ulcers

Answer 1 – **Arterial insufficiency**. There are a number of factors that support the likelihood of arterial insufficiency. They are: location of ulcer over the lateral malleolus; the depth of the ulcer (exposing the tendons); the past history (50 pack year and hypertension suggest he is an arteriopath). **Lymphatic stasis**: lymphatic ulcers are rarely that deep. **Peripheral neuropathy** usually appears on pressure areas of the feet and ankles. **Venous insufficiency**: venous ulcers are associated with oedema, and are usually on the medial side and shallower. **Vitamin B12 deficiency** is a cause of neuropathy.

Q6 Essential or Secondary Hypertension

Answer 2 – **Offer diuretics and check renal function in 2 weeks' time**. This man has a high BP reading and has brought evidence of home BP readings averaging over 135/85 mmHg. Furthermore, he has type 2 diabetes. The current revision of the NICE guidance (www.nice.org.uk/guidance/ng136) recommends that, for those aged < 80 with diabetes, doctors should offer lifestyle advice and discuss starting drug treatment. Furthermore, in those with diabetes, an **ACE inhibitor** or ARB is recommended as first-line therapy. He is over 40, and his BP is not over 180/120 mmHg with high-risk features, and therefore **specialist evaluation** is not required. Home BPs are sufficient to diagnose poorly treated hypertension – there is no need for **24-hour ambulatory BP monitoring**.

Q7 Myocardial Infarction

Answer 1 – **Acute myocardial infarction**. Although there are in fact a number of potential diagnoses, myocardial infarction is the most likely here, given the nature of the pain, the risk factors and the observations. **Precordial catch syndrome** is a sharp left-sided chest pain, often worse on movement or breathing. It is more common in younger people but can occur at any age. It is typically transient, lasting seconds or minutes. **Pericarditis** causes a similar pain, but is often worse with lying down and better leaning forward. Neither of these fits the description here. **Aortic dissection** is typically a tearing pain radiating to the back; this is certainly possible, and is one of the most often missed diagnoses, but is not the most likely diagnosis here. **Pulmonary embolus** is another potential diagnosis here, but typically causes more pleuritic pain, and is associated with reduced saturations. Again, it is commonly missed and should be considered, but is not the most likely diagnosis. Correcting **potassium** in this instance has no bearing on the prognosis.

Q8 Peripheral Vascular Disease

Answer 5 – **Patient to stop smoking**. This is a question of what has the most influence on progression of peripheral vascular disease at this late stage. While **control of cholesterol**, **diabetes** and **BP** does play a part, the most significant risk factor is his smoking. Note, when talking about tobacco consumption: 1 g is roughly equivalent to 1 cigarette, so he smokes the equivalent of around 100 a week, or 15 a day.

Q9 Painful Swollen Leg

Answer 3 – **Duplex ultrasonography**. Clinical suspicion of deep vein thrombosis (DVT): the patient has symptoms consistent with DVT, including pain, swelling, and tenderness in the calf. His elevated D-dimer (2.4 mcg/mL) further supports the suspicion of DVT, although D-dimer is not specific and can be elevated in other conditions. Duplex ultrasonography is the first-line imaging modality for diagnosing DVT because: it is non-invasive, widely available and cost-effective, and it combines B-mode imaging (to visualise thrombus and vein anatomy) and Doppler flow assessment (to evaluate blood flow in the veins). **CT venography** is rarely used for DVT diagnosis due to the invasive nature, contrast-related risks and higher radiation exposure. It may be considered in complex or inconclusive cases. **Direct venography** was once considered the gold standard, but is now rarely used because it is invasive, involves radiation and requires intravenous contrast, which carries a risk of nephrotoxicity or allergy. **Magnetic resonance imaging** (MRI): MRI venography can detect DVT but is not routinely used as a first-line investigation due to limited availability, higher cost and the need for patient cooperation during the procedure. **Plethysmography** evaluates venous outflow but is not commonly used for diagnosing DVT due to lower sensitivity and specificity compared to duplex ultrasonography.

Q10 Right Heart Valve Disease

Answer 5 – **Tricuspid regurgitation due to right ventricular dysfunction**. Tricuspid regurgitation is a murmur that is loudest in inspiration. It is associated with signs of right heart failure, and becomes more common with age and lung disease. Pacing leads are placed on the right side of the heart (except in exceptional circumstances) and therefore do not cause **mitral regurgitation**, but can cause tricuspid regurgitation. **Mitral regurgitation due to age-related degeneration** is possible, but it typically causes a murmur which is loudest in expiration, due to increased venous return from the pulmonary veins. **Pulmonary regurgitation** causes an early diastolic murmur. **Triscuspid regurgitation due to rheumatic fever as a child** could be a possibility, but it would be unusual to present at the age of 87.

Q11 Varicose Veins

Answer 1 – **Compression hosiery**. Compression hosiery is the most appropriate first-line management in the absence of skin changes or other complications. It causes symptomatic relief, and is non-invasive, easy to use and effective.

Duplex ultrasound is a diagnostic tool looking at severity – it is not an intervention that would change management. **Laser therapy** and **vein stripping** are not indicated at this stage. **Lifestyle advice** would not manage her symptoms at this stage.

Q12 Infective Endocarditis

Answer 2 – **Bacterial endocarditis.** Ascending aortic dissection is usually a dramatic event that presents with a very short history of severe pain, rather than a gradual decline over time. **Cardiac tamponade** can present with a more gradual history, but patients tend not to look well, and it does not cause valve dysfunction (although it may coexist). **Rheumatic fever** is rare in the UK, due to the availability of antibiotics. It also tends to present with fever and painful joints. It is more common in children and rare in adults. A **ruptured papillary muscle** tends to cause sudden-onset shortness of breath due to mitral regurgitation which typically produces a loud pansystolic murmur heard best at the apex. Endocarditis is the most likely answer given the insidious presentation, regurgitant murmur and raised inflammatory markers.

Q13 Vasovagal Syncope

Answer 3 – **Discharge with education about the importance of hydration and avoidance of triggers.** This is a classic history of vasovagal syncope. Around 50% of people will faint at some stage in their life, and it is a benign condition. The history, absence of findings on examination and ECG are reassuring. Such patients do not need **admission** or **further investigations.** They do not need **referral to neurology.** They do not need **referral to a cardiologist** unless this is a frequent problem which has not responded to lifestyle measures and is impacting on quality of life.

Q14 Heart Murmurs

Answer 2 – **Aortic stenosis.** The combination of symptoms and signs makes aortic stenosis the most likely diagnosis. Aortic stenosis typically causes an ejection systolic murmur heard best in the aortic area (the upper right sternal edge). It is associated with shortness of breath on exertion, angina and, when very severe, syncope, particularly on exertion. **Aortic incompetence** is a diastolic murmur, as is **mitral stenosis. Mitral incompetence** does cause breathlessness but is typically a pansystolic murmur heard best in the mitral area. Both aortic stenosis and mitral regurgitation are loudest in expiration (right-sided murmurs are typically loudest in inspiration). **Innocent flow murmurs** are less common with age and with symptoms.

Q15 Venous Ulcers

Answer 4 – **Venous insufficiency**. There are a number of pointers here to venous insufficiency. Venous ulcers are typically around the medial malleolus, shallow and sloughy, and there is often haemosiderin discolouration of the surrounding skin. **Arterial insufficiency**: arterial ulcers are usually painful, and deep (punched out). **Lymphatic stasis** is uncommon and typically due to infection or trauma. **Peripheral neuropathy** causes ulcers on the plantar surfaces of the feet. **Vitamin B12 deficiency** can cause neuropathy, but rarely ulcers.

Q16 Chest Pain

Answer 3 – **Myocardial infarction**. In a 60 year old man with these symptoms, myocardial infarction is always going to be a probable diagnosis. **Aortic coarctation** does not present acutely in adulthood, although it rarely may be discovered when investigating a patient for hypertension. **Aortic dissection** is possible and has to be considered, but it is less common than myocardial infarction. Pain is typically described as tearing and commonly radiates to the back. **Pericarditis** tends to cause pain over the left side of the chest, is sharp, and is worse on inspiration or movement. A **right-sided pneumonia** would not tend to present so acutely and would be associated with right-sided pleuritic chest pain more commonly than epigastric pain.

Q17 Cold, Painful, Pale, Pulseless Leg/Foot

Answer 2 – **Fixed mottling of the skin**. Irreversible ischaemia refers to tissue death or necrosis due to prolonged lack of blood supply. Fixed mottling of the skin takes place over a longer period of time and is an indication of underlying necrosis. **Hair loss over the shin** can occur with chronic ischaemia due to reduced blood flow over a prolonged period, but it is not a sign of irreversible ischaemia. **Pain at rest** and **absence of pedal pulses** will occur in acute ischaemia. **Yellow discolouration with thickening of the nail of the hallux** is more common in chronic ischaemia – but does not indicate irreversibility.

Q18 Hypertension

Answer 2 – **Add an ACE inhibitor**. His BP is above target (135/85) and he has albuminuria. Therefore, some intensification of therapy is required. **Continuing with the present medication and dosing and reviewing in 3 months** is thus wrong. Comparative reviews suggest that a combination of calcium channel blockers and ACE inhibitors is the best when there is microalbuminuria. Thus, adding an ACE inhibitor is preferable to **adding a thiazide diuretic, changing the amlodipine to another calcium antagonist** or **increasing amlodipine to 10 mg**. Of note, patients tend to experience fewer side effects when using a combination of lower-dose antihypertensives.

Q19 Palpitations

Answer 4 – **Supraventricular tachycardia**. This trace shows a narrow complex tachycardia at a rate of 216 bpm. It is most likely to be a supraventricular tachycardia, particularly when taken together with the history. The complexes are narrow so it is not a **ventricular tachycardia**. Furthermore, it is regular, and therefore it is not **atrial fibrillation**. It could be **atrial flutter**, but in a young person, not on medication, with no other medical issues, this is less likely, and the rate is wrong (the underlying flutter rates in younger people tend to be around 300 bpm, although it can be slower in older people or in those on medication, such as flecainide). At 216 bpm, it is unlikely to be **sinus** rhythm at rest or, indeed, on exertion.

Q20 Aneurysms, Ischaemic Limb and Occlusions

Answer 2 – **CT angiography lower limbs**. The clinical vignette for this question points to a potential acutely ischaemic foot (potentially from a popliteal aneurysm) and the phrasing of 'most appropriate investigation' is asking for the investigation that is most definitive in terms of diagnosis and planning management. A CTA will not only confirm ischaemia – it will also provide all the information required to plan an emergency surgical approach. Although a **USS arterial duplex** would be useful in the elective setting, it is unlikely to be available as an emergency, particularly out of hours. An abnormal **ABPI** or **transcutaneous oxygen pressure** in the left foot would further increase clinical suspicion of acute ischaemia, but it will not be able to guide management. An **X-ray of the left leg** will not be able to provide evidence of ischaemia in the foot and is also not specific enough to detect all popliteal aneurysms.

Q21 Aortic Dissection

Answer 1 – **Arrange CT angiogram of aorta**. This is a history concerning for aortic dissection. The patient has a history of hypertension that has not been controlled. Normal chest X-ray and ECG do not rule out a dissection. The wide pulse pressure and murmur at the left sternal border suggest aortic regurgitation. It would be worth checking a BP on both arms, but the absence of differential BP readings also does not rule out dissection. You must have a high index of suspicion to make the diagnosis of aortic dissection. In this case, a CT angiogram of aorta was performed and revealed a Type A aortic dissection. **CT pulmonary angiogram**: pulmonary embolism is unlikely as the primary cause since the patient has hypertension, no significant respiratory distress, and no strong risk factors. **Continue treatment for acute coronary syndrome**: treating as ACS without ruling out aortic dissection risks worsening the condition with anti-coagulation. **Discharge with medical management for NSTEMI**: aortic dissection is a life-threatening emergency, and discharge without definitive imaging could be fatal. **Echocardiogram**: while useful for detecting complications, transthoracic echocardiography is not the gold standard for diagnosing aortic dissection – CT angiography is preferred.

Q22 Arrhythmias

Answer 4 – **Supraventricular tachycardia**. The most likely diagnosis is supraventricular tachycardia (SVT). **Atrial fibrillation** typically presents with an irregularly irregular rhythm and is less common in a young, healthy individual without structural heart disease. **Complete heart block** would present with bradycardia (not tachycardia), as the atria and ventricles beat independently, and the ventricular escape rhythm is slow. **Panic attack** can cause palpitations and tachycardia but is less likely to produce a heart rate as high as 220 bpm. **Ventricular tachycardia** would typically present with a wide complex tachycardia on ECG and is less common in a structurally normal heart, particularly in a young individual.

Q23 Cardiac Arrest

Answer 1 – **Bilaterally absent N20 somatosensory evoked potential**. The bilateral absence of N20 somatosensory evoked potentials > 24 hours after the return of spontaneous circulation is associated with unfavourable neurological outcome in the comatose survivors of out-of-hospital cardiac arrest. The negative predictive value of this test is almost 100% with almost 0% false negative results. Bilateral absence of N20 as a finding is reliable for neurological prognosis only when the pathway of the sensory stimulus to the brain remains intact – i.e. in the absence of brainstem, upper cervical spine and posterior fossa pathology (haemorrhage, infarct, oedema). While **EEG showing partial complex seizure activity** suggests brain dysfunction, seizures alone do not definitively indicate a poor prognosis. An **NSE > 30 mcg** suggests neuronal injury but lacks specificity, with higher thresholds (e.g. > 60 mcg/L) being more predictive. **Not opening eyes to voice or painful stimuli** is concerning but not sufficient for prognostication, as some patients recover from prolonged coma. Lastly, the **ongoing need for respiratory and cardiovascular support** reflects severity but does not reliably distinguish between reversible and irreversible brain injury.

Q24 Deep Vein Thrombosis

Answer 2 – **Score = 1**. This question requires the student to go through each point in the table. 'Nothing else of note' means no cancer, previous DVT, paralysis. Calf swelling is > 3 cm (= 1 point). No swollen veins; pitting oedema is bilateral; there is no swelling in the thigh, no tenderness in the deep veins, no history of being bedridden, no obvious alternative diagnosis. Adding that up – answer = +1.

Q25 Gangrene

Answer 1 – **Intravenous antibiotics**. The patient's chronic foot ulcer with erythema, swelling, pus and X-ray findings of periosteal reaction and cortical thinning are indicative of osteomyelitis, a serious infection of the bone, likely secondary to her diabetic foot ulcer. Intravenous antibiotics are the most appropriate course of action to ensure adequate tissue penetration and to effectively manage the bone infection. Empirical IV antibiotics covering Staphylococcus aureus and gram-negative organisms should be started promptly, pending culture results. **Oral antibiotics** may be insufficient to penetrate bone tissue adequately, especially in a chronic and severe infection such as osteomyelitis. **Silver sulfadiazine dressing** is beneficial for superficial wound care but cannot treat a deep bone infection. **Surgical intervention** may be required if there is necrotic tissue or abscess formation, but the initial step is to control the infection with IV antibiotics. **Topical antibiotics** are ineffective for osteomyelitis and are inappropriate in the presence of systemic infection signs.

Q26 Ischaemic Heart Disease

Answer 3 – **Myocardial infarction**. The character and radiation of the pain, described as central dull crushing pain, is a classical description of cardiac-sounding chest pain. Pleuritic chest pain, which would be consistent with a **pulmonary embolism** (PE), is usually described as sharp pain worse on inspiration, and **pericarditis** causes chest pain that is sharp and relieved on leaning forward. Although the patient had pain after heavy lifting, which could be consistent with **musculoskeletal pain** (MSK), this is a distraction, as MSK pain is usually described as sharp localised pain and is often reproducible on palpation of the affected area. The patient also has multiple cardiac risk factors, normal oxygenation (making **COPD** and PE less likely) and a key finding of ST elevation localised to the inferior leads on the ECG, making myocardial infarction the most likely diagnosis and correct answer.

Q27 Mitral Valve Disease

Answer 4 – **Mitral stenosis**. Although mitral stenosis is becoming less common in the UK, it is important to consider in patients from countries with greater incidences of rheumatic disease. Mitral stenosis can progress to acute decompensation, such as pulmonary oedema, and physiological changes which occur during pregnancy can precipitate these symptoms in patients previously asymptomatic.

Q28 Cardiac Failure

Answer 1 – **Cardiac amyloid**. This patient has presented with heart failure syndrome (breathlessness, peripheral oedema, raised BNP). The echocardiogram shows a normal ejection fraction; therefore, this is a presentation of heart failure with preserved ejection fraction (HFpEF). He has had a previous myocardial infarction; however, the echo findings are not in keeping with an **ischaemic cardiomyopathy**. In an ischaemic cardiomyopathy you would expect to see impaired left ventricular systolic function, regional wall motion abnormalities and a reduced ejection fraction. Similarly, the ejection fraction would be reduced in a **dilated cardiomyopathy**. **Hypertrophic cardiomyopathy**, **hypertensive heart disease** and cardiac amyloid can all cause left ventricular hypertrophy and HFpEF. His speckled myocardium and small QRS complexes are typical findings of cardiac amyloid (alongside the proteinuria), making this the correct answer.

Q29 Myocarditis

Answer 2 – **Myocarditis**. Whilst the patient presents with chest pain, there are no significant ischaemic changes reported on his ECG and his age goes against this. **Acute coronary syndrome** is unlikely in a young, otherwise healthy patient with no risk factors and no ischaemic ECG changes. A **pulmonary embolism** is improbable given the **negative D-dimer** and lack of significant respiratory distress. **Pericarditis** often presents with pleuritic chest pain and pericardial rub, but it typically does not cause such a **markedly elevated troponin**. **Pneumonia** is also unlikely as the primary issue, given the absence of fever, cough or lung findings, although it could coexist with myocarditis.

Q30 Pericardial Disease

Answer 2 – **Admit, request echocardiogram, start colchicine and ibuprofen**. The symptoms and investigations suggest pericarditis, likely due to a viral cause. According to the ESC guidelines, all patients require an echo to look for a pericardial effusion. First-line treatment is with aspirin/NSAIDs and colchicine. This patient had a subacute course, tachycardia and slightly low BP and would warrant further assessment rather than quick discharge. A **CT scan and corticosteroids** are unnecessary initially, as steroids are generally reserved for refractory or autoimmune cases. **Corticosteroids upfront** can increase recurrence risk and are not first-line. **Discharging with colchicine and follow-up** is inappropriate given the potential risk of complications. **Discharging with only ibuprofen** without confirming effusion status is unsafe, as pericardial tamponade must be excluded first.

Q31 Unstable Angina

Answer 5 – **Normal troponin cardiac biomarkers**. The other responses contribute to a higher MACE risk in this patient. A normal troponin value implies there is no myocardial injury or necrosis and thus predicts better prognostic outcome. Nevertheless, the presence of high-risk features described in this patient would contribute to a higher MACE score. An early invasive strategy would therefore be recommended in this patient. **Age** is an indication for admission, as older patients have higher cardiovascular risk. **Cardiovascular risk factors** such as diabetes, smoking and family history significantly increase the likelihood of coronary artery disease. **Dynamic ECG changes** suggest ongoing myocardial ischaemia, making an invasive approach necessary. **A history of highly suspicious cardiac angina** further reinforces the need for urgent management.

Q32 Blackouts and Faints

Answer 4 – **Hypertrophic cardiomyopathy**. Undetected hypertrophic cardiomyopathy (HCM) is the most common cause of sudden cardiac death (SCD) in young athletes. This autosomal dominant condition has an overall prevalence of roughly 0.1% in the general population and is characterised by an increase in left ventricular thickness, which can lead to left ventricular outflow tract (LVOT) obstruction. In a large case series of SCD in 1,866 young athletes, HCM was found to be the cause of death in approximately 40% of cases. **Long QT syndrome** increases the risk of arrhythmias but typically causes syncope or SCD during emotional stress rather than endurance exercise. **Aortic dissection** is rare in young individuals without hypertension or connective tissue disorders and would present with severe chest or back pain. **Dilated cardiomyopathy** is more associated with heart failure rather than exertional sudden death. **Brugada syndrome** causes SCD but is more likely during rest or sleep rather than exercise.

Q33 Cardiorespiratory Arrest

Answer 1 – **Put out an emergency arrest call**. This is the first action to be taken when cardiorespiratory arrest is diagnosed. Early notification and mobilisation of the cardiac arrest team would ensure the prompt arrival and presence of the team at scene. **Start chest compressions** is not entirely correct as the initiation of chest compression should start immediately after the diagnosis of cardiac arrest and the emergency arrest call / call for help. **Start rescue breaths** is not the correct next step as rescue breaths are not the first action on diagnosis of cardiac arrest in adults – although it is the first action in paediatric patients. **Try to clarify the CPR status of this patient** is not correct as, in an emergency, the clarification of CPR status of the patient may not be possible or readily available. Therefore, unless it is already known from before that the patient is not for CPR, starting CPR is the right approach until the uncertainty around the CPR status of the patient is clarified. When in doubt/uncertainty regarding CPR status, start CPR until a senior member of the team (usually the cardiac arrest team leader) clarifies the CPR status. Diagnosis of cardiorespiratory arrest is clinical, and the confirmation of the cardiac arrest rhythm is done with the use of a defibrillator monitor. Always start CPR and aim for application of a defibrillator as soon as possible. Therefore, **Try to find a monitor / ECG device to check the cardiac rhythm as soon as possible** is not the correct answer.

Q34 Limb Claudication

Answer 5 – **105/150**. The ABPI is calculated using the best possible systolic BP recordings. Irrespective of which leg ABPI is measured in, both upper limb SBPs are measured, and whichever is the highest is taken as the denominator. The same applies to the numerator – check both dorsalis pedis and posterior tibial systolic pressure and use the highest SBP for the calculation. Therefore, left leg ABPI = 0.7: Higher of the left ankle systolic BPs (posterior tibial or dorsalis pedis) / Higher of the brachial systolic pressures (right or left arm).

Q35 Low Blood Pressure

Answer 5 – **Pulmonary embolus**. The most appropriate answer to this clinical question is pulmonary embolus. This man has recently undergone orthopaedic surgery resulting in a period of immobility. It is widely accepted that a total hip replacement is a high-risk procedure for the development of a venous thromboembolism (VTE) in the post-operative recovery period. He describes shortness of breath and pleuritic chest pain, both of which are common symptoms associated with a pulmonary embolus. Additionally, his observations suggest a potential respiratory issue, as he has been noted to have hypoxia and tachypnoea in the context of hypotension. On review of the alternative diagnoses, there is no cardiac-sounding chest pain described in the history or ECG features of ischaemia, making **acute coronary syndrome** less likely. The operation was uncomplicated, with no clinical deterioration occurring in the first 24–48 hours post-operatively, suggesting acute **haemorrhage** is unlikely. There is nothing in the history or past medical history that implies this man is at risk of developing a **pneumothorax** – for example COPD, asthma or chest wall injury. **Pneumonia** is a possibility and should be considered as a differential diagnosis. However, the patient is afebrile and pulmonary embolism is a better fit for the clinical picture presented.

Q36 Peripheral Oedema and Ankle Swelling

Answer 3 – **Deep vein thrombosis**. **Acute heart failure**, **chronic congestive heart failure** and **nephrotic syndrome** are unlikely as these tend to cause bilateral leg swelling, although it can be more prominent in one leg. **Sepsis** is less likely; although cellulitis can indeed cause unilateral leg swelling and redness, as well as tenderness to palpation, which could then lead to sepsis, there are no other clues in the history that the person has sepsis – that is, there is no mention of a temperature, hypotension or tachycardia. Therefore, deep vein thrombosis is the best answer for the information given.

Q37 Shock

Answer 2 – **Insert a chest drain**. As per the ATLS® algorithms/ guidelines, needle decompression of the tension pneumothorax should be followed by insertion of the chest drain. **Allow her to discharge herself**: a patient who is becoming anxious and shouting can indicate hypoxia due to worsening of a tension pneumothorax which needs emergency treatment rather than discharging home! **Order a CXR to check for resolution of the pneumothorax**: investigations should not delay the treatment in these cases. **Start 2 L of oxygen via nasal cannula**: these patients need high-flow oxygen via a non-rebreathing mask. **Start vasopressors to improve BP**: vasopressors are indicated in distributive shock (anaphylactic/ septic/neurogenic shock), not in obstructive shock (tension pneumothorax / cardiac tamponade).

Child Health

Q38 Attention Deficit Hyperactivity Disorder

Answer 1 – **ADHD**. Although **Tourette syndrome** involves tics, these need to be complex motor tics associated with vocalisations, not suggested in the scenario, and Tourette syndrome is much less prevalent than ADHD. **Autism spectrum disorder** is not characterised by fidgety behaviour or lack of concentration. **Lead toxicity** can cause behaviour problems in children but this would not be likely, and other symptoms would be present. **Dyspraxia** can occur alongside ADHD but is principally a problem of coordination.

Q39 Autism Spectrum Disorder

Answer 1 – **A qualitative impairment in reciprocal social interaction**. The diagnostic criteria for autism spectrum disorder include a qualitative impairment in reciprocal social interaction, so this is true. **Emotionally determined selectivity in verbal communication** is just a description of mood-dependent verbal responsiveness, and not a diagnostic criterion for ASD. Although this young patient has struggled in the transition from primary to secondary school, this is not a necessary condition for the diagnosis to be made (although there is a desire for sameness which means that change is often perceived as a threat). **The presence of challenging behaviour** is not a diagnostic requirement of ASD, and neither is **intellectual impairment**.

Q40 Cerebral Palsy and Hypoxic-Ischaemic Encephalopathy

Answer 4 – **Spastic hemiplegic cerebral palsy**. Increased tone and brisk reflexes are signs of spasticity, and as these are identified in both the left upper and lower limbs but not the right upper or lower limb, the pathology is hemiplegic in nature (affecting just one half of the body). **Athetoid cerebral palsy** tends to present with abnormal writhing movements, while **ataxic cerebral palsy** is characterised by poor coordination. **Spastic paraplegic cerebral palsy** would affect all four limbs, while **spastic diplegic cerebral palsy** would only affect the lower limbs or upper limbs bilaterally (most commonly the lower limbs).

Q41 Croup

Answer 5 – **Keep her settled with mum and administer an oral dose of dexamethasone and antipyretics before admitting for close observation**. This child has a classic history for croup. The fact that she has inspiratory stridor and some intercostal recession at rest but remains alert puts her in the Moderate Severity category. The priority should be keeping her settled and comfortable, giving her some steroid treatment preferably in the form of oral dexamethasone (which has been shown to be less likely to lead to rebound symptoms than prednisolone) and observing her in case of deterioration. **A neck and chest X-ray to look for foreign body inhalation** is unnecessary, as the presentation is typical for viral croup rather than a sudden-onset obstruction. **Urgent senior paediatric, anaesthetic and ENT review with IV antibiotics** would be appropriate for epiglottitis, but this child is alert, not drooling, and has a classic croup presentation. **A thorough throat examination** is not advised, as it could distress the child and worsen airway obstruction. **Giving prednisolone and allowing discharge** is inappropriate, as dexamethasone is preferred, and stridor at rest warrants inpatient observation.

Q42 Behavioural Difficulties in Childhood

Answer 3 – **Send an urgent referral to secondary care for assessment**. Referral to secondary care is correct as according to the NICE guidelines if a child or young person's behavioural problems are suggestive of ADHD and are having an impact on their development or family life. Within a community setting, primary care practitioners should not **make a diagnosis of ADHD** or **start methylphenidate**. Offering group-based ADHD-focused support **is helpful but should follow a formal diagnosis rather than precede it. Tell the patients not to worry** is wrong as the parents are concerned and therefore you should offer support and advice on how to help their child.

Q43 Cystic Fibrosis

Answer 3 – **50%**. CF is an autosomal recessive condition, meaning that a child needs to inherit the p.Phe508del CF-causing mutation from both of their parents in order to be homozygous and therefore have the CF phenotype. In this scenario, the child will definitely inherit one disease-causing allele from the mother, as the mother is homozygous for the CF mutation (p.Phe508del). The father is heterozygous, so there is a 50% chance that the child will inherit two copies of the CF causing p.Phe508del mutation. Therefore, there is a 50% chance the child will have CF.

Q44 Abnormal Development / Developmental Delay

Answer 1 – **Fragile X genetic testing**. The combination of symptoms in the boy is indicative of fragile X syndrome, including a characteristic facial appearance, autism-like behaviours and poor speech development, and genetic testing would confirm diagnosis. A **microarray-based comparative genomic hybridisation** would be appropriate first line if the combination of symptoms did not indicate a specific diagnosis, but also fragile X is not picked up by microarray alone. **Thyroid function tests** are carried out in newborn screening, and hypothyroidism presents with feeding difficulties, jaundice, sleepiness and constipation, and tends to be diagnosed earlier. Similarly, some inherited metabolic disorders identified by testing **urine organic acids** tend to present neonatally, with poor feeding, vomiting and faltering growth, and are often identified in newborn screening. An **MRI brain** is useful for identifying intracranial structural abnormalities, not commonly associated with this disorder.

Q45 Down Syndrome

Answer 2 – **A choice of amniocentesis or chorionic villus sampling**. As the woman is in her 11th week of pregnancy, she can be offered prenatal genetic diagnosis by chorionic villus sampling or amniocentesis and informed of the risks. Amniocentesis cannot be performed until 15 weeks, meaning she would have longer to wait for results. **A blood test for Robertsonian translocations**: Robertsonian translocations are not a common cause of Down syndrome and fetal testing is a priority. **A nuchal translucency scan** is used in screening and would have been included in her combined test. **A fetal echocardiogram** could detect a heart defect but it is not diagnostic for Down syndrome and fewer than half of people with Down syndrome have congenital heart disease. **An MRI scan of the pelvis** has no role in diagnosing chromosomal abnormalities.

Q46 Congenital Abnormalities

Answer 2 – **20-week ultrasound scan**. The 20-week ultrasound scan is the anomaly scan and in routine practice will provide the most accurate diagnosis of any neural tube defects. While a neural tube defect may be diagnosed at the **12-week ultrasound scan**, this would not rule out a defect. The **combined test** and **quadruple test**, and **nuchal translucency measurement**, are all used to assess the chances that the fetus has a chromosomal abnormality.

Q47 Epiglottitis

Answer 5 – **Urgently assembling an appropriate team to manage him, including an experienced anaesthetist, ENT surgeon and paediatrician**. The sudden onset of symptoms of fever, throat pain, inability to swallow and drooling in the context of an unvaccinated child are concerning for epiglottitis. Your priority is to secure his airway and to avoid distressing him as this may provoke a sudden worsening of his condition. In order to assess and manage him safely, you need an experienced team around you with the skills to secure his airway via intubation or front of neck access if required.

Inserting a cannula in order to administer a third-generation cephalosporin: although giving intravenous antibiotics is an important part of his management, this is very likely to distress him so should be avoided until his airway is secure. **Moving him onto the examination couch in order to do a full assessment** and **examining his throat to identify the cause of his symptoms**: you should not move him away from his mother or try to examine his throat for the same reasons; this can be done at the time of intubation. Finally, **discussing with his mother the importance of vaccinating children**: the reasons for him not being vaccinated should be sensitively explored and education provided at an appropriate time, when the child is safe and the family can engage.

Q48 Febrile Convulsion

Answer 1 - **Admit to paediatrics**. She has had a complex febrile convulsion given that she has had two seizures within 24 hours. This means that she should be referred to paediatrics and is likely to be admitted for observation. As she has completely recovered, examination is normal and there are no red flags, it is unlikely that she has a serious underlying infection. However, the cause of the infection is yet to be identified. **Continuing observations in the emergency department and then discharging** would be appropriate for a **single simple febrile seizure**, but recurrent seizures require inpatient assessment. **Discharging immediately with advice** is unsafe, as the child has had multiple seizures in a short time. **Obtaining an MSU and prescribing empiric antibiotics** is unnecessary unless there are signs of a UTI, and antibiotics do not prevent febrile seizures. **Routine outpatient follow-up** is not the immediate priority; inpatient monitoring is needed first.

Q49 Measles

Answer 2 – **Measles**. The small pinpoint ulcerations in the mouth (Koplik spots) are pathognomonic of measles. **Chickenpox** presents with a vascular rash, not earache and not Koplic spots. Measles presents with the above; history of travel and lack of immunisation also support the possibility of measles. **Mumps** presents with swelling in the salivary glands. **Rubella** has mild rash and lymphadenopathy. **Toxoplasmosis** can present with fever and fatigue, but not Koplic spots.

Q50 Mesenteric Adenitis

Answer 5 – **Mesenteric adenitis**. Fever and mild abdominal signs in a young child should raise suspicion of mesenteric adenitis. The condition may mimic **appendicitis** and require surgery. Appendicitis is likely to produce more localising signs in a child aged 7. The history is too short to be consistent with **Crohn's disease. Meckel's diverticulitis** is much less common and typically presents with symptoms such as vomiting, rectal bleeding or a palpable mass. None of these features is described in the scenario, making Meckel's diverticulitis less likely. **Irritable bowel syndrome** is uncommon in this age group and is a chronic functional disorder rather than an acute condition.

Q51 The Sick Child

Answer 2 – **150 ml bolus of 0.9% saline.** This child should be managed using the ABCDE approach – Airway: patent; Breathing: whilst his respiratory rate is a little high, there are no other signs of respiratory compromise; Circulation: lethargy, dry mucous membranes and poor skin turgor are signs of dehydration. Their eyes are not sunken as this is usually a late sign. This child has multiple features of shock – raised heart rate, prolonged capillary refill time, low systolic BP – and needs a fluid bolus before we think about maintenance fluids, hence **30 ml 10% dextrose** is incorrect. Fluid boluses should not contain dextrose – ruling out **150 ml bolus of 0.9% saline + 5% dextrose** and **500 ml 0.9% saline + 5% dextrose at 52 ml/hour** – and are now advised to be 10 ml/kg, ruling out **300 ml bolus of 0.9% saline**.

Q52 Mumps

Answer 4 – **12 months**. In the NHS childhood vaccination schedule in the UK, the first MMR dose is given at 12 months. At **2 months**, babies receive the 6-in-1, rotavirus and MenB vaccines, and at **3 months** the second dose of 6-in-1 and rotavirus vaccines, and the pneumococcal vaccine. There are no scheduled **6 months** vaccines (the third round of vaccines is given at 4 months and includes 6-in-1 and MenB vaccines). At **3 years and 4 months** – the 'pre-school' vaccines – children receive the second dose of the MMR vaccine and a 4-in-1 pre-school booster. Some children are recommended to have extra vaccines, such as BCG if their patients are born in countries with high rates of TB. Some children with severe illness and chronic health conditions may have individualised regimes. As a rule, babies born prematurely receive their vaccines as scheduled from their date of birth, not their corrected age based on expected date of delivery.

Q53 Non-accidental Injury

Answer 5 – **Non-accidental injury**. The description does not sound consistent with a **birthmark**. The baby is clinically well and afebrile making **meningococcal sepsis** unlikely. **Henoch–Schönlein purpura** is unlikely due to her age. The proposed mechanism of injury occurring as **accidental bruising** during a nappy change would be an unlikely one. The Child Protection Companion (RCPCH) states 'Bruises in babies and pre mobile babies should raise concern about abuse, or risk of subsequent abuse, and needs careful evaluation.' Answer 5 is therefore correct.

Q54 Rubella

Answer 4 – **Starts behind the ears and on the face, then spreads over the whole body**. The rash of rubella classically starts behind the ears and on the face, then spreads to the whole body. It fades after 2 days and it is unusual for it to last more than 3 days. This can be important to ascertain to suspect the diagnosis, as it is very dangerous for women who are pregnant and susceptible to rubella to be exposed. It does not follow the pattern of the other rashes described.

Starts on the trunk and spreads to the extremities: many rashes can start on the trunk and spread to extremities, such as urticaria and non-specific viral infections. **Affects the hands and feet only**: conditions such as pompholyx eczema or palmoplantar psoriasis affect only the hands and feet. **Causes Koplik spots in the mouth prior to the main rash developing**: Koplik spots are white spots, often with a red background, which occur in the mouth due to measles. They develop before the measles rash occurs on the rest of the body and are pathognomonic of measles. **Causes painful lesions in the mouth and genitals**: rubella does not cause painful lesions.

Q55 Whooping Cough

Answer 1 – **2 days**. Whooping cough is a highly contagious disease, and is particularly dangerous to babies under 3 months old. Exclusion from school helps reduce the spread of the disease, so is required for patients with suspected or confirmed cases. After antibiotics have been started, the patient is still infectious for **2 days**. After this time, they can return to school and usual activities if they are well enough.

Q56 Biliary Atresia

Answer 4 – **Refer to a specialist centre for operation**. BA is a very rare paediatric condition and needs specialist management once a clinical diagnosis is considered. **CT scan** entails radiation exposure and is less sensitive for biliary pathology and hence is not the right step. **Endoscopic retrograde cholangio-pancreatography** is an invasive second-line test when the ultrasound scan appears normal. **Phototherapy** is indicated in neonatal hyperbilirubinaemia – however, once an obstructive cause like BA is suspected, any treatment like this would delay the diagnosis and potentially have a negative impact on surgical treatment. **Refer to a transplant unit for liver transplantation**: referral without full work-up is not advisable. Urgent referral to a specialist paediatric unit will ensure early investigation and timely diagnosis and treatment, with good expected outcome.

Q57 Henoch–Schönlein Purpura

Answer 3 – **4–6 weeks**. HSP is self-limiting in a majority of cases and one would expect symptoms to have resolved within 4–6 weeks. Appropriate follow-up monitoring of BP and urinalysis should be performed regularly as renal involvement is present in 50% of cases and may present weeks to months later. Patients and their families should be warned to remain vigilant for red flag features, including severe pain, macroscopic haematuria, neurological or abdominal complications, and that recurrences may occur within 6 months in around one-third of cases.

Q58 Kawasaki Disease

Answer 1 – **Coronary arteritis**. Coronary arteritis is correct as this 3 year old boy has a clinical diagnosis of Kawasaki disease considered. Kawasaki is an acute vasculitis with the main risk being the development of coronary aneurysms. This is why it is important to consider Kawasaki disease and ensure prompt treatment to reduce the risk of complications. **All other options**: none of the other answers is a known complication of Kawasaki disease.

Q59 Pyloric Stenosis

Answer 5 – **Hypochloraemic hypokalaemic metabolic alkalosis**. Pyloric stenosis leads to the loss of hydrochloric acid (HCl) and potassium (K+) through vomiting, resulting in hypochloraemia (low chloride levels) and hypokalaemia (low potassium levels). Metabolic alkalosis occurs due to the loss of gastric acid (HCl), leading to an increase in blood pH. The other options (1, 2, 3 and 4) do not fit the clinical picture described and are not associated with pyloric stenosis. Therefore, answer 5 is the most likely blood biochemistry result in this case.

Q60 Child Abuse

Answer 1 – **Mental health, substance misuse, domestic violence**. It is recognised that there are risk factors for child abuse and the amalgamation of parental mental health issues or learning disability, substance misuse and domestic violence is a strong predictor of adverse long-term impact on children. The Child Protection Companion (RCPCH) states that 'research indicates that, with adequate support, parents who are experiencing a single problem are often able to be effective and loving parents and present little risk of significant harm to children'. They further state that 'There is considerable evidence that many parents also experience other difficulties and it is the multiplicative impact of combinations of factors that have been found to increase the risk of harm to children. The combination of parental mental illness, learning disability and problem substance misuse coexisting with family disharmony and violence is the best predictor of adverse long-term effects on children.' **All other options are** therefore incorrect.

Q61 Crying Baby

Answer 4 – **Parental reassurance with consideration of prolonged period of observation**. The baby in this scenario appears well, has no red flags in the history, a normal examination and normal observations with no fever. It is very normal for babies to cry and, although challenging for parents, requires reassurance when there are no other concerns. A period of observation can help support parents and provide evidence that there is nothing serious underlying. **Partial septic screen and commence intravenous antibiotics**: a septic screen would only be indicated if the child appeared unwell, there were signs of serious infection or observations were abnormal, for example the presence of fever and tachycardia. **CT head** would only be required if there were signs of non-accidental injury or the baby had abnormal neurology. There are no features of significant GORD (pain with feeds, refusing feeds, poor weight gain) or cow's milk protein allergy (rash, bloody stool, poor weight gain) to indicate the need to **commence omeprazole** or **commence dairy- and soya-free trial for mum**. There is no evidence omeprazole reduces crying.

Q62 Family History of Possible Genetic Disorder

Answer 5 – **2 in 3**. There is no history that she has been adopted (so not **1 in 25**). Both parents must have been heterozygous (they are well, but had a child with cystic fibrosis). At conception, she had 1 in 4 chance of cystic fibrosis (CC), 2 in 4 chance of being a carrier (Cc) and 1 in 4 of not inheriting any cystic gene (cc). In this case, assume that she did not inherit the condition – i.e. she is not homozygous cystic (CC). This means that she has 2 in 3 chance of being a carrier (Cc) and 1 in 3 of not inheriting any cystic gene (cc), so **all other options** are incorrect.

Q63 Infant Feeding Problems

Answer 4 – **Reassure parents and advise his symptoms should improve with age**. The child in this scenario is described as well appearing, is gaining weight, and has none of the red flags. The vomiting after feeds is an isolated issue and it is therefore appropriate to reassure the parents that this is likely due to immature oesophageal sphincter function. It would not be correct to **commence omeprazole and refer for paediatric opinion** as omeprazole does not reduce vomiting and is only indicated if significant GORD is suspected. There are no additional symptoms such as bloody stool or rash to suggest cow's milk protein allergy and therefore no indication to **advise mother to try a soya- and dairy-free diet**. To **request a barium swallow** would only be indicated in cases where very severe GORD or aspiration was suspected. **Advise changing to formula feeding with thickener**: thickener is again a treatment for GORD, which is not the underlying diagnosis as the patient has isolated vomiting, which can be normal in infants due to the immature oesophageal sphincter.

Q64 Neonatal Death or Cot Death

Answer 1 – **Bed sharing** is a known risk factor for sudden unexpected death in infancy (SUDI), as it increases the risk of accidental suffocation or overlaying, particularly when multiple individuals share the same sleep surface. **Breastfeeding** is protective against SUDI, not a risk factor. **Room sharing** (but not bed sharing) is recommended as it reduces SUDI risk. Being a **second-born infant** does not increase the risk of SUDI. An **uncomplicated pregnancy** does not contribute to increased risk.

Q65 Learning Disability

Answer 4 – **Fragile X syndrome**. **Autism Spectrum Disorder** (ASD): while some symptoms of social anxiety and repetitive behaviours can overlap with Fragile X syndrome, ASD typically presents with a broader range of symptoms, including communication challenges and restricted interests. It is not characterised by distinctive physical features such as a long face and large ears. Intellectual disability is not always present in ASD. **Attention deficit hyperactivity disorder** (**ADHD**) primarily involves symptoms of inattention, hyperactivity and impulsivity. While individuals with Fragile X syndrome may exhibit attention difficulties, ADHD does not account for the specific physical features and social anxiety commonly seen in Fragile X. Intellectual disability is not a specific feature of ADHD. **Down syndrome** is characterised by intellectual disability, distinctive facial features and some health issues such as heart defects. However, it does not typically present with the social anxiety and repetitive behaviours associated with Fragile X syndrome. **Williams syndrome** is characterised by distinct facial features, including a broad forehead, small upturned nose and wide mouth. People with Williams syndrome tend to have a highly social and outgoing personality, which contrasts with the social anxiety often seen in Fragile X syndrome. Additionally, Williams syndrome is not typically associated with repetitive behaviours or intellectual disability to the extent seen in Fragile X.

Q66 Prematurity

Answer 4 – **Optimal cord clamping, gentle ventilatory support, maintain normothermia, and consider surfactant administration.** Optimal cord clamping reduces risk of necrotising enterocolitis and intraventricular haemorrhage. Gentle lung inflation followed by non-invasive ventilatory support is most appropriate initially, with consideration for surfactant if signs of respiratory distress. Keeping preterm babies normothermic is strongly associated with improved outcomes. **Prompt cardiopulmonary resuscitation for bradycardia, avoidance of hypothermia, early administration of resuscitation drugs**: preterm babies with bradycardia will almost always respond to effective lung inflation. It is very unusual for CPR or resuscitation drugs to be required, and these should not be considered until effective ventilation has been established. **Immediate intubation to administer surfactant**: babies born before 32 weeks do not all require surfactant routinely. This should be a clinical decision (indications include respiratory distress, respiratory acidosis or high oxygen requirement). **Non-invasive ventilatory support to ensure lung inflation, and withdrawal of active care if baby fails to respond**: 29 weeks prematurity is not at the limit of viability, and full resuscitation and active care would be appropriate. **Avoidance of optimal cord clamping, but non-invasive ventilatory support**: optimal cord clamping is particularly beneficial in preterm babies, reducing the risk of IVH, NEC and death.

Q67 Pubertal Development

Answer 3 – **Constitutional delay of growth and puberty.** This explains around 60% of male cases of delayed puberty. However, this is a diagnosis of exclusion and other causes must be considered. **Kleinfelter's syndrome** is highly unlikely, as males with this condition are typically tall, with a below-average IQ. A **CNS tumour** should always be considered – in this instance, there is a history of headaches, but there are no red flags highlighted, headaches are not progressing having been present for a long time, and there is no focal neurology. An MRI could still be considered. An **acquired gonadal**

defect is unlikely without a known medical cause – e.g. previous trauma, chemotherapy or infection such as mumps. **Delayed puberty secondary to an underlying medical condition** should also be considered, and baseline investigations for conditions which may be asymptomatic should be completed, including thyroid function, coeliac screen and inflammatory markers.

Q68 Dysmorphic Child

Answer 5 – Turner **syndrome**. Patients with Turner syndrome often present with primary amenorrhoea due to premature ovarian failure; however, adrenarche is controlled by the adrenal gland so occurs independently. Up to 50% have a cardiac anomaly – these patients will usually be detected in the neonatal period and can be treated with growth hormone and oestrogen and progesterone replacement therapy. **Congenital hypothryoidism** is now almost always detected in the neonatal period thanks to the newborn blood spot test – adequately treated patients should have normal growth and puberty. Patients with **DiGeorge syndrome** and **Down syndrome** go through normal puberty. **Klinefelter syndrome** occurs in males. While onset of puberty is at the normal age, testes remain small and most patients will suffer from testicular failure with azoospermia, reduced hair growth and gynaecomastia.

Q69 Vaccination

Answer 1 – **All of them**. Egg allergy does not stop any vaccination, except in the case of previous anaphylaxis which necessitated admission to the intensive care unit. MMR is not made with egg. There is no justification for giving MMR as separate vaccines, so **all other options** are incorrect.

3 Dermatology

Q70 Acute Rash

Answer 1 – **Administer intramuscular antibiotics**. The history suggests meningococcal disease which is a medical emergency. Immediate antibiotics are required and a single intramuscular dose of benzylpenicillin is first-line treatment, given as proximally as possible. This can be given while waiting for hospital transfer which should not be delayed. 1 is therefore the correct answer. **Administer rectal diazepam** is incorrect; rectal diazepam is not indicated in this scenario. **Cannulate and set up fluids**: cannulation and fluids may be part of treatment but would not be the first action. **Give oral paracetamol to bring down the temperature**: oral paracetamol can be used for fever but in this scenario she is refusing fluids and has signs of acute meningococcal disease which requires immediate antibiotics and hospital transfer. **Reassure the parents and wait for the ambulance**: an ambulance should be arranged, and treatment should be started as soon as possible while waiting for the ambulance. Reassurance is unlikely to be helpful here as the child is severely ill.

Q71 Acne Vulgaris

Answer 1 – **Isotretinion**. According to NICE guidance, first-line options for acne include topical adapalene, **topical benzoyl peroxide**, topical clindamycin or **topical azelaic acid**. These topical preparations can be used in combination with one another or individually. If these options fail, second-line treatment options include either oral lymecycline 408 mg or **oral doxycycline** 100 mg once daily. This patient has tried topical treatments as well as oral antibiotics, to no avail. Therefore, the next line of treatment would include management with isotretinoin. Isotretinoin is routinely given for 4 months at a dose of 0.5–1 mg/kg per day. **Laser treatments** are not available on the NHS and are only useful for acne scarring and not in cases of active acne.

Q72 Atopic Dermatitis and Eczema

Answer 3 – **Antimetabolite**. Methotrexate inhibits the enzyme dihydrofolate reductase, essential for the synthesis of purines and pyrimidines. Methotrexate (MTX) is an antimetabolite most used in chemotherapy, and as an immunosuppressant in autoimmune diseases. **Alkylating agents** are compounds that react with electron-rich atoms in biologic molecules to form covalent bonds. Examples include cisplatin and cyclophosphamide. Daunorubicin and doxorubicin are **anthracyclines**, which are antibiotics derived from streptomyces bacteria. Vinblastine is an example of a **vinca alkaloid**, a type of drug that blocks cell growth by stopping mitosis. **Xanthine oxidase inhibitors** are predominantly used in the prevention and treatment of gout associated with hyperuricaemia.

Q73 Cutaneous Fungal Infection

Answer 4 – **Skin scraping and microscopy using KOH**. The superficial nature of these infections, combined with the lack of evidence that there is systemic involvement, rules out a blood test (either **blood culture** or **Beta-D-mannan antigen test**). A **skin culture** might not be useful as fungi can be natural residents of the skin and a **urease test** would not help in the diagnosis. KOH skin preparations are a common method for the diagnosis of superficial skin infections.

Q74 Basal Cell Carcinoma

Answer 3 – **Mohs micrographic surgery**. **Reassure and discharge** would not be the appropriate option in this scenario, as this lesion will likely grow, ulcerate and bleed, therefore a margin-controlled excision via Mohs micrographic surgery (MMS) would be the most appropriate choice. MMS is a tissue-sparing, precise method of skin cancer removal. The main advantage is that it offers precise microscopic control of the entire tumour margin while maximising conservation of healthy tissue, with the best cosmetic outcomes. Mohs surgery is particularly suitable for the central face, eyelids/canthi, eyebrows, nose, lips, chin, ear and periauricular area. Pulsed CO_2 **laser** can be effective in ablating superficial basal cell carcinomas (BCCs) but is not a proposed treatment option under the NHS and would not be suitable for nodular variants. **Two cycles of cryotherapy**: cryosurgery and **curettage and cautery** are alternative treatment options for low-risk BCCs but are not preferred for nodular subtypes. Moreover, cryosurgery can cause hypertrophic scarring and permanent pigment alteration, which would not be the best outcome for the patient in the clinical vignette.

Q75 Scarring

Answer 1 – **Keloid scarring**. The most likely diagnosis is Keloid scarring. The earlobe is a common site for the formation of keloid scars associated with ear piercings. Keloids have a high recurrence rate following surgical excision. **Keratoacanthomas** are rapidly growing skin tumours with a central keratinous plug. **Lipomas** are slow growing like keloids, but are soft in texture and not associated with trauma or surgery. **Sebaceous cysts** may be found on the ear but are fluctuant, often with an identifiable punctum. **Squamous cell carcinomas** are slow growing, often in sun-exposed sites, typically have an ulcerated centre, and may be associated with regional lymphadenopathy.

Q76 Cellulitis

Answer 2 – **Commence appropriate oral antibiotics**. The patient has cellulitis, given the erythematous, warm and tender swelling of his calf with proximal spread, and should be treated with **oral antibiotics** (e.g., flucloxacillin) as he is systemically well. **Admitting for a fasciotomy** is unnecessary as there is no indication of compartment syndrome or necrotising fasciitis. **A CT pulmonary angiogram or ventilation/perfusion lung scan** is not required, as there are no signs of pulmonary embolism (e.g., dyspnoea, pleuritic chest pain, hypoxia). **Reassurance alone** is inappropriate, as untreated cellulitis can progress to systemic infection, particularly in a patient with poorly controlled diabetes, which increases the risk of complications.

Q77 Contact Dermatitis

Answer 5 – **Type IV**. Type IV cell-mediated hypersensitivity reactions are caused by Th1 cells secreting cytokines, which activate macrophages and cytotoxic T cells and can cause macrophage accumulation at the site. The most common forms of this include contact dermatitis and the tuberculin reaction. **Type I** hypersensitivity reactions are caused by IgE-mediated hypersensitivity. It causes localised and systemic anaphylaxis, seasonal allergies including hayfever, and food allergies (such as those to peanuts and shellfish). **Type II** hypersensitivity reactions are IgG-mediated cytotoxic hypersensitivity reactions. A common example is seen in transfusions of a mismatched blood type. **Type III** hypersensitivity reactions are also known as immune complex-mediated reactions. The most common forms of this are seen in glomerulonephritis, rheumatoid arthritis and systemic lupus erythematosus. **Complex-mediated** is another term for Type III.

Q78 Cutaneous Warts

Answer 3 – **Recommend topical salicylic acid paints**. Topical salicylic acid paints are the recommended first-line treatment for those with cutaneous warts as they are well tolerated by patients and are readily accessible. **Cryotherapy** is second line as this can be uncomfortable and cause scarring. **Watch and wait** is not appropriate here as the patient is embarrassed about his warts. **Immunotherapy** is incorrect as this is more expensive and is reserved for recurrent, more complex, warts. **Surgical excision under local anaesthetic** is not first line when effective, more conservative treatments are available.

Q79 Urticaria

Answer 2 – **Increase fexofenadine to 180 mg four times a day**. According to NICE guidance, if triggers can be identified, they should be avoided in the first instance. Once thorough investigations have been performed and a clear diagnosis of urticaria is made, a non-sedating antihistamine (for example cetirizine, fexofenadine or loratadine) can be offered for up to 6 weeks. **Start prednisolone 30 mg daily for 10 days** – if symptoms are severe, a short course of oral steroids can be given in conjunction. If there is inadequate response to the first-line antihistamine treatment, a switch to a different antihistamine could be considered; however, the recommendation is to increase the dose of antihistamine to up to four times a day (off-label use). Other options thereafter include leukotriene receptor antagonists (such as montelukast or zafirlukast) and topical anti-pruritic agents such as topical menthol or calamine lotion. **Start flucloxacillin 1 g four times a day for 7 days / Start ibuprofen 400 mg three times a day**: antibiotics such as flucloxacillin and non-steroidal anti-inflammatory agents are not indicated in the management of urticaria.

A **dairy-free diet** is not indicated, as there is no evidence of food allergy or intolerance triggering the urticaria.

Q80 Head Lice

Answer 2 – **Head lice**. Head lice infestation is also called *Pediculosis capitis*, which is the infection of the human scalp and the head hair by the head louse (*Pediculus humanus capitis*). It can affect all ages across the world but is a common problem in girls who share hairbrushes, beds and clothing. Head lice are abundant in school-age children in the UK and usually present with itching, irritability, trouble sleeping, scratching, crusting, scaling and head sores. Generally, nits are easy to see as white grains on the hair shaft. **Atopic dermatitis** would present with **dry, scaly skin and widespread itching**, but not visible nits. **Scalp folliculitis** causes **pus-filled lesions** rather than white grains. **Scalp psoriasis** presents with **thick, silvery scales**, typically without persistent itch or nits. **Tinea capitis** (fungal infection) can cause scalp irritation and hair changes, but it usually has **patchy hair loss, scaling or inflammation**, rather than visible nits.

Q81 Malignant Melanoma

Answer 5 – **Superficial spreading melanoma**. Superficial spreading melanoma is the most common form of melanoma, accounting for approximately 70% of all melanomas. It often develops on an existing mole, which is described in this clinical scenario. This type of melanoma can be found anywhere but is most found on the trunk in males and legs in women. **Nodular melanomas** account for 10–15% of melanomas and are often raised and firm to touch. They grow and spread rapidly and are often associated with a poor prognosis. The lesion is described as 'macular' in this scenario, therefore 'nodular' melanoma is an unlikely diagnosis. The lesion is also described as pigmented, making the **amelanotic melanoma** subtype an unlikely diagnosis. Most patients with **lentigo maligna melanoma** are older than 40 years, and the peak age of diagnosis is between 60 and 80 years. Unlike superficial spreading melanoma, lentigo maligna is not related to the number of melanocytic naevi (moles) or atypical naevi and tends to occur on the face. **Acral lentiginous melanoma** is commonly seen in Asians and Africans and is found on the palms, soles, tongue and nails.

Q82 Impetigo

Answer 5 – **Topical application of fusidic acid. Hospitalisation for intravenous antibiotics** – according to NICE guidance, impetigo should be referred to secondary care if the patient is systemically unwell or immunocompromised, which is not the case in this scenario, therefore intravenous antibiotics will likely not be necessary. In all patients with uncomplicated impetigo, you could consider prescribing topical hydrogen peroxide 1% cream, fusidic acid 2% or mupirocin 2%. The length of course can be increased to 7 days if required, based on clinical judgement, depending on the severity and number of lesions. Children and adults should stay away from school and other childcare facilities or work until lesions are healed, dry and crusted over, or 48 hours after initiation of antibiotics. **Hospitalization for IV antibiotics** is unnecessary as the child is systemically well. **Topical steroids** would not treat the bacterial infection and may worsen impetigo. **No treatment** is inappropriate, as impetigo is contagious and requires management. **Oral flucloxacillin** is reserved for **extensive or severe** impetigo, but this case can be managed with topical antibiotics alone.

Q83 Psoriasis

Answer 4 – **Guttate psoriasis**. Guttate psoriasis is a form of acute psoriasis described as a shower of small, pink-red, scaly 'raindrops' lesions. Guttate psoriasis typically develops 1–2 weeks after a streptococcal infection of the upper respiratory tract – particularly tonsillitis – or other sites, such as perianal streptococcal dermatitis. Beta-haemolytic streptococci can directly stimulate skin-homing T-cell proliferation in the tonsils. **Chronic plaque psoriasis** is common, but often does not present acutely, after an upper respiratory tract infection, as described in this clinical vignette. The lesions are described as 'pinpoint' and there is no mention of an 'unwell' patient with generalised 'erythema', making **erythrodermic psoriasis** an unlikely option. There is no mention of the palms and soles and there is no nail involvement, making **palmoplantar psoriasis** an unlikely choice. **Flexural psoriasis** is relatively common, but the vignette clearly states the lesions are widespread.

Q84 Scabies

Answer 5 – **Topical permethrin 5% cream once weekly for 2 weeks**. According to NICE guidance, the first-line treatment for scabies is permethrin 5% cream to be used on day 1 and day 7 of treatment. It is also recommended that all members of the patient's household, their sexual partners within the past month, and any other close personal contacts (even if asymptomatic) should be treated. Bedding, clothing and towels should be decontaminated by washing at a high temperature (at least 60 °C) and drying in a hot dryer, or dry-cleaning, or by sealing in a plastic bag for at least 72 hours. Secondary infections can be treated with topical or systemic antibiotics, such as **oral flucloxacillin**, although clinical features for a superadded infection are not described in this clinical scenario. If symptoms persist despite two courses of treatment with topical permethrin, oral ivermectin can be used. A post-scabietic itch is expected to last up to 4 weeks after eradication; this can be treated with crotamiton 10% cream. **Oral B12 and folate supplementation**, **oral prednisolone** and **oral fexofenadine** are not treatment options proposed by NICE guidance.

Q85 Petechial Rash

Answer 4 – **Immune thrombocytopenia**. The answer is immune thrombocytopenia, which presents with isolated low platelets – it often follows a viral infection. Usually the patient is well with non-blanching petechiae. **Acute leukaemia** usually presents with an unwell child, with other cytopenias, and with blast cells. It would be unusual to have this in an otherwise well child. **Haemolytic uraemic syndrome** usually follows an episode of bloody diarrhoea; there is no haemolytic anaemia. **Henoch–Schönlein purpura** has a rash on the lower extremities, possibly with abdominal pain, arthritis and renal involvement, but not low platelets. **Sepsis** causing petechiae would invariably come with an unwell child.

Q86 Squamous Cell Carcinoma

Answer 3 – **Immunosuppression**. Common risk factors for cutaneous squamous cell cancers (SCCs) include increased age, male gender, previous skin malignancies, actinic keratoses, outdoor occupation or recreation, smoking, Fitzpatrick skin type I–II, previous cutaneous injuries such as thermal burns or ulcers, inherited syndromes such as xeroderma pigmentosum, exposure to arsenic, and immune suppression due to disease or medications. Organ transplant recipients have an increased chance of developing cutaneous SCCs due to the high level of immunosuppression they are on. Given the fact that this patient has had an organ transplant and is on immunosuppressants such as prednisolone and azathioprine, he is at a much higher risk of developing non-melanoma skin cancers than the general population.

Excessive sun exposure is a major risk factor for skin cancer, but he reports generally covering up outdoors. **Family history** is more relevant for **melanoma**, but his lesion is more suggestive of **SCC** rather than melanoma. **Pesticide exposure** has not been strongly linked to **cutaneous malignancies**. **Smoking** increases the risk of SCC, but immunosuppression plays a much greater role, especially in transplant recipients.

Q87 Viral Exanthema

Answer 2 – **Erythema infectiosum**. Erythema infectiosum (Fifth disease) is caused by parvovirus B19 and mainly affects the cheeks with sparing of the nasal ridge. It is followed by lace-like or network-pattern erythema on the trunk and limbs. **Chickenpox** presents with a **vesicular rash** in different stages of healing, not a lace-like pattern. **Herpes virus infection** (e.g. herpes simplex or varicella) causes **localized vesicles**, not a widespread erythematous rash. **Pityriasis rosea** begins with a **herald patch**, followed by a Christmas-tree distribution rash, rather than a facial rash. **Scabies** presents with **intensely pruritic burrows and papules**, usually in **intertriginous areas**, not a slapped cheek or lace-like rash.

Q88 Bites and Stings

Answer 2 – **Admit to a general medical ward for observation and referral to immunology specialist**. This woman has suffered an anaphylactic reaction to the bee venom after having been sensitised by the previous sting. She has been administered adrenaline and should attend the medical ward for observation. She should also be referred to an immunologist for further testing. **Administering oral antihistamines and sending her home** is inappropriate, as antihistamines do not prevent life-threatening reactions. **Admitting to ITU** is unnecessary, as she has improved with IM adrenaline and is haemodynamically stable. **Sending her home with advice to return if unwell** does not account for the risk of delayed reactions. **Simply advising GP follow-up for an EpiPen** without specialist referral and ED observation is inadequate, as anaphylaxis requires urgent hospital evaluation.

Q89 Burns

Answer 4 – **5400 mLs**. The Parkland formula is a widely used method for estimating fluid requirements in burn patients to prevent hypovolaemic shock. It considers both the patient's weight and the extent of the burns to provide an appropriate fluid volume for initial resuscitation. The formula's 4 mL/kg/% TBSA is designed to replace fluid losses due to the increased capillary permeability and fluid shifts that occur following significant burn injuries. Half of the fluid should be given in the first 8 hours. Formula for first 8 hours is 2 x 36 x 75 = 5400 mLs.

Q90 Folliculitis

Answer 5 – **Topical benzoyl peroxide**. This is most likely a solitary inflammatory pustule (mild acne vulgaris), which is best managed with topical benzoyl peroxide, an antimicrobial and keratolytic agent. **Incision and drainage** is reserved for larger, fluctuant abscesses rather than small pustules. **No management** is inappropriate as mild acne can worsen without treatment. **Oral flucloxacillin** is not necessary for a single non-severe lesion unless there are signs of spreading infection (e.g. cellulitis). **Surgical excision** is excessive and not indicated for a simple pustule.

Q91 Chronic Rash

Answer 1 – **Patch test**. A **skin biopsy** would not be the first choice in diagnosing contact dermatitis. RAST tests are not first line in diagnosing contact dermatitis. A **radioallergoabsorbance test** (RAST) with a particular allergen may be performed to measure allergen-specific IgE in the patient's serum, although a negative test result does not rule out protein contact dermatitis. RAST tests and **serum IgE** are used for food and pet allergies rather than contact dermatitis secondary to exposure to chemicals, which is the likely case in this scenario, given she is a hairdresser. The clinical picture could signify a skin infection, and **skin swab for MC&S** would be useful as part of this patient's work-up. However, a patch test would be the most 'relevant' investigation as it can identify an irritant that this patient could potentially avoid.

Q92 Nail Abnormalities

Answer 1 – **Multiple site biopsy followed by surgical excision**. Acral lentiginous melanomas are commonly seen in Asians and Africans and are found on the palms, soles, tongue and nails. Hutchinson's sign, periungual extension of brown-black pigmentation from longitudinal melanonychia onto the proximal and lateral nailfolds, is an important indicator of subungual melanoma. Biopsy of a lesion suspicious of acral lentiginous melanoma should remove a long ellipse of skin, or there should be several biopsies taken from multiple sites, as a single site could miss a malignant focus. **Obtain a nail clipping**: nail clippings and scrapings are useful in the diagnosis of fungal infections but are not indicated in the work-up for a melanoma. **Treat with cryotherapy**: cryotherapy is not indicated here and is more useful when suspecting a diagnosis of a myxoid cyst or a viral wart. The patient does not demonstrate signs for an overt bacterial infection or paronychia therefore to **treat with penicillin-based antibiotics** would not be the correct choice here. **Reassurance and discharge** would be dangerous, as melanoma requires early intervention.

Q93 Pressure Sores

Answer 1 – **Exposure of deep structures, e.g. bones or tendons**. Pressure sores are usually divided into 4 grades. Grade 1 – **non-blanchable erythema of intact skin**; grade 2 – **erythema with partial-thickness skin loss which involves the epidermis** and superficial part of the dermis; grade 3 – **full-thickness skin loss exposing subcutaneous fat** and involving epidermis and dermis; grade 4 – destruction of deep tissues and even the fascial layers, and exposing muscles, tendons, bones, etc.

Formation of eschars is not a defining feature, as eschar can appear at different stages.

Q94 Pruritus

Answer 2 – **Aqueous menthol 1% cream and non-sedating antihistamines**.

A course of oral prednisolone or **topical steroids and an emollient**: topical and oral prednisolone are often treatments for pruritus secondary to an underlying dermatosis. **Referral to dermatology for consideration of UVB therapy**: UVB therapy can be used in generalised pruritus of unknown origin but tends to be a second-line treatment option. **Topical capsaicin cream** can be useful, particularly in pruritus secondary to nerve damage, such as brachioradial pruritus.

Q95 Skin or Subcutaneous Lump

Answer 3 – **Sebaceous cyst**. From the findings, the most likely diagnosis is sebaceous cyst although there is no mention of the punctum. This is not always seen in a sebaceous cyst. The management is excision under local anaesthesia. A **dermoid cyst** is usually congenital and commonly found in **midline locations**, often deeper and less associated with skin fixation. **Melanoma** is a pigmented lesion, usually changing in shape, size or color, rather than a firm subcutaneous swelling. **Seborrhoeic keratosis** appears as a waxy, stuck-on, pigmented lesion, not a subcutaneous mass. **A wart** is a small, rough epidermal lesion, typically not presenting as a deep swelling.

Q96 Skin Ulcers

Answer 2 – **Pyoderma gangrenosum**. The classic presentation of an ulcer – with undermined edges, induced by an injury that is now worsening, with a violaceous border – is classic for pyoderma gangrenosum. It frequently is associated with an internal disease or condition. Some common associations include inflammatory bowel disease, malignancy and hepatitis. A **basal cell carcinoma** is often described as a pearly-white lesion with raised borders and arborising vessels, on a sun-exposed area such as the face. **Squamous cell carcinomas** (SCCs) can appear as scaly red patches, open sores, rough, thickened or wart-like skin, or raised growths with a central depression. At times, SCCs may crust over, itch or bleed. **Venous ulceration** is often exudative, shallow, and the painful ulcers have 'sloping' edges that do not heal easily. They do not typically present with a violaceous hue. Rashes due to **vasculitis** typically present with a purpuric/petechial widespread rash that appears as 'bleeding points' under the skin.

Q97 Skin Lesion

Answer 4 – **Lipoma**. A lipoma is a soft, mobile, rubbery, non-tender subcutaneous swelling that develops slowly over years, making it the most likely diagnosis in this case. An **abscess** would be tender, erythematous and often fluctuant, which this lesion is not. An **epidermoid cyst (sebaceous cyst)** is firmer, often has a central punctum, and may become inflamed or infected. A **ganglion** typically occurs near joints or tendons, especially on the wrist, rather than the back of the neck. **Skin abscess** is not consistent with this painless, long-standing lesion.

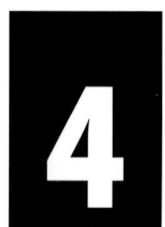

Ear, Nose and Throat

Q98 Stridor

Answer 5 – **Urgent ENT and ITU involvement**. This history is suggestive of acute epiglottitis – the child is unwell, drooling, and has not received vaccination against Haemophilus influenza B, the most likely causative organism. **Examine pharynx using tongue depressor**: agitation and distress can worsen respiratory compromise and, since attempts to examine have not been tolerated by the child, persisting in doing so is unwise and may cause a rapid clinical deterioration. **Bloods for FBC, U&E, CRP**: the same is true for painful interventions such as phlebotomy, and **administering high-flow oxygen via reservoir facemask** in a 3 year old is also likely to increase upset. This child is too unstable to safely transfer for a **chest X-ray** and needs urgent input from specialty services such as anaesthetics, ITU and ENT in order to secure the airway prior to undertaking further diagnostic procedures and interventions.

Q99 Rhinosinusitis

Answer 5 – **Reduction or loss of sense of smell lasting 12 weeks**. The diagnostic criteria for *chronic* rhinosinusitis are nasal blockage or nasal discharge, plus or minus facial pain or pressure, plus or minus reduction or loss of sense of smell lasting more than *12 weeks*. Other signs and symptoms can include headache, halitosis, fatigue, otalgia, cough and teeth or jaw pain. **None of the other options** meets the 12-week diagnostic criterion for chronic rhinosinusitis.

Q100 Epistaxis

Answer 1 – **Anterior ethmoid artery**. The correct answer is anterior ethmoidal artery, which is a branch of the internal carotid artery. The **lateral nasal artery** and **superficial temporal artery** are branches of the external carotid artery. **Anterior sphenopalatine artery**: the sphenopalatine artery does contribute to Kiesselbach's plexus but does not have an anterior or posterior branch. The **ophthalmic artery** gives rise to the anterior and posterior ethmoid arteries, but it itself is not a direct contributor.

Q101 Ménière's Disease

Answer 2 – **Dysdiadochokinesia**. The correct answer is dysdiado-chokinesia, which is the inability to perform rapid alternating movements and is associated with cerebellar lesions. **All other options** are signs and symptoms which can present in patients with Ménière's disease.

Q102 Obstructive Sleep Apnoea

Answer 3 – **Obesity**. The distribution of fat in the mandibular and facial area as well as the upper respiratory region in the presence of relaxed muscles during sleep causes narrowing of the upper respiratory tract. Other risk factors include male sex, smoking, alcohol, family history, hypothyroidism, adenotonsillar hypertrophy, sleeping supine and craniofacial abnormalities. **Asthma** is not a major risk factor for OSA, though both conditions can coexist. **Female sex** is associated with lower OSA prevalence compared to males, though risk increases after menopause. **Sleeping prone** does not increase OSA risk; supine sleeping is more problematic due to gravitational airway collapse. **Thyroidectomy** may lead to hypothyroidism, which can contribute to fatigue, but it is not a direct risk factor for OSA.

Q103 Otitis Media

Answer 1 – **Mastoiditis**. Mastoiditis is a complication which can occur in otitis media. **Paralysis**, **visual loss** and **stroke** are highly unlikely unless there is intracranial involvement in the form of a brain abscess or seizures. **Parapharyngeal abscesses** are not related to otitis media.

Q104 Infectious Mononucleosis

Answer 3 – **Full blood count and Monospot test**. A full blood count would allow us to assess inflammatory markers that would be raised due to infection. A Monospot test is specific for EBV infection and thus would allow us to effectively diagnose infectious mononucleosis. Although **arterial blood gases** would allow us to assess the patient's current levels of O_2, CO_2 and pH, the patient is not in any respiratory distress at present and as such this would be an inappropriate investigation. Although **chlamydia screen** and **throat swab** would allow us to rule out chlamydia or any other microbiological aetiologies as a differential, a full blood count should typically be the first-line investigation. Lastly, **ultrasound of the neck** would not be advisable at this stage.

Q105 Otitis externa

Answer 3 – **Staphylococcus aureus**. Although earache and muffled hearing are quite non-specific symptoms, the examination findings of erythema of the ear canal and exudate (or discharge) suggest inflammation of the lining of the external ear canal, leading to a diagnosis of otitis externa. The short history makes fungal infection unlikely. The commonest cause of bacterial otitis externa is staphylococcus aureus. **Haemophilus influenza B** and **streptococcus pyogenes** are common causes of acute otitis media. **Aspergillus niger** is a fungal cause of otitis externa but typically presents with black spores and chronic symptoms rather than acute bacterial infection. **Treponema pallidum** is the bacteria responsible for syphilis – this is not a common cause of ear infections.

Q106 Dizziness

Answer 3 – **Posterior circulation ischaemia**. This patient has features in keeping with a posterior circulation cerebrovascular event. He is demonstrating signs and symptoms of acute disequilibrium such as dizziness, nausea, vomiting and unsteadiness, as well as focal neurological sequelae including visual and cerebellar signs. He also has atrial fibrillation which puts him at an increased risk of a stroke. This patient requires an urgent CT head to determine management of his stroke. With **Ménière's disease**, you would expect vertigo associated with nausea, tinnitus, fullness of the ear and hearing loss, but no focal cerebellar signs. For **benign paroxysmal positional vertigo**, you would expect episodic vertigo provoked by head movements which resolves when the head is kept still, and, again, no cerebellar signs. **Vestibular neuritis** usually presents with sudden, spontaneous, severe vertigo, and is preceded by an upper respiratory tract infection. **Postural hypotension** normally involves a change in posture, which provokes pre-syncope.

Q107 Ear and Nasal Discharge

Answer 3 – **Pseudomonas aeruginosa**. The condition described is malignant (necrotising) otitis externa which is most commonly caused by infection with Pseudomonas aeruginosa. This requires urgent referral to secondary care for intravenous antibiotics, CT scan and ENT review. **Haemophilus influenzae** is associated with **otitis media**, not malignant otitis externa. **Herpes simplex** can cause Ramsay Hunt syndrome but presents with vesicles and facial nerve palsy, which are absent here. **Staphylococcus aureus** is a common cause of typical bacterial otitis externa, but it is less likely to cause necrotizing infection. **Streptococcus pneumoniae** is a leading cause of otitis media, not external ear infections.

Q108 Tonsillitis

Answer 1 – **Epstein–Barr virus**. The correct answer is Epstein–Barr virus, which causes infectious mononucleosis. This can be investigated using a Monospot test – if positive, there is a risk of splenomegaly, and patients must be advised to avoid contact sports. **Paramyxovirus** causes mumps. **Parvovirus B19** causes Fifth's disease or 'slapped cheek syndrome' and affects the paediatric population. **Hepatitis A virus** causes fever and jaundice. **Herpes zoster virus** is associated with chickenpox and shingles (if reactivated later).

Q109 Hearing Loss

Answer 3 – **Otosclerosis**. Otosclerosis is common in females of young age, and is associated with family history. Hearing loss can be exaggerated following pregnancy. Pure tone audiogram usually shows low-frequency hearing loss. **Congenital cholesteatoma** usually presents with ear discomfort or hearing loss in teenage years. Tinnitus is not common. Examination reveals a white mass behind an intact tympanic membrane. Diagnosis is confirmed by CT scan. **Impacted wax** can cause a blocked feeling and some degree of hearing loss, and occasionally tinnitus. Can occur at any age. No associated family history. **Superior semi-circular canal dehiscence** usually presents with chronic disequilibrium or vertigo, made worse by sound (Tulio phenomenon), and autophony. **Traumatic perforation of the tympanic membrane** follows a history of trauma, associated with pain or discomfort or bleeding from the ear. It can result in hearing loss, depending on the size of the perforation.

Q110 Hoarseness and Voice Change

Answer 1 – **2-week-wait referral to ENT**. There are several red flag symptoms within the history (neck lump, otalgia, persistent dysphonia) which should alert the clinician to a potential malignant cause. The patient should therefore be urgently referred for specialist assessment. An **MR scan of the neck** may be undertaken during staging imaging (more commonly a CT), but should not delay a referral to ENT. **Antireflux treatment** is not appropriate as reflux alone would not explain the neck lump and progressive worsening symptoms. **Thyroplasty** is a surgical intervention for vocal cord paralysis, not indicated without a confirmed diagnosis. **Voice therapy** is useful for benign voice disorders, but this patient needs urgent cancer exclusion first.

Q111 Sore Throat

Answer 5 – **Streptococcal tonsillitis**. The fever pain score is 3 (no fever but enlarged purulent tonsils). We would treat this as tonsillitis as patient is on immunosuppressant drugs and, because of that, the threshold for treatment is lower than in a healthy patient. **Glandular fever** is common in a younger population although exceptions occur. **Herpes simplex infection** can cause painful ulcerative pharyngitis but typically presents with oral vesicles or ulcers rather than simple exudate. **Laryngitis** presents with hoarseness rather than tonsillar exudate.

Q112 Nasal Obstruction

Answer 1 – **2-week fast-track referral to ENT**. In this case, the clinician needs to suspect sinonasal malignancy and refer to a specialist. The key points in the patient's history are unilateral epistaxis and nasal obstruction, with a fleshy mass on the anterior rhinoscopy. Smoking is also a risk factor. **All the other answers** are not suitable management options, and empirical treatment in this scenario may cause unnecessary delays in diagnosis and treatment.

Q113 Acoustic Neuroma

Answer 3 – **Magnetic resonance imaging**. The correct answer is magnetic resonance imaging (MRI) of the internal auditory meatus and brain. This provides information on the anatomy, size and characteristics of the neuroma and helps with planning the management. **Pure tone audiometry** should be done to assess the extent of hearing loss but is not the gold-standard investigation. **Computed tomography** will not provide the same depth of information. **Flexible nasoendoscopy** and **nerve function tests** are not indicated.

Q114   Benign Paroxysmal Positional Vertigo

Answer 4 – **Dix–Hallpike test**. The correct answer is Dix–Hallpike test, which is used to provoke vertigo and torsional nystagmus in patients with BPPV. **Allen's test** is used to assess collateral arterial blood supply into the hands and is commonly used where endovascular access is required. **Ortolani's test** is to assess for congenital hip dislocation or developmental dysplasia of the hip. **Buerger's test** is used to assess for arterial insufficiency in the lower limb. **Active compression test** is for the shoulder.

Q115   Painful Ear

Answer 5 – **Urgent referral to rheumatology**. Giant cell arteritis is a medical emergency and includes risk for serious complications such as blindness if not acted upon quickly. Vision loss can occur in one in five patients if diagnosis is confirmed. Best way to confirm the diagnosis is by taking a temporal artery biopsy but sometimes it can be negative. **Routine referral to ophthalmology or rheumatology** is inappropriate, as delayed treatment increases the risk of irreversible blindness. **Treating with steroids and reviewing in 1 week** is risky, as the patient needs urgent specialist input. **Urgent ophthalmology referral** is appropriate if vision loss is already present, but rheumatology referral is the best next step for diagnosis and long-term management.

Q116   Snoring

Answer 4 – **Referral to sleep apnoea clinic**. History is suggestive of obstructive sleep apnoea and management is further assessment with overnight pulse oximetry, and once OSA is confirmed, treatment will be CPAP. Treatment for OSA is optimising the weight and CPAP, but **referral for gastric bypass surgery** is necessary when initial conservative measures do not help to reduce the weight.

OSA can cause cardiovascular complications and so further management is usually indicated. **Prescribe sleeping tablets for him and his wife**: this is not appropriate, because the patient is not being treated for the underlying cause. **Reassuring without treatment** is unsafe, as untreated OSA can lead to hypertension, cardiovascular disease and accidents. **Urgent ENT referral** is unnecessary at this stage, as first-line assessment is through a sleep clinic, and ENT intervention is considered later if surgical airway correction is needed.

Q117 Speech and Language Problems

Answer 1 – **2-week-wait referral to ENT**. Refer urgently to ENT for a fibre-optic laryngoscopy to assess for potential cancerous changes. Red flag indications include changes to voice, emerging dysphagia (swallowing problems), pain on swallowing and unilateral discomfort in throat and ear. **All other options** are incorrect as these represent secondary, onward referrals or actions following initial diagnosis.

Q118 Swallowing Problems

Answer 4 – **Peritonsillar abscess**. The acute presentation makes **malignancy**, where symptoms tend to present more insidiously, very unlikely, as well as young age. There is no mention of a **foreign body** in the history given. The acute presentation, pyrexia and presence of lymphadenopathy all point towards an infective cause. The key symptom that makes the diagnosis more likely to be a peritonsillar abscess over **glandular fever** and **supraglottitis** is the significant trismus. Supraglottitis does not affect the oral tissues and glandular fever does not commonly produce severe trismus. Another clue to help aid diagnosis may be pain being felt more significantly on one side compared to the other.

Q119 Vertigo

Answer 3 – **Ménière's disease**. The patient is presenting with the typical triad of symptoms – of vertigo lasting for more than 30 minutes, fluctuating hearing loss and tinnitus. Fullness in the ear usually occurs in Ménière's disease. In **vestibular labyrinthitis**, vertigo is of sudden onset and is severe, usually lasting for a few days and improving with time. There may be hearing loss and tinnitus. There is no fluctuating hearing loss or feeling of fullness in the ear. **Acoustic neuroma** is a benign tumour in the vestibulo-cochlear nerve, which usually presents with unilateral hearing loss or tinnitus or both, and without a feeling of fullness in the ear. It is uncommon for it to present with vertigo. So, it is unlikely to be acoustic neuroma. With **benign paroxysmal positional vertigo**, vertigo is provoked by head movements and, unlike in Ménière's disease, it lasts for a few seconds to minutes. It does not present with hearing loss or tinnitus. **Otitis** media presents usually with ear pain, a blocked feeling and some degree of hearing loss. It does not present with vertigo, unless it has resulted in complications such as mastoiditis, etc.

Q120 Tinnitus

Answer 1 – **Repeat the scan in 9 months' time**. Wait and watch is commonly followed for patients with acoustic neuroma, unless the patient presents with a large tumour and with pressure symptoms. Patients usually have interval scan between 6 and 12 months to monitor the size of the growth. **Extending the MRI to the whole CNS** is unnecessary unless there is suspicion of neurofibromatosis type 2 (bilateral schwannomas). **Stereotactic radiosurgery** is usually considered for larger, growing or symptomatic tumours, but is not first-line for a small, stable lesion. **Surgical resection via retrosigmoid or translabyrinthine approach** is typically reserved for larger tumours (> 2 cm), progressive hearing loss or brainstem compression. Since this patient is asymptomatic aside from tinnitus, watchful waiting with MRI surveillance is the best option.

Q121 Anosmia

Answer 5 – **Nifedipine**. Anosmia is a possible side effect of nifedipine. **Doxycycline** is an antibiotic which can be used for the treatment of bacterial sinusitis. **Intranasal steroids** and **loratadine** can be used as a treatment for nasal mucosal inflammation. Anosmia is not listed as a side effect of lisinopril.

Endocrine

5

Q122 Addison's Disease

Answer 1 – **Admit to hospital urgently**. This patient has primary adrenal insufficiency (Addison's disease) given her hyperpigmentation, hypotension, hyponatraemia and low morning cortisol with elevated ACTH. This may be due to reactivation of tuberculosis. She also has hypoglycaemia and renal impairment, which are concerning signs of an adrenal crisis, requiring urgent hospital admission for IV hydrocortisone and fluid resuscitation. **Adrenal biopsy** is not needed for diagnosis, as adrenal insufficiency is confirmed biochemically. **ACTH stimulation testing** is useful in stable cases but is not needed in a critically unwell patient with already confirmed adrenal failure. **Prescribing hydrocortisone** is necessary but should be done urgently in a hospital setting with IV replacement. **Tuberculostatic medication** may be needed if active TB is confirmed, but the immediate priority is treating adrenal insufficiency.

Q123 Dehydration

Answer 4 – **Immediate 250 ml Hartmann's and reassessment**. This patient is clinically dehydrated – you can tell this from the history, the examination, the observations and the blood results. They require fluid resuscitation. Due to the patient's heart failure, you should go about this cautiously, with repeated fluid reassessment, hence immediate 250 ml Hartmann's and reassess is the correct answer.

2.5 L Hartmann's prescribed over 48 hours is wrong as the patient needs much earlier reassessment before such a large volume is given. **Encourage oral fluids** – the patient is unable to take oral fluids due to vomiting, so this is inappropriate. **Immediate 500 ml 0.9% NaCl followed by 1 L Hartmann's over 2 hours** could be dangerous as 0.9% NaCl is likely to worsen the hypokalaemia. **Immediate 500 ml 0.9% NaCl followed by 1 L Hartmann's over 2 hours**: given the hypokalaemia, potassium should be replaced. In A&E or on the ward, this should be slow and cautious, at a rate of 10 mmol/hour. Over 20 mmol/hour, cardiac monitoring and a central line should be considered with the patient being on the high dependency unit or intensive care unit. Therefore, 40 mmol KCl over 1 hour would be dangerous, so this option is incorrect.

Q124 Diabetes Insipidus

Answer 2 – **Complete nephrogenic diabetes insipidus**. This patient has polyuria, polydipsia, hypernatraemia, high plasma osmolality and very low urine osmolality, which strongly indicate diabetes insipidus (DI). Given his history of long-term lithium use, nephrogenic DI is the most likely cause, where the kidneys become resistant to antidiuretic hormone (ADH). His high plasma copeptin (23.5 pmol/L) confirms that ADH secretion is intact, ruling out central DI, while his very dilute urine osmolality (170 mosm/kg) is consistent with complete nephrogenic DI, as the kidneys fail to respond to ADH, leading to excessive water loss and an inability to concentrate urine.

Complete central DI is ruled out by his high copeptin levels, as central DI would show low ADH production. **Partial nephrogenic DI** would present with a higher urine osmolality (> 300 mosm/kg) due to some residual renal response to ADH. **Partial central DI** is also unlikely, as it would have low copeptin levels. **Primary polydipsia** would present with low plasma osmolality, which is not seen here.

Q125 Cushing's Syndrome

Answer 5 – **Urinary free cortisol 2765 nmol/day**. A markedly elevated 24-hour urinary free cortisol (UFC) is highly suggestive of Cushing's syndrome, as UFC directly measures unbound, biologically active cortisol over time, avoiding fluctuations seen in serum cortisol levels. **Dexamethasone suppression test (1 mg) showing serum cortisol of 35 nmol/L at 8 a.m.** suggests adequate suppression, making Cushing's unlikely. **Normal morning salivary cortisol but low midnight cortisol** does not fit Cushing's, as Cushing's patients lose the normal diurnal variation and typically have high midnight cortisol. **A random afternoon serum cortisol of 96 nmol/L** is non-diagnostic, as cortisol varies throughout the day. **A 9 a.m. serum cortisol of 600 nmol/L** is within the normal range and does not confirm Cushing's.

Q126 Diabetes Mellitus Type 1 and 2

Answer 3 – **Measurement of capillary blood ketones**. The patient has diabetes as random blood glucose is > 11.1 mmol/L and he is symptomatic. **Check urgent HbA1c**: although an Hba1c would usually be done, this would only serve to confirm the diagnosis of diabetes, but would not change his immediate management. His age and BMI place him in an indeterminate risk group for type 1 versus type 2 diabetes but the relatively short history of osmotic symptoms is suggestive of possible type 1 diabetes and the vomiting is concerning that he may be developing diabetic ketoacidosis (DKA). The most important next step therefore is to check his blood ketone level as DKA is potentially life threatening and needs to be diagnosed and treated quickly. **Arrange urgent plasma C-peptide**: a plasma C-peptide is unlikely to be helpful in this situation. **Start metformin**: metformin is used as first-line treatment in a well patient with type 2 diabetes and therefore would not be appropriate here. **Refer to diabetes team**: referral would be appropriate, but not before establishing whether the patient has DKA and starting treatment.

Q127 Electrolyte Abnormalities

Answer 1 – **Hypercalcaemia secondary to primary hyperparathyroidism**. The calcium is raised with a non-suppressed PTH. PTH may not always be classically elevated in cases of primary hyperparathyroidism. About 20% of people with significant disease can have high calcium and normal PTH levels. Phosphate is low. These are common findings seen in primary hyperparathyroidism. Her symptoms also fit with this diagnosis. **Renal failure secondary to renal stones**: renal stones and osteoporosis are common complications of primary hyperparathyroidism and, in addition to the symptoms and her relatively young age, are indications for surgical treatment. **Hyperkalaemia** is mild and not the primary issue, as it is likely related to her hyponatraemia or medication use, rather than causing her symptoms. **Hypophosphataemia** is present but is a consequence of PHPT rather than an independent diagnosis. **Hypovolaemic hyponatraemia** is unlikely as the patient does not have clear signs of dehydration or significant sodium loss.

Q128 Diabetic Ketoacidosis

Answer 2 – **Prescribe 0.9% normal saline along with a fixed-rate intravenous insulin infusion**. Initial treatment for DKA should include 0.9% normal saline along with an intravenous infusion of insulin. This should be prescribed as a fixed-rate infusion (0.1 units/kg/hour) rather than a variable-rate infusion. **All other options** are incorrect. Bolus doses of intravenous insulin are not recommended. Although patients should continue with their usual long-acting insulin subcutaneously, this should be given alongside the fixed-rate insulin infusion.

Q129 Hypercalcaemia of Malignancy

Answer 3 – **Rehydrate with intravenous fluids for 24 hours**. First-line treatment for a moderate to severely raised calcium is intravenous fluids. If, after 24 hours of rehydration, calcium remains elevated, then second-line treatments such as bisphosphonates could be considered if the patient has a known or suspected underlying malignancy. **Zoledronate (4 mg IV) and pamidronate (60 mg IV)** are **bisphosphonates**, used to lower calcium levels, but should only be given after adequate hydration, as they can worsen kidney function. **Calcitonin 100 units SC every 8 hours** is used for severe, symptomatic hypercalcaemia (> 3.5 mmol/L) or when rapid calcium reduction is needed, but it is not the first step. **Treating with IV fluids and a loop diuretic** is outdated, as loop diuretics should not be used unless there is fluid overload, as they can worsen dehydration

Q130 Hyperlipidemia

Answer 2 – **Hypertriglyceridemia-induced pancreatitis**. Epigastric pain radiating to the back, amylase levels of more than 4 times the upper limit of normal, triglycerides levels above 10 mmol/L. **Cholecystitis** is unlikely as the ultrasound shows a normal biliary tree, and there is no right upper quadrant tenderness or gallstones. **Myocardial infarction** is doubtful despite a mildly elevated troponin, as ECG is normal and the pain pattern aligns more with pancreatitis. **Pneumonia** is not supported by the absence of respiratory symptoms or lung findings on chest X-ray. **Ruptured aortic aneurysm** is unlikely due to the absence of hypotension, shock or a pulsatile abdominal mass.

Q131 Hypoglycaemia

Answer 3 – **Administer orally 15–20 g fast-acting carbohydrate**. The patient has developed symptomatic hypoglycaemia. You can assume this is due to insulin treatment as he has type 1 diabetes.

The immediate priority is therefore to correct the low blood glucose. As he is conscious and compliant, he should be given 15 to 20 g of fast-acting glucose in the form of a sugary drink such as Lucozade (make sure it is the sugar-containing version), fruit juice (200 ml carton), dextrose tablets (3–5) or glucose gel. **Administer intramuscular 1 mg glucagon / Administer intravenous 10% glucose at 200 ml over 15 minutes**: glucagon or intravenous dextrose would only be indicated if he was confused, non-compliant or unable to take oral treatment because of reduced conscious level or inability to swallow. **Arrange urgent chest X-ray / Urgently take blood cultures and administer paracetamol**: a CXR and blood cultures would also be indicated in due course as he has a temperature and a cough, but these can wait until the immediate problem of hypoglycaemia has been corrected.

Q132 Hyperosmolar Hyperglycaemic State

Answer 4 – **Prescribe 0.9% sodium chloride over 1 hour along with a fixed-rate intravenous insulin infusion.** Fluid replacement in patients with HHS should always start with 0.9% sodium chloride. If insulin is required immediately (due to the presence of ketones), it should be given as a fixed-rate infusion (0.05 units/kg/hour), not as a variable rate or as a subcutaneous injection. Therefore, **all other options** are incorrect.

Q133 Polydipsia (Thirst)

Answer 2 – **Diabetes mellitus**. This man has a random blood glucose > 11.1 mmol/L, together with typical symptoms diagnostic of diabetes mellitus. His symptoms are most likely due to elevated blood glucose levels. **Alcohol excess** is unlikely as he only drinks occasionally, and his symptoms are better explained by hyperglycaemia. **Diabetes insipidus** typically presents with **severe polyuria and dilute urine** rather than hyperglycaemia. **Hyponatraemia (131 mmol/L)** is mild and unlikely to be the primary cause of his symptoms, as it is likely secondary to osmotic diuresis from hyperglycaemia. **Psychogenic polydipsia** is less likely given his **weight loss and hyperglycaemia**, which strongly point towards diabetes.

Q134 Hyperparathyroidism

Answer 3 – **Parathyroid hormone**. A raised calcium has been confirmed on two occasions. None of the medications the patient is taking is commonly associated with hypercalcaemia. The next recommended test is therefore a PTH to help determine the cause of the raised calcium. Further investigations will depend on whether PTH is normal/raised or suppressed. **CT thorax, abdomen and pelvis** is used to investigate malignancy-related hypercalcaemia, but malignancy is less likely without symptoms such as weight loss, bone pain or a markedly elevated calcium level. **Myeloma screen** is indicated in suspected multiple myeloma (which can cause hypercalcaemia), but the absence of renal dysfunction, anaemia or bone pain makes this less likely. **Serum ACE** is used for sarcoidosis, but hypercalcaemia due to granulomatous disease is typically associated with elevated vitamin D, which should be checked first. **Vitamin D** deficiency can cause secondary hyperparathyroidism but would not cause isolated hypercalcaemia, making it a less appropriate initial investigation.

Q135 Hyperthermia and hypothermia

Answer 2 – **Assess the patient using an ABCDE approach, apply blankets and a bear hugger, commence warmed intravenous infusion, and consider sepsis six treatment and analgesia.** This patient has moderate hypothermia, likely secondary to her long lie. **Assess the patient using an ABCDE approach, and consider whether this could be serotonin syndrome or neuroleptic malignant syndrome**: she is acutely unwell and requires urgent ABCDE assessment and initiation of treatment. Serotonin syndrome and neuroleptic malignant syndrome present with hyperthermia, so are not relevant in this case. **Assess the patient using an ABCDE approach, give paracetamol, perform an electrocardiogram and give a stat dose of atropine**: atropine is not indicated without severe adverse features of bradycardia (shock, syncope, myocardial infarction or heart failure). **No immediate action and admitting for monitoring** would delay critical interventions in a potentially life-threatening situation. **Starting intravenous antibiotics immediately without further assessment** is inappropriate, as her presentation suggests hypothermia as the primary concern, and infection should be evaluated systematically rather than assumed.

Q136 Hypothyroidism

Answer 1 – **High TSH and low T4.** In primary hypothyroidism, TSH is raised whilst the T4 levels are low. The pituitary release of TSH is increased in response to falling levels of thyroid hormones via a negative feedback loop. **All other options** are incorrect.

Q137 Obesity

Answer 1 – **Cholestasis**. Orlistat should not be prescribed to people with chronic malabsorption syndrome or cholestasis as dietary absorption of fat is already impaired in these people. **All the other conditions** are not contraindicated – and all may be improved with weight loss associated with orlistat.

Q138 Hypoparathyroidism

Answer 5 – **Omeprazole**. Omeprazole is associated with hypomagnesaemia. This in turn suppresses PTH secretion leading to hypocalcaemia. Magnesium must be replaced otherwise any improvement in calcium will be transient. **Bendroflumethiazide** is associated with hypercalcaemia. **Atorvastatin**, **bisoprolol** and **lisinopril** are not commonly associated with calcium disorders.

Q139 Thyrotoxicosis

Answer 5 – **At least 6 months**. Current guidance in the UK recommends that women should wait at least 6 months after treatment to become pregnant.

Q140 Pituitary Tumours

Answer 1 – **Intravenous hydrocortisone and aggressive fluid resuscitation**. This patient has pituitary apoplexy and adrenal crisis due to severe ACTH deficiency (tachycardia, hypotension, renal impairment, vomiting, hyponatraemia and hyperkalaemia). **All the options listed** above are potentially correct but the best next thing to do is to give intravenous hydrocortisone and fluids to resuscitate her while other measures are being arranged. Treatment should not be delayed till investigations are available since it is a life-threatening condition.

Q141 Thyroid Nodules

Answer 1 – **Inferior to the cricoid cartilage**. Being able to palpate the isthmus is a key clinical skill as a thyroid examination starts at that point. You will first need to palpate the cricoid cartilage as the isthmus lies inferior to it. Palpating **inferior to the hyoid bone** and **inferior to the thyroid cartilage** are too superior; palpating **inferior to the sternum** is too inferior, and palpating **lateral to the thyroid cartilage** is too superior and lateral as the isthmus is located at the midline.

Q142 Fatigue

Answer 1 – **Chronic fatigue syndrome**. This is the most likely diagnosis as the patient has described symptoms of persistent fatigue, post-exertional malaise, unrefreshing sleep and difficulty concentrating. All these symptoms have persisted for over 4 months, making the diagnosis of chronic fatigue syndrome most likely. Moreover, bloods are normal, confirming suspicions that the fatigue is unlikely to be linked to an underlying biochemical cause. Although **depression** might present with fatigue, there is no mention of low mood or anhedonia, making it less likely. Although **lymphoma** could present with painful lymphadenopathy, the patient has denied any weight loss or fevers in keeping with this diagnosis, and there are no signs of lymphadenopathy on examination, nor any abnormalities on blood test results. **Infectious mononucleosis** and **Lyme disease** are both less likely diagnoses without the relevant infection histories, as well as with the negative Monospot and Borreliosis blood tests.

Q143 Weight Gain

Answer 4 – **Gliclazide**. Gliclazide is an insulin secretagogue that works via the sulphonylurea receptor on the pancreatic beta cell to stimulate insulin secretion. It has been associated with weight gain of 3.6 to 4.2 kg, particularly when used as first-line treatment. **Atenolol** can cause mild weight gain by reducing metabolic rate, but its effect is less pronounced than sulfonylureas. **Dapagliflozin**, an **SGLT2 inhibitor**, is more likely to cause **weight loss** due to increased urinary glucose excretion. **Atorvastatin** and **Ramipril** have no effect on weight.

Q144 Gynaecomastia

Answer 3 – **Make an urgent referral to the 2-week-wait clinic for suspected breast cancer**. The presence of a unilateral mass and nipple change in a man over 50 are red flags for breast cancer, therefore it should be treated as suspicious and should be referred via a 2WW pathway. This should not be delayed whilst arranging additional investigations. **Advising weight loss** is inappropriate as, although obesity is a risk factor for gynaecomastia, the presence of a firm mass with nipple changes is concerning for malignancy. **Waiting 2 weeks to review** risks delaying diagnosis and treatment in a potentially serious condition. **Testing for prolactin and gonadotrophins** is useful in suspected gynaecomastia but is not the priority when malignancy is suspected. **Urgent MRI** is not the first-line investigation, as mammography and ultrasound with biopsy are the preferred diagnostic tools for suspected male breast cancer.

Q145 Weight Loss

Answer 3 – **Hyperthyroidism**. The patient is likely to have hyperthyroidism, possibly from Graves' disease. Positive pointers include signs and symptoms of hyperthyroidism and signs suggestive of thyroid eye disease. Management plan would involve a thyroid function test, thyroid autoantibodies including TSH receptor antibodies, referral to the endocrinologist and ophthalmologist and consideration for use of beta-blockers and anti-thyroid medication such as carbimazole. **Addison's disease** typically presents with postural hypotension, hyperpigmentation and electrolyte disturbances (hyponatraemia, hyperkalaemia), which are absent here. **Fibromyalgia** does not cause weight loss, tremors or tachycardia. **Lymphoma** can present with night sweats and weight loss but would typically cause lymphadenopathy rather than diffuse thyroid enlargement with eye signs. **Underlying infection** could cause fatigue and weight loss, but the presence of goitre, tremor and proptosis strongly suggests a thyroid disorder.

Gastrointestinal

6

Q146 Vitamin B12 and/or Folate Deficiency

Answer 3 – **Vitamin B12**. The clinical presentation is consistent with megaloblastic anaemia secondary to vitamin B12 deficiency, as described for this topic. **Vitamin A** deficiency primarily presents as night blindness. **Vitamin B5**, pantothenic acid, is ubiquitous in all diets and specific deficiency is unreported. **Vitamin C** deficiency results in scurvy due to defective collagen formation, notably in bone and connective tissue. **Vitamin E** refers to a range of related compounds which are rarely absent from the diet. Deficiency is usually secondary to malabsorption of fat which would lead to a change in stool consistency and colour; furthermore, symptoms are primarily neurological.

Q147 Acute Cholangitis

Answer 5 – **Ultrasound abdomen**. It is the easiest and simplest investigation, and can rule out the commonest causes, such as gall stones. **Contrast-enhanced CT abdomen and pelvis**: this is more invasive and involves radiation exposure. It is useful in detecting malignancies, abscesses or pancreatitis, but is not the first-line investigation for suspected biliary obstruction. **Endoscopic retrograde cholangiopancreatography** (ERCP) is primarily a therapeutic procedure, not a diagnostic imaging modality. It is used to remove bile duct stones or place stents, but is not typically the first investigation. **Magnetic resonance cholangiopancreatography** (MRCP) is excellent for detailed imaging of the biliary and pancreatic ducts without using contrast. However, it is more expensive and less available than ultrasound, making it more suitable as a follow-up investigation after ultrasound if needed. **Non-contrast CT abdomen and pelvis**: like the contrast-enhanced CT, this is less effective at detecting biliary pathology compared to ultrasound, and involves unnecessary radiation without adding significant value as the initial test.

Q148 Alcoholic Hepatitis

Answer 2 – **Aspartate transferase : alanine transaminase (AST: ALT) ratio ≥ 2.** AST (aspartate aminotransferase) is produced by mitochondria in hepatocytes, skeletal muscle, and cardiac, brain, pancreatic and kidney tissue, while ALT (alanine aminotransferase) is produced only by hepatocytes. In AH, AST levels in blood increase due to mitochondrial damage and ALT activity is inhibited, resulting an AST:ALT > 2. **A Maddery discriminant function ≤ 13**: a Maddery discriminant function (Maddrey score) can be used to estimate mortality risk and disease severity in AH. It is calculated as follows: DF = (4.6 x [prothrombin time (sec) – control prothrombin time (sec)]) + (serum bilirubin mg/dL). A Maddrey score > 32 would be suggestive of AH with a high chance of short-term mortality. However, it is important to note that a high AST:ALT ratio is not specific to alcoholic hepatitis, and so a diagnosis should be confirmed with additional tests. **Jaundice** is a clinical manifestation of liver disease that results from the accumulation of bilirubin in the blood and tissues, leading to a yellowing of the skin and eyes. While jaundice is commonly associated with AH, it is not a specific sign for this condition. Jaundice can occur in many other liver diseases, such as viral hepatitis, autoimmune hepatitis, primary biliary cholangitis and drug-induced liver injury. Therefore, a diagnosis of AH cannot be based solely on the presence of jaundice, but must take into account other clinical, laboratory and imaging findings, as well as a detailed history of alcohol use. **Spider naevi** (spider angiomata) are vascular lesions that consist of a central arteriole surrounded by smaller radiating vessels. While spider naevi are commonly associated with AH, they are not a specific sign for this condition. Spider naevi can occur in many other liver diseases, such as viral hepatitis, primary biliary cholangitis, and cirrhosis of various etiologies. **Tender hepatomegaly** can be indicative of liver inflammation and is a common feature of AH. However, it is not a specific sign for this condition as it can also occur in other types of hepatitis, such as viral or autoimmune hepatitis and fatty liver disease. Therefore, a diagnosis of AH cannot be based solely on the presence of tender hepatomegaly, but must take into account other clinical features and laboratory findings, including an elevated AST:ALT ratio, as well as a history of heavy alcohol use.

Q149 Peritonitis

Answer 5 – **Perforated peptic ulcer**. Points in favour of peptic ulcer are: sudden-onset abdominal pain; long-term use of NSAIDs; abdominal tenderness; and SIRS response such as tachycardia, hypotension, pyrexia. In **ischaemic colitis**, patients will present with colicky abdominal pain, tenderness and cramping associated with rectal bleeding and diarrhoea. **Acute pancreatitis** will present with epigastric pain which radiates to the back, which worsens on lying flat and improves with sitting up and bending forward. There may be history of recent endoscopic retrograde cholangiopancreatography or patient may be known to have gallstones, which are risk factors of acute pancreatitis. In **decompensated liver cirrhosis**, patient will present with abdominal distension, ascites, jaundice, encephalitis and upper GI bleed. **Metformin sensitivity** causes abdominal pain and diarrhoea, but does not cause pyrexia and is normally more chronic.

Q150 Anal Fissure

Answer 4 – **Fibre supplement with stool softener**. This would manage the symptoms and soften and form the stool to be less painful when being passed.

Abdominal ultrasound would give very limited information about the bowel. **Botox injection** would be used if topical ointment and diet assistance did not improve the situation. It would not tackle any underlying dietary issues. **CT colonography scan** would provide full information about the large bowel and associated structures and is better tolerated by patients than a colonoscopy but, unless there are any red flags, this would not be the next step. **No further management needed**: this would not tackle any underlying dietary issues.

Q151 Ascites

Answer 1 – **Broad-spectrum intravenous antibiotics and spironolactone**. This scenario describes a patient with ascites secondary to decompensated liver cirrhosis from alcohol excess. The abdominal pain and fever should cause concern for possible spontaneous bacterial peritonitis (SBP), which is confirmed with the results of the ascitic tap having a large number of white cells, which are mostly neutrophilic. Broad-spectrum IV antibiotics and spironolactone is correct as it involves diuretics to manage the ascites and treats the SBP with broad-spectrum antibiotics (e.g. tazocin or cefotaxime). Antibiotics are initiated even before any bacteria are identified (often takes hours–days for these results) to avoid deterioration of the patient's condition. The diuretics would aim to counter the neuro-hormonal response to portal hypertension and relieve the ascites. **Give ACE inhibitor + spironolactone**: this does include spironolac-tone (aldosterone inhibitor) which can help the ascites, but the ACE inhibitor could cause hypotension or cause an acute kidney injury, best avoided in this acute setting. **Intravenous 0.9% saline infusion + analgesia (paracetamol + codeine)** is incorrect. Analgesia is import-ant for pain, but doesn't address the SBP or ascites. Codeine is often avoided due to side effects of constipation which can precipitate hepatic encephalopathy. Intravenous saline is likely to worsen the ascites due to the sodium load and retention of water. Intravenous fluids may be warranted if the patient was haemodynamically unstable (especially if septic) but should be used cautiously. **Pabrinex infusion** is very important for those reliant on alcohol to prevent complications such as Wernicke's encephalopathy. It would also be prudent to initiate benzodiazepines to prevent alcohol with-drawal whilst an inpatient, but this should be used very cautiously in patients who are encephalopathic. **Therapeutic paracentesis** may be needed at some point during this patient's stay. At this stage, they are not significantly dyspnoeic and it would be sensible to try to relieve ascites with diuretics in the first instance. If this was to fail or the patient started splinting his diaphragm and became very dyspnoeic, then a drain would be warranted.

Q152 Acute Pancreatitis

Answer 3 – **Serum amylase or lipase**. Elevated levels of serum amylase or lipase are classic laboratory findings in acute pancreatitis. **Arterial blood gas** (ABG): while ABG might be useful in assessing the patient's overall condition, it is not specifically indicative of pancreatitis. **Magnetic resonance cholangiopancreatogram** (MRCP) is a useful imaging modality for visualising the pancreatic and bile ducts, but it may not be the most appropriate initial investigation for this patient. It is more commonly used for evaluating chronic pancreatitis or sus-pected biliary obstruction, rather than acute pancreatitis. **Ultrasound scan of abdomen**: while ultrasound can be useful in diagnosing pancreatitis by visualising gallstones or pancreatic inflammation, it may not be as sensitive or specific as serum amylase or lipase levels in the acute setting.

X-ray of abdomen: X-ray is generally not useful in diagnosing pancreatitis. It may reveal non-specific findings such as ileus or non-specific bowel gas patterns but is unlikely to provide a definitive diagnosis of pancreatitis.

Q153 Cholecystitis

Answer 5 – **Ultrasound scan** will give a full clinical picture. If the US is inconclusive, then proceed with a magnetic resonance cholangiopancreatography.

CT abdomen would not show the biliary tree in sufficient detail. **Erect chest X-ray** would be the initial investigation if perforation was expected. **Magnetic resonance cholangiopancreatography** is not indicated at this stage – only if the ultrasound is inconclusive. **No further investigation**: this would not give a full clinical picture as the imaging is crucial to see any stones and impact on the biliary system.

Q154 Malnutrition

Answer 1 – **Calculate her BMI and complete a MUST score.** Although this patient is in a higher risk category for malnutrition (as she is over 65 years old), there is no indication from the information given to suggest that she is currently malnourished. Therefore, the first step would be to screen using her BMI and MUST score. **Take blood tests to assess for micronutrient deficiency**: if she is deemed to be at risk of malnutrition, or is malnourished, then further blood tests may be taken to assess for micronutrient deficiencies and she may be advised to **switch to fortified meals**, and then she could be **prescribed oral food supplements**, if she is able to eat and drink normally. **Commence enteral nutrition via a nasogastric tube**: enteral feeding would only be used if she was unable to tolerate oral nutrition, or was unable to maintain nutrition with oral intake.

Q155 Cirrhosis

Answer 1 – **Anti-mitochondrial antibodies**. These are highly specific for primary biliary cirrhosis. **Anti-smooth muscle antibodies** are associated with other autoimmune hepatitis. **Ceruloplasmin level** checks for Wilson's, **hepatitis B surface antigen** for hepatic cirrhosis, **serum ferritin level** for conditions such as haemochromatosis or is a marker for inflammation.

Q156 Colorectal Tumours

Answer 4 – **Refer for colonoscopy as part of 2-week-wait**. This gives a full clinical picture. Patient may have a hereditary disease such as familial adenomatous polyposis, which would need urgent intervention. **CT colonoscopy** is not as good as direct colonoscopy as samples cannot be taken and there is an associated radiation risk. Assessing **genetic markers** would not be indicated at this stage. It would only be available if tissue had been taken from the father/grandmother. **Proctoscopy** would not give any information concerning the colon – where any tumour is likely to be. **Watch and wait, reviewing the patient in 2 months' time if still symptomatic**: this option would allow for any pathology to increase in size.

Q157 Coeliac Disease

Answer 5 – **Tissue transglutaminase 2**. If coeliac disease is suspected, the serology for total IgA and tTG is the first-choice investigation. **Anti-gliadin antibody** was used historically but is no longer recommended due to its lower sensitivity and specificity compared to tTG–IgA. **Endomysial antibody** (EMA) is also highly specific for coeliac disease but is more labour intensive and expensive than tTG–IgA. It is often used as a confirmatory test if the tTG–IgA is positive.

While a **full blood count** (FBC) may reveal anaemia, which is common in coeliac disease due to malabsorption, it is not diagnostic or specific for coeliac disease.

Human leukocyte antigen (HLA): HLA-DQ2 and HLA-DQ8 testing can help rule out coeliac disease if negative, but is not used as a first-line test because it is less practical and more costly. Almost all individuals with coeliac disease will have one of these HLA types, but many people with these HLA types do not develop coeliac disease.

Q158 Constipation

Answer 4 – **No other management needed at the moment**. The history and examination findings are in keeping with a presentation of opioid-induced constipation. This patient has no symptoms consistent with bowel obstruction or perforation. There is nothing in the history and examination to suggest this patient is critically unwell, sick or dying. **Admission to hospital for administration of intravenous fluids**: there is no evidence of dehydration or systemic illness that would necessitate hospital admission or intravenous fluids. Her observations and blood tests are normal. **Arrange CT colonoscopy scan**: there is no indication for a CT colonoscopy at this point, as the constipation is most likely opioid-induced, and there are no red flags for a more serious underlying condition, such as bowel obstruction or malignancy. **Change her treatment escalation plan to avoid**

future admission: this would be inappropriate given that her current condition does not suggest a need to alter her treatment escalation plan, especially since she is on a full resuscitation plan.

There is no indication for an **urgent referral to colorectal surgeon**. The situation appears to be a straightforward case of opioid-induced constipation.

Q159 Appendicitis

Answer 4 – **Normal WCC and CRP**. A normal WCC and CRP 12 hours from onset of symptoms have a good negative predictive value. A negative pregnancy test helps rule out ectopic pregnancy as the cause of her symptoms. A **normal ultrasound** does not rule out appendicitis. **Absence of vomiting**: not all patients present with vomiting, but most have anorexia and nausea. A **low-grade fever** (< 38) is common with appendicitis. **Normal pulse**: the pulse can be normal.

Q160 Diverticular Disease

Answer 3 – **Contrast CT abdomen**. **Blood cultures** are vitally important but are part of the sepsis six. **Chest X-ray**: projection imaging is 2D. On a chest X-ray, the patient would need to be sat up for 10 minutes prior to the X-ray in an erect position for the free air to show under the diaphragm. This would show a perforation but not an abscess or mass. **MRI abdomen** is slower and gives less information than a contrast CT scan. **Ultrasound scan** would show an abscess or mass but is difficult in larger patients. On its own it would not give enough information.

Q161 Gallstones and Biliary Colic

Answer 5 – **Ultrasound abdomen**. FBC may give a clue of underlying inflammation, LFTs may indicate whether there is any biliary obstruction, and USS is a standard radiological investigation to confirm the diagnosis. Other investigations may also be needed according to the findings of these three tests, but they are not done regularly. **CT scan of abdomen** is less sensitive for gallstones and is not the preferred initial test. **Intraoperative cholangiogram** is used during surgery to assess the bile ducts but is not an initial diagnostic tool. **Magnetic resonance cholangiopancreatography** (MRCP) is more useful if common bile duct obstruction or choledocholithiasis is suspected, but there is no evidence of jaundice or abnormal liver function here. **Plain abdominal radiograph** is not useful in diagnosing gallstones, as most are radiolucent and would not be visible.

Q162 Pancreatic Cancer

Answer 2 – **Biliary stent**. Although the other interventions may be needed as part of the patient's cancer treatment, it is important to address the obstructive jaundice first. A surgical intervention such as a **Whipple procedure (pancreaticoduodenectomy)** or **cholecystectomy** are treatments for localised pancreatic or gallbladder cancer and they wouldn't be performed in someone with metastatic disease. **Commence chemotherapy**: chemotherapy is likely to be considered for the treatment of metastatic pancreatic cancer but cannot be considered in patients until the obstructive jaundice is treated and they have sufficient recovery of the liver function. When considering chemotherapy, other factors also need to be considered, such as the patient's wishes, fitness and comorbidities. **Antibiotics** may have a role if there is any sign of biliary sepsis.

Q163 Gastric Cancer

Answer 3 – **Gastric carcinoma**. Gastric cancer is the most likely – it causes nausea, anorexia and weight loss. Iron deficiency results from chronic blood loss. Risk factors are age and smoking. The lymph node is Virchow's node which is a sign of metastatic spread. **Atrophic gastritis** typically presents with chronic gastritis symptoms and lacks the acute signs of malignancy such as weight loss and a palpable lymph node. **Duodenal ulcer** usually presents with epigastric pain relieved by eating, and it does not typically cause weight loss or a palpable lymph node. **Oesophageal carcinoma** can present with similar systemic symptoms, it typically causes dysphagia (difficulty swallowing) as a prominent symptom.

Pancreatic carcinoma often presents with jaundice, abdominal pain, and sometimes a palpable mass, but not typically with a supraclavicular lymph node.

Q164 Gastro-oesophageal Reflux Disease

Answer 4 – **Gastro-oesophageal reflux disease**. Heartburn is the common presenting complaint for GORD. Presence of risk factors such as smoking, alcohol intake, obesity supports the diagnosis. Acidic taste in the mouth suggests the presence of gastric juice in oral cavity during regurgitation. While **cardiac ischaemia** can cause chest pain, the characteristics of the pain in this case (burning, associated with acid taste, worse when lying down) are more typical of GORD, rather than angina or heart-related pain. **Costochondritis** causes chest pain due to inflammation of the costal cartilage but does not typically involve the burning sensation, acid regurgitation or the positional component related to GORD. While **gastric cancer** can cause abdominal pain, weight loss and other symptoms, it is far less common and typically presents with more severe or progressive symptoms than described here. **Sinus congestion** can cause post-nasal drip and throat irritation, but it does not typically cause retrosternal burning pain or acid regurgitation.

Q165 Haemorrhoids

Answer 4 – **Grade III**. Haemorrhoids that prolapse (cross the dentate line) via defaecation or valsalva manoeuvre, however, need to be reduced manually. Remember that grade III requires manual reduction, whereas **grade II** reduces spontaneously. Haemorrhoids that remain in the rectum are classified as **grade I**. Those that remain prolapsed and cannot be reduced are classified as **grade IV**. **Grade 0** does not exist.

Q166 Inflammatory Bowel Disease

Answer 5 – **Ulcerative colitis**. The patient has the symptoms of IBD, negative tests for **coeliac disease** and **Gastroenteritis**, and no psychiatric symptoms of anorexia nervosa. Positive faecal calprotectin level and UC is more common in non-smokers. **Crohn's disease** is possible but usually presents with more systemic symptoms (e.g. perianal disease, fistulas or strictures) and often skip lesions on imaging. **Diverticulosis** generally causes painless bleeding in older individuals and does not cause chronic diarrhoea with mucus.

Q167 Hepatitis

Answer 1 – **Acute viral hepatitis**. The presentation is most consistent with acute hepatitis, with very elevated hepatocellular enzymes, which suggests liver cell damage. Liver tenderness on palpation is common with acute hepatitis. The elevated ALT is suggestive of liver cell damage – rather than **haemolysis secondary to glucose-6-phosphate dehydrogenase deficiency**, **Crigler–Najjar syndrome** or **Gilbert's syndrome**. The level is too high for chronic damage such as would follow **liver cirrhosis**.

Q168 Hiatus Hernia

Answer 4 – **Hiatus hernia**. **Lung abscess** usually presents with a productive cough, fever and sweats. Chest X-ray shows consolidation with a cavity containing an air fluid level. Upper endoscopy is more diagnostic in **gastric cancer**. If the patient has lung metastasis, it may be seen in chest X-ray. **Emphysema** manifests as hyperinflated lungs in plain X-ray. Retrocardiac opacity with air fluid level in the background of chronic heartburn should arouse the suspicion of hiatus hernia. Abdominal pain and vomiting could be symptoms of obstructed hernia. Pleural effusion is a collection of fluid in the pleural space and is suggested by increased density at the costophrenic angle. **Haemomediastinum**, as the name represents, is the presence of blood in the mediastinum. This is usually related to chest trauma, rupture of the thoracic aorta, aorta or vertebral artery, or a tumour. Non-traumatic cases are rare. X-ray shows widened mediastinum, with straight, smooth and sharply defined margins.

Q169 Hernias

Answer 3 – **Positive cough impulse.** The presence of an expansile cough impulse is almost diagnostic of a hernia. **Multiple palpable lumps** and a **firm consistency** can be seen in various other causes of abdominal masses and will not necessarily be a defining characteristic of a hernia. Similarly, the presence of a **previous surgical scar over the mass**/lump will not confirm the presence of an incisional hernia. **Rebound tenderness** is a sign of peritonitis most commonly seen in acute appendicitis and is not associated with hernias.

Q170 Irritable Bowel Syndrome

Answer 3 – **Hyoscine**. An antispasmodic would be a first-line option for a patient with IBS who could not manage their symptoms with diet and lifestyle changes alone. **Loperamide**, as an anti-motility agent, would not be appropriate for a patient with constipation-dominant IBS. **Amitriptyline** and **citalopram** are second-line therapies for patients who have not been helped by laxatives, loperamide or antispasmodics. **Linaclotide** is a prosecretory agent used for moderate to severe IBS but is typically reserved for cases that do not respond to lifestyle and fibre modifications.

Q171 Hyposplenism/Splenectomy

Answer 2 – **Encapsulated bacterial**. These patients are suspectable to infections caused by encapsulated microorganisms because splenectomy patients are deficient of B cells that produce IgM, which promotes clearance of polysaccharide-encapsulated bacteria as the polysaccharide capsule itself impairs bacterial opsonisation and hence prevents phagocytosis. They are advised to seek help early following any flu-like illnesses as they are susceptible to overwhelming post-splenectomy infection. They will need lifelong antibiotics for bacterial infections. Vaccination is important to all splenectomy patients as they are immune compromised. **Covid-19** risk is not specifically increased due to splenectomy, though general immune function may be slightly affected. **Fungal infections** are more commonly seen in immunocompromised patients (e.g. those with HIV or chemotherapy-induced neutropenia). **Helminth infections** are more associated with poor sanitation and travel exposure rather than asplenia. **Protozoal infections** such as malaria are a risk in endemic areas, but asplenia does not specifically predispose to them beyond a higher severity risk in cases of Plasmodium infection.

Q172 Gastrointestinal Perforation

Answer 5 – **Small or large bowel**. Fixed portions of the bowel (e.g. proximal jejunum and distal ileum) are more susceptible to injury than mobile portions. Functional closed loops of bowel can sustain single or multiple blow-out perforations of their anti-mesenteric border, due to raised intra-luminal pressure. The **anus** is unlikely to be perforated as a result of a high-speed collision, as it is fixed. Perforation of the anus usually occurs via direct trauma, e.g. insertion of a foreign object. The **appendix** is unlikely to be perforated as the result of a high-speed collision, as it is protected by other loops of bowel.

The risk factors for **hypopharynx** occurring are mainly related to oesophageal catheterisation or trachea intubation. The patient would present with neck pain, odynophagia, torticollis or retrosternal pain. Perforation of the **oesophagus** is usually the result of an endoscopic procedure, variceal disruption, tumour erosion or excessive vomiting. There is no history of this.

Q173 Abdominal Distension

Answer 2 – **Decompensated liver disease**. Risk factors of excessive alcohol intake, stigmata of chronic liver disease (icterus, spider naevi) and presence of ascites on examination make decompensated liver disease the most likely explanation for this patient's presentation. The clinical features are not in keeping with **small bowel obstruction, functional bloating, colorectal cancer or small intestinal bacterial overgrowth**.

Q174 Infectious Colitis

Answer 1 – **Campylobacter jejuni**. Campylobacter jejuni is the most likely pathogen causing this patient's infectious colitis, as it is a common cause of bacterial gastroenteritis associated with travel and is known to cause bloody diarrhoea. **Escherichia coli, Clostridium difficile** and **norovirus** cause diarrhoea but it is less likely to be bloody. Clostridium difficile usually follows prolonged courses of antibiotics. **Coxiella burnetii** is the cause of Q fever, which is not associated with diarrhoea.

Q175 Infectious Diarrhoea

Answer 2 – **Advise patient to stay home, drink fluid and get plenty of rest**. Overall, the best course of action is to advise the patient to stay home, drink plenty of fluids and get rest. If their symptoms worsen or persist for more than a few days, they should seek medical attention. The patient's symptoms suggest that they may have acquired an infection, likely from their recent trip to South Asia. **Isolate the patient**: this may be necessary in certain cases, but it is not warranted in this situation as the patient is not exhibiting severe symptoms and is not known to have a highly contagious disease. **Admit to the hospital**: likewise, hospital admission is not necessary in this case as the patient's symptoms are mild. **Prescribing broad-spectrum antibiotics**: without knowing the specific type of infection, this can lead to antibiotic resistance and other complications. **Collect a faecal sample and send for microbiological culture**: this is a good option to determine the exact cause of the illness, but it is not necessary in this case as the patient's symptoms are mild and they can recover with rest, fluids and supportive care.

Q176 Intestinal Ischaemia

Answer 2 – **Mesenteric artery embolus**. The short history, episode of diarrhoea, background of atrial fibrillation and pain out of proportion with examination are all associated with acute arterial embolus, therefore this is the most likely cause. Management initially involves ABCDE assessment and resuscitation. A CT angiogram is likely to be the most useful next investigation if available and if the patient is haemodynamically stable. **Mesenteric vein thrombosis** would typically present with a more insidious history. There may be a history of VTE or causes of a hypercoagulable state (factor V Leiden, Protein C deficiency). The patient may be younger and the pain normally unrelated to food. **Non–occlusive ischaemia** is more likely in the presence of a condition causing decreased cardiac output, such as septic shock, cardiogenic shock or acute heart failure. It may also be seen in patients who have had abdominal surgery – for example, aortic aneurysm repair.

In **mesenteric artery thrombosis**, you would expect patient risk factors for atherosclerosis, such as smoking, diabetes, high cholesterol, cardiac history. The history is commonly acute-on-chronic with pre-existing abdominal symptoms, often related to food. **Chronic colonic ischaemia** may be due to atherosclerosis or hypoperfusion of another cause. It is common in elderly, comorbid patients and would not present as an emergency like in this scenario.

Q177 Intestinal Obstruction and Ileus

Answer 4 – **Nasogastric tube insertion and observe on ward**. This is the correct answer as the patient is presenting with acute abdominal pain, nausea, vomiting, abdominal distension and tachycardia, which could suggest a possible blockage of the intestine. This requires immediate medical attention, and the patient needs to be resuscitated with fluids and a nasogastric tube for decompression of the abdomen. **Reassure the patient and send her home following fluid replacement**: this is incorrect as it does not address the underlying cause of the patient's symptoms. **Abdominal angiogram** and **colonoscopy** are probably irrelevant and there are better investigations at a later stage. **Direct straight to the theatre for bowel resection**: this is incorrect as it is too invasive and should only be considered if less invasive measures have failed.

Q178 Change in Bowel Habit

Answer 3 – **CT colonography**. The patient has multiple comorbidities and a long-standing cardiac history. Use anti-coagulants and lower the risk of perforation.

Colonoscopy: reference standard; not advised in patients with long-standing cardiac and mobility issues. **CT colonography** is better tolerated and has similar outcomes. **Flexible sigmoidoscopy** is not sufficiently complete to investigate altered bowel habit and positive FIT. **Capsule colonoscopy** is currently only available in pilot trusts and not utilised nationwide. A **water-soluble enema** is no longer advised unless needed for patients with potential perforation and who are high risk for exploratory surgery.

Q179 Intussusception

Answer 1 – **Abdominal ultrasound**. Abdominal ultrasound has high sensitivity and specificity when performed by an experienced sonographer. **Chest X-ray** is not useful in diagnosing intussusception but may be done if perforation is suspected. **CT chest, abdomen and pelvis**, **gastroscopy** and **diagnostic peritoneal lavage** would not be appropriate first-line investigations.

Q180 Malabsorption

Answer 1 – **Colestyramine**. The main differential is between recurrence of Crohn's disease and bile acid diarrhoea following her terminal ileal resection. Reassuring investigations and improving weight make active Crohn's disease less likely and so **infliximab** is unlikely to improve symptoms. Bile acid diarrhoea is therefore the most likely cause and can be treated empirically with bile acid binders such as colestyramine. A **gluten-free diet trial** is a treatment for coeliac disease which would need confirming first with either strongly positive serology or duodenal biopsies. **Pancreatic enzyme replacement** is a treatment for pancreatic exocrine insufficiency. **Mesalazine** is a treatment for colitis and not indicated here.

Q181 Liver Failure

Answer 1 – **Alcoholic hepatitis**. The presentation of jaundice, right upper quadrant tenderness and disorientation suggest acute liver failure with a hepatic encephalopathy. This is supported with hyperbilirubinaemia and high prothrombin time. The AST/ALT ratio > 2 suggests alcoholic hepatitis, and is not characteristic of any of the other causes. **Ascending cholangitis** usually presents with a fever (Charcot's triad – fever, jaundice, right upper quadrant pain) or Reynolds' pentad (Charcot's triad plus shock and altered mental status). **Biliary obstruction** (e.g. due to gallstones or malignancy) would cause significantly raised alkaline phosphatase (ALP) and gamma-glutamyl transferase (GGT), which are only mildly elevated here. **Hepatitis C** rarely presents as acute liver failure and is more commonly chronic and asymptomatic in early stages. **Paracetamol overdose** typically causes severely elevated ALT and AST (often > 1000 IU/L), whereas this case follows the enzyme pattern of alcohol-related liver disease.

Q182 Necrotising Enterocolitis

Answer 3 – **Haemodynamic resuscitation**. This question assesses the ability of the candidate to manage a critically unwell patient. The child has got necrotising enterocolitis. All options are part of management; here, the best next step is to be determined. Investigations are critical in guiding the treatment, but patient should be stable enough to have these investigations, therefore the best next step is hemodynamic resuscitation. The patient will need **Abdominal X-ray** and to have **blood gases** tested but, in this scenario, haemodynamic resuscitation takes precedence. **Intravenous antibiotics** are essential for treating NEC but should be administered after initial resuscitation. **Surgical review** is necessary if there are signs of perforation or peritonitis, but immediate stabilisation takes precedence before surgical intervention.

Q183 Diarrhoea

Answer 5 – **Urgent transfer to the surgical assessment unit**. The patient's presentation with severe abdominal pain, intermittent bloody diarrhoea, fever, tachycardia, hypotension and localized tenderness with guarding in the left iliac fossa suggests a potentially serious and acute intra-abdominal condition. The combination of these symptoms raises concerns for conditions such as acute diverticulitis with possible complications (e.g. perforation or abscess), ischaemic colitis or other serious surgical pathologies. The **2-week-wait referral to the colorectal team** is for non-urgent cases suspected of having colorectal cancer or other chronic conditions. This patient requires immediate assessment, not delayed referral. **Oral co-amoxiclav**: while antibiotics may be part of the treatment for conditions such as diverticulitis, oral antibiotics are not sufficient given the severity of the symptoms, and initial management should be in a hospital setting with intravenous antibiotics if needed. **Oral loperamide**: this anti-diarrhoeal medication is contraindicated in the presence of bloody diarrhoea and potential bowel obstruction or severe colitis, as it can worsen the condition. While **stool culture** may be useful to identify an infectious cause, it does not address the immediate need for surgical evaluation and is not the next most appropriate step.

Q184 Oesophageal Cancer

Answer 5 – **Pneumonia. Dumping syndrome** is a late complication of oesophagectomy. **Anastomotic stricture** is also a late complication of oesophagectomy. **Anastomotic leak** usually occurs within the first 2 weeks after oesophagectomy but affects 6 in 100 people (6%). **Conduit necrosis** is a rare but very serious complication and its incidence is roughly 1–3%. Pulmonary complications such as **pneumonia** are the most common early complications post-oesophagectomy, occurring in 16–67% of patients.

Q185 Peptic Ulcer Disease and Gastritis

Answer 1 – **1 month PPI trial and review after 4 weeks. Referral for upper GI endoscopy**: patient does not have alarm symptoms necessitating urgent endoscopy, even though he is over 55 years. Helicobacter pylori has been excluded already. The priority is to provide a trial of treatment and assess response; if he has ongoing symptoms, he is likely to be offered a referral for gastroscopy. Despite the jaundiced tinge to his eyes, his LFTs are normal which indicates the absence of hepatitis / liver failure. His drinking habit is a risk factor for cancer of the upper GI tract, and needs addressing. Hepatitis A is particularly common in low- and middle-income countries with poor sanitary conditions. Helicobacter pylori exclusion and PPI trial are the first steps of management on algorithm. **Send him home with antacids and lifestyle advice and review after 4 weeks**: the patient should not be sent home with antacids only for 4 weeks without investigating differential diagnosis. **Abdominal CT scan** is not warranted at this stage, as there are no red flag symptoms (e.g. weight loss, anaemia, persistent vomiting). **Blood tests including hepatitis screening and serum lipase** are unnecessary, as there is no indication of liver disease or pancreatitis.

Q186 Jaundice

Answer 2 – **Ascending cholangitis**. This patient has risk factors for gallstones (45, fertile, raised BMI). In the absence of jaundice, the most likely diagnosis would be **acute cholecystitis**. However, combination of RUQ pain, fever and jaundice, otherwise known as the Charcot's triad, is in keeping with a diagnosis of cholangitis. The presence of fever suggests an acute inflammatory process, which is less likely with **Gilbert's disease** and **fatty liver disease**. **Pancreatic carcinoma** often presents as painless jaundice associated with red flag symptoms such as weight loss and loss of appetite.

Q187 Perianal Abscesses and Fistulae

Answer 3 – **Incision and drainage**. Perineal abscess should be first treated by incision and drainage. **Antibiotics** can be given after this. **Fistulectomy** should be offered only after confirmation of an existing fistula. **Laxatives** may be helpful in patients with history of constipation. **Topical glyceryl trinitrate ointment** is useful in anal fissures, but has no use in perineal abscess.

Q188 Viral Gastroenteritis

Answer 1 – **Arrange emergency admission to hospital**. From the vignette, it appears this patient probably has norovirus. Due to her comorbidities, she has many risk factors for dehydration. Looking at the clinical picture and this patient's observations, she likely has severe dehydration and should be admitted to hospital for close monitoring of renal function and careful administration of intravenous fluids. **Place the patient into isolation, encourage oral intake and review in 24 hours**: if the patient was not displaying signs of dehydration, this could be considered. **Commence a beta-blocker and anti-coagulation for atrial fibrillation**: the patient is not known to be in atrial fibrillation, therefore an ECG would be required for a formal diagnosis before this could be considered. **Collect a stool culture**: this could be indicated if the residential home is able to manage a norovirus outbreak, but would not be the first step in this patient's immediate management. **Commence loperamide to stop diarrhoea**: this is not indicated.

Q189 Viral Hepatitides

Answer 5 – **He has previously had a hepatitis B infection, which has resolved**. The serology results show HBsAg negative (no active infection), anti-core antigen positive (evidence of past infection) and anti-HBs positive (immunity, either from past infection or vaccination), indicating a resolved hepatitis B infection with immunity. **Chronic hepatitis B infection** would require a positive HBsAg for more than 6 months. **Acute hepatitis B infection** would typically show HBsAg positive and anti-HBc IgM positive. **Vaccination without prior infection** would show anti-HBs positive but anti-core negative (vaccines do not generate anti-core antibodies). **Never having had a hepatitis B infection or vaccination** would show negative HBsAg, anti-HBc and anti-HBs.

Q190 Volvulus

Answer 2 – **Flexible sigmoidoscopy and flatus tube**. The clinical assessment has confirmed a likely case of volvulus. The most appropriate treatment for this closed loop obstruction is decompression with a sigmoidoscopy and flatus tube. **All other options**: these would not correct the closed loop obstruction and therefore could lead to perforation of the bowel.

Q191 Acute Abdominal Pain

Answer 2 – **Pregnancy test**. Lower right-sided abdominal pain, nausea, vomiting and reduced appetite could indicate several conditions, including appendicitis, gastrointestinal issues, gynaecological problems or UTI. Given the patient's age and gender, it is crucial to consider ectopic pregnancy as this is a potentially life-threatening condition. Now the question appears slightly false as, when urine is taken from a patient, they would probably do **urinalysis** while waiting for the pregnancy test. But pregnancy test is more 'essential' than urinalysis. **Troponin** is a test to diagnose cardiac issues – she has none of the right symptoms. **Liver function tests** may point to liver-related issues but that is unlikely with these symptoms. **Ultrasound** would be very useful – but it is a next step.

Q192 Bleeding from Lower GI Tract

Answer 2 – **CT angiogram**. The patient has signs of active bleeding and observations that suggest haemodynamic compromise, therefore the key is to act urgently. Thus, a **plain CT**, which is a diagnostic investigation, is not correct; furthermore, a plain scan without contrast is poor at finding a bleeding point. According to the guidelines published by Oakland, and the associated scoring system, this patient would score at least 10 and therefore warrants an urgent CT angiogram to identify a source of bleeding. At this point, a decision can be made regarding which therapeutic intervention, including **all other options** on the list, is indicated.

Q193 Vomiting

Answer 5 – **Nasogastric tube insertion**. The key to this question is which intervention to perform *first*. The brown offensive-smelling vomitus is likely faeculent vomiting secondary to bowel obstruction, and urgent NG decompression of the GI tract can prevent fatal aspiration. Fluid resuscitation should be performed, as the clinical examination reveals signs of dehydration. The combination of intravenous resuscitation and NG decompression is often referred to as 'drip and suck'. As bowel obstruction is assumed, **administration of metoclopramide** could cause perforation due to its prokinetic effect, and as such should be avoided. **Blood transfusion** has no clear role in this patient, as there is no obvious evidence of bleeding (vomitus description in keeping with faeculent vomiting rather than coffee-ground vomiting), and no mention of low haemoglobin. Eventual **transfer to theatre** for this patient may be required, for treatment of his presumably obstructed inguinal hernia – however, he should be resuscitated appropriately prior to this. His tachycardia may improve with fluid resuscitation. **Intravenous antibiotics** may be indicated in this patient; however, the first and most important step is decompression and resuscitation.

Q194 Bleeding from Upper GI Tract

Answer 4 – **Immediate activation of the major haemorrhage protocol**. This patient presents with a major haemorrhage, as evidenced by their haemodynamic instability despite adequate fluid resuscitation. Whilst the other answers may be correct in some circumstances, activation of the major haemorrhage is the most important next step in management, which is what the question is asking. Patients with major variceal bleeding such as this should undergo endoscopy as soon as they have been stabilised, rather than within 24 hours. **Further 1 L intravenous crystalloid**: further intravenous fluids may be appropriate; however, this patient has already received a large volume, and any more fluids should accompany the major haemorrhage bundle of blood products. **CT angiogram** can be useful when the source of bleeding cannot be identified endoscopically, but is not usually a first-line investigation. **Intravenous vitamin K 10 mg** may be appropriate if coagulation is deranged as a result of nutritional deficiencies, but will not stop the bleeding or stabilise the patient in the short term.

Q195 Change in Stool Colour

Answer 4 – **Oesophagogastroduodenoscopy**. This patient has features of an upper gastrointestinal bleed. She has been on iron tablets, which tend to cause darkening of the stool towards a black colour, commonly with associated constipation. Being on iron tablets can sometimes make it hard for melaena to be identified, but considering this patient's stools became more loose and were described as sticky, this is more in keeping with true melaena. Melaena describes the features of blood which has been digested, causing it to have classically 'tar-like' appearances: liquid consistency, black, shiny and sticky. For the blood to have been digested, the bleeding source is often in the upper gastrointestinal tract (oesophagus, stomach or duodenum), although this is rarely seen in bleeds from the caecum or ascending colon. This patient's bloods not only show anaemia, but also a disproportionate rise in the urea compared to the creatinine which, again, points towards an upper GI bleed. The history of osteoarthritis may mean that the patient takes non-steroidal anti-inflammatory drugs (NSAIDs) which are associated with peptic ulceration. **Colonoscopy** or **flexible sigmoidoscopy** would be a sensible option if the patient described haematochezia (fresh blood passed per rectum). A **stool culture** is helpful when patients have haematochezia, as infections (salmonella, shigella or campylobacter) can cause bloody diarrhoea, but not typically melaena. A **faecal calprotectin** can screen for bowel inflammation and is useful for investigation or monitoring of inflammatory bowel disease (IBD), which is less likely in this scenario.

Q196 Food Intolerance

Answer 4 – **Serum IgE blood test**. This is the correct answer as the patient presented with features suggestive of an IgE-mediated food allergy which has the potential to be life-threatening. A serum IgE blood test would be the most appropriate next step in his management to identify the presence of specific IgE antibodies. Providing an epinephrine auto-injector should be considered as life-saving treatment can be administered rapidly. An **oral food challenge** is incorrect as this should only be considered in appropriately controlled medical settings and is not appropriate as an initial step due to potential risk of anaphylaxis.

Provide reassurance and discharge home: this is incorrect due to the presence of concerning clinical features from the history and examination. **Review in 2 weeks with a food diary**: this is inappropriate as it risks delayed diagnosis and increased allergen exposure. A **trial elimination diet** is incorrect as, without confirmation of specific IgE antibodies and access to an epinephrine auto-injector, this is not recommended in potential IgE-mediated food allergy.

Q197 Chronic Abdominal Pain

Answer 3 – **Refer the patient for a 2-week-wait colonoscopy**. The patient has unexplained weight loss, abdominal pain and a positive FIT; therefore a 2-week wait referral should be considered. He also has a change in bowel habit which is an additional red flag for bowel cancer. Other pointers include potentially unhealthy diet which is a risk factor for bowel cancer. **Prescribe an antispasmodic**: antispasmodics would be useful in irritable bowel syndrome. **Recommend dietary modifications and lifestyle changes**: useful if irritable bowel syndrome is suspected; however, other diagnoses have not yet been excluded. **Stool microscopy** would be useful if gastroenteritis was suspected; however, there is no history of vomiting, no fever, no recent travel, no blood in stool, and loose stools would be expected to be more frequent. **Urinalysis**: there are no urinary symptoms or loin pain, making urological pathology unlikely.

Q198 Decreased Appetite

Answer 3 – **Diabetic ketoacidosis**. High blood sugar and ketones in urine favour the diagnosis of diabetic ketoacidosis. All of the listed conditions can cause the symptoms described in the first half of the question. However, the symptoms described in the second half of the question, along with the lab findings, point towards DKA as the most likely diagnosis. **Acute mesenteric ischaemia** typically presents with severe abdominal pain out of proportion to examination findings and is not associated with hyperglycaemia or ketonuria. **Acute pancreatitis** would present with epigastric tenderness and elevated lipase/amylase, which are not mentioned here. **Infectious gastroenteritis** can cause vomiting, but it does not explain the hyperglycaemia, ketonuria or metabolic acidosis. **Ureteric colic** would present with severe, colicky flank pain and haematuria, which are absent in this case.

Q199 Faecal Incontinence

Answer 1 – **Damage to the external anal sphincter**. Third- or fourth-degree tears during vaginal deliveries can lead to injury to the anal sphincters, particularly the external anal sphincter, compromising its ability to maintain continence. This is supported by studies such as a systematic review by Wilson et al. (2020), which found that obstetric anal sphincter injuries significantly increased the risk of faecal incontinence. **Damage to the internal anal sphincter** or **damage to the puborectalis** is unlikely as these typically result in different patterns of incontinence. **Damage to the rectoanal**

inhibitory reflex is less likely as it is associated with neurologic conditions rather than obstetric trauma. **Rectocele** primarily causes symptoms related to obstructed defaecation rather than faecal incontinence.

Q200 Lump in Groin

Answer 5 – **Request an urgent surgical review**. The patient's age, gender and BMI place him at high risk of an inguinal hernia. He has red flag symptoms (pain, loose stools) for strangulation, which requires urgent surgical review. His weight loss is long-standing and a likely red herring. **Refer to the sexual health clinic**: his recent history of unprotected sex should prompt discussion on sexual health screening regardless; however, his symptoms of pain and loose stools are not suggestive of infective lymphadenopathy as the likely cause. **Reassuring and safety-netting** is inappropriate as a strangulated hernia requires immediate intervention. **Screening for blood-borne viruses** may be relevant given his unprotected oral sex exposure but is not the priority in this acute setting. **Ultrasound with Doppler** may confirm strangulation but should not delay an urgent surgical review, which is the most time-sensitive and critical step.

Q201 Melaena

Answer 1 – **Bleeding oesophageal varices**. The patient has metabolic risk factors and works in the hospitality industry with daily alcohol availability. The presentation with melaena, followed by haematemesis, suggests a cause proximal to the ligament of Trietz. Thrombocytopaenia is an indicator of splenic sequestration of platelets associated with portal hypertension due to cirrhosis of the liver (though non-cirrhotic causes are recognised). **Colonic carcinoma** typically causes lower GI bleeding (bright red blood or occult blood in stool) rather than haematemesis and melaena. **Gastric carcinoma** can cause upper GI bleeding but usually presents more insidiously with weight loss and anaemia rather than sudden massive bleeding. **Haemorrhoids** cause painless bright red rectal bleeding, not melaena or haematemesis. **Mallory–Weiss tear** causes self-limiting haematemesis, often after repeated vomiting, and does not usually result in significant haemodynamic instability.

Q202 Abdominal Mass

Answer 3 – **Intussusception**. Intussusception is one of the surgical emergencies where a portion of the bowel telescopes into the lumen of an adjoining segment leading to intestinal obstruction. It is most common in infants between 6 and 9 months old. If left untreated, it may lead to bowel necrosis, perforation, peritonitis and death. It is believed to be associated with preceding viral infection resulting in enlarged Peyer's patches acting as a 'lead point'. It commonly presents with a classical triad of intermittent abdominal pain, vomiting and passage of redcurrant jelly stool. A sausage shaped mass may be felt in the right hypochondrium. Quick resuscitation, bowel decompression and reduction of intussusception are important. **Choledochal cyst** is a congenital dilation of the bile ducts, typically presenting with jaundice, abdominal pain, and a right upper quadrant mass, but not with bloody stool or the severe pain pattern seen here. **Hydronephrosis**: this refers to dilation of the renal pelvis due to obstruction of urine flow and can cause abdominal mass and pain, but it does not cause bloody stools or the acute pain pattern seen here. **Viral hepatitis** may present with jaundice, malaise and liver enlargement, but it is unlikely to cause the symptoms described in this case, especially the bloody stool. **Wilms tumour** is a paediatric kidney cancer that may present with an abdominal mass, but it does not typically cause bloody stools or the acute pain episodes seen with intussusception.

Q203 Nausea

Answer 5 – **Ondansetron**. Substantial unintentional weight loss over a short period of time should be immediately concerning for undiagnosed malignancy. The examination findings of cachexia and palpable nodules in his umbilicus and left supraclavicular fossa should be concerning specifically for GI malignancy – describing a Sister Mary Joseph Nodule, and Virchow's node, respectively. Centrally acting antiemetics should help to settle this patient's symptoms, whilst endoscopic and radiological investigations are performed. **Metoclopramide** and **domperidone** should be avoided until you are sure there is no evidence of obstruction (e.g. gastric outflow obstruction in this case – nausea after eating may be caused by delayed gastric emptying). **Amitriptyline** has no role in nausea; **levomepromazine** can cause antimuscarinic effects with cyclizine.

Ondansetron is the answer as it has no interaction with cyclizine and acts centrally.

Q204 Perianal Symptoms

Answer 5 – **Topical glyceryl trinitrate**. This is correct as the patient likely has an anal fissure; this will help relax the anorectal muscles and relieve the pain. **Mebendazole** is incorrect – it would be used to treat threadworms, a common parasitic infection in children. **Oral antibiotics** is incorrect, as there is no evidence of infection; this would be appropriate for an anorectal abscess. **Rubber band ligation** is incorrect, as it is more likely an anal fissure, due to the pain, whereas this would be correct for haemorrhoids. **Surgical haemor-rhoidectomy** is incorrect, and would only be appropriate for large external haemorrhoids.

The correct answer is topical glyceryl trinitrate as the patient likely has an anal fissure from the history of constipation and blood on wiping. As the questions asks for the most appropriate *initial* man-agement, this is a good starting point as it is best to approach management in the order: conservative, medical and surgical options.

Q205 Rectal Prolapse

Answer 1 – **Commence a trial of laxatives and arrange colorectal surgical review**.

This patient has a clinical diagnosis of a rectal prolapse. There is no clinical evidence of bowel obstruction, so an **urgent CT scan of her abdomen** is not indicated. Ultimately, this patient needs to be reviewed by the colorectal team and ideally should not be discharged without the prolapse being reduced first. She can then be considered for surgical management on a semi-elective basis, provided she is fit enough. It would be appropriate to trial some laxatives and offer advice about dietary fibre in the meantime. If there are any red flags for malignancy, the patient should also have an urgent '2-week-wait' colorectal referral. **Giving an enema and asking the GP to follow up** is insufficient, as it does not address the underlying cause or long-term management. **Manually attempting to reduce the prolapse** is not appropriate unless it is acutely incarcerated and causing ischae-mia. **Routine outpatient colorectal referral** may delay necessary intervention, and inpatient assessment ensures timely management.

Q206 Organomegaly

Answer 3 – **Schistosomiasis**. The scenario is typical for schistosomia-sis. **Amoebic abscess** of the liver can cause symptoms such as fever, abdominal pain and hepatosplenomegaly. However, it causes neither eosinophilia nor blood in the urine. **Malaria** can cause symptoms such as fever, fatigue and abdominal pain, but it typically presents with cyclic fevers, not persistent symptoms over 3 months. Additionally, hepatosplenomegaly is less commonly associated with malaria compared to other diseases like schistosomiasis. **Tuberculosis** would present with respiratory symptoms, not hepatosplenomegaly. **Typhoid** gives abdominal pain and fatigue – but typically presents with high fever.

7 General Duties

Q207 Adverse Drug Effects

Answer 1 – **The medication should be suspected as causing an adverse drug reaction.** The Yellow Card system encourages a low threshold for reporting, and suspicion alone is a valid cause for reporting. It is not a requirement that **the medication should be under the black triangle monitoring scheme, should have prescription-only status** or **should already have proven causality.** The **medication should not be a vaccine**: biological agents and vaccines may cause adverse reactions and do fall under the reporting scheme.

Q208 Disease Prevention/Screening

Answer 1 – **A negative result makes the condition less likely.** In a highly Sensitive test, a Negative result will effectively rule Out the condition in question – this can be remembered as 'SnOut'". **The test is prone to producing false negatives:** such a test will have very few false negatives. **A positive result makes the condition more likely:** a positive result may indeed rule in but does not necessarily do so. It is in the context of a highly Specific test that a Positive result effectively rules In a condition – this can be remembered as 'SpPin'. A highly sensitive test will have few false negatives and so few cases of the condition are missed. **The test has a high positive predictive value:** the more sensitive a test, the greater is its negative (as opposed to positive) predictive value. **The test is unlikely to produce false positives** is incorrect, as sensitivity does not measure the false-positive rate.

Q209 Metastatic Disease

Answer 5 – **Surgery to remove right kidney followed by adjuvant chemotherapy.** Treatment should be aimed at removal of the primary tumour if possible, plus addressing any secondary tumour burden thereafter. This latter may be done in several ways guided by factors such as prognosis, treatment side effects and patient preference. **Blood transfusion followed by referral to urology** is not necessary unless the patient has severe anaemia or active bleeding. **Chemotherapy followed by surgery to remove the liver mass** is incorrect, as RCC is poorly responsive to traditional chemotherapy, and nephrectomy is typically prioritised. **Chemotherapy followed by surgery to remove the right kidney** is incorrect because nephrectomy is generally the first step unless the patient is not fit for surgery. **Surgery to remove the liver mass followed by adjuvant chemotherapy** is incorrect, as nephrectomy is the primary treatment for RCC, and liver metastases are often treated with systemic therapy rather than surgery.

Q210 Fit Notes

Answer 5 – **Unfit for work for 6 weeks**. This question is looking for an understanding of when a fit note is required for duration of sickness (> 5 days), and also for an appreciation of job role in relation to what may require a fit note. In this question the patient is a manual labourer working in a contaminated and dangerous environment. **Fit for work** and **May be fit for work with workplace adaptations** are clearly incorrect as these options are completely unreasonable. **Unfit for work for 2 weeks and GP to review** is incorrect as it is a waste of the patient's time and NHS resources to ask the GP to review, given that the orthopaedic team know she will be non-weight bearing for 6 weeks. **May be fit for work with amended duties** is also incorrect as this fails to appreciate her job, most aspects of which she will frequently be precluded from, and makes no reference to the dangerous environment she works in. Thus, 'Unfit for work for 6 weeks' is the best option as this gives the patient certainty, and does not require further appointments to re-sign the fit note or review her unfit-for-work status.

Q211 Multi-organ Dysfunction Syndrome

Answer 5 – **Persistent, uncontrolled systemic inflammation**. Systemic inflammatory response syndrome (SIRS) is a condition that can arise from a variety of severe clinical insults, including pancreatitis, which is the case in this scenario. SIRS involves a widespread inflammatory response throughout the body, which, if uncontrolled, can lead to multiple organ dysfunction or failure.

MODS occurs when the body's response to this widespread inflammation becomes dysregulated, leading to the failure of multiple organ systems. The transition from SIRS to MODS is typically driven by persistent and uncontrolled systemic inflammation. In this case, the woman's pancreatitis initiated SIRS, which then escalated into MODS. The most common and well-recognised mechanism for this progression is the ongoing inflammatory response that cannot be adequately controlled, resulting in widespread organ damage.

Infection spread to multiple organs could potentially cause MODS, but there is no specific indication from the question that an infection has spread. The scenario describes the progression as part of the inflammatory process, rather than an infection per se. **Inadequate fluid resuscitation** could exacerbate the condition, particularly in the setting of sepsis or severe dehydration, but it is not the primary mechanism for the progression from SIRS to MODS. **Genetic predisposition to organ failure** and **Delayed immune response** could play a role in the individual's susceptibility to developing MODS, but the most direct and common cause in this clinical context is the persistent, uncontrolled systemic inflammation.

Q212 Sepsis

Answer 2 – **Commence intravenous fluid resuscitation**. According to sepsis six, initial management of sepsis is 'give oxygen, give intravenous antibiotics, give intravenous fluid and take blood culture, measure urine output, measure lactate level'. Intravenous fluid should be commenced first – it is the correct answer.

Blood capillary glucose measurement is not a criterion on sepsis six. Do not **estimate urine output**: this must be measured accurately. Intravenous antibiotics should be commenced, not **oral antibiotics**. **Oxygen titrated to achieve an oxygen saturation 92–94%**: target oxygen saturations > 94% (88–92% if at risk of carbon dioxide retention – e.g. in COPD (Chronic Obstructive Pulmonary Disease)). So all other options are incorrect.

Q213 Acid-Base Abnormality

Answer 2 – **Metabolic acidosis with partial respiratory compensation**. A pH of 7.16 is an acidosis, which rules out **metabolic alkalosis with respiratory compensation** and **respiratory alkalosis with no compensation**. The pCO_2 is low; its level therefore does not make sense with the pH and we can deduce that the acidosis is metabolic. This is confirmed by the high lactate and low base excess and rules out **respiratory acidosis with partial metabolic compensation**. As the pH is abnormal, this is not a compensated picture and we can rule out **metabolic acidosis with full respiratory compensation**.

Q214 Delirium

Answer 1 – **CAM**. The Confusion Assessment Method (CAM) is a tool for identifying delirium. It has more than 90% sensitivity. A positive or negative result depends on four criteria: acute onset and fluctuating course; inattention; disorganised thinking; altered levels of consciousness. The CAM is considered to indicate delirium if both features 1 and 2 are present, with at least one of features 3 or 4. **CURB-65** is used to assess severity and mortality risk in community-acquired pneumonia, not cognitive impairment. **Glasgow Blatchford score** is for assessing upper gastrointestinal bleeding severity and need for intervention. **HEART** score is used for risk stratification in acute coronary syndrome (ACS). **PESI score** is for prognosticating pulmonary embolism (PE) severity and mortality risk.

Q215 Drug Overdose

Answer 1 – **Amitriptyline.** Amitriptyline is a tricyclic antidepressant and therefore has anticholinergic effects. This explains his elevated heart rate, dry oral cavity, dilated pupils, drowsiness and urinary retention leading to a palpable bladder. **Cocaine** use could lead to an elevated heart rate and dilated pupils, but is associated with agitation rather than drowsiness and wouldn't account for the dry oral cavity or urinary retention. **Diazepam** overdose would cause drowsiness, but not account for the other signs and symptoms. **Fentanyl** overdose would also cause drowsiness, but the patient's pupils would be constricted. **Paracetamol** overdose would not cause dilated pupils, dry oral cavity or urinary retention.

Q216 Death and Dying

Answer 2 – **End of life care should be offered and promptly instituted**. This patient has incurable disease and is clearly nearing the end of life. Further distressing interventions (e.g. **bilateral chest drains** or an **echocardiogram**) should be avoided. **Refer for dialysis**: dialysis is interventional and would be highly distressing. **Give intravenous calcium chloride 20 ml of 10%, with 10 units of insulin and dextrose**: calcium chloride would be at a dose of 10 ml of 10% but would only be of short-lived cardio-protection. End of life care is appropriate and should be quickly arranged. Sensitive communication and whole patient management is key.

Q217 Deteriorating Patient

Answer 5 – **Set up a 0.9% saline solution**. Following an ABCDE assessment, under C (circulation), you would notice that this lady is significantly hypotensive. Therefore, the most appropriate next course of action would be to start intravenous fluids to improve her BP before moving on. You would also likely **request a senior review**, **arrange full blood count** and possibly **arrange admission to ITU**. However, these would all come following your initial assessment and implementation of acutely life-saving treatments. **Arrange sedation**: sedating this patient would be high risk and should only be done by a senior clinician when appropriate.

Q218 Mental Capacity Concerns

Answer 5 – **Invite the patient to sign a consent form**. Capacity is context-dependent and this lady passes a four-stage test for capacity with regard to the proposed treatment in question. Other parties do not need to be consulted and no legal procedures need be invoked. **Consulting an independent mental-capacity advocate** is unnecessary, as she has demonstrated capacity to make this decision. **Continuing without consent** is unethical and illegal, as informed consent is always required. **Discussing the procedure with the lasting power of attorney (LPA) and asking them to consent** is incorrect because an LPA can only make decisions if the patient lacks capacity, which is not the case here. **Asking the patient's son to consent** is inappropriate, as family members cannot give consent unless they are an appointed LPA, and in this scenario, the patient can consent for herself.

Q219 Driving Advice

Answer 5 – **Remind the patient of their duty to inform the DVLA**. In this circumstance, it is important to remind the patient of their legal responsibility to inform the DVLA and stop driving immediately. It is prudent to give the patient the benefit of the doubt initially, as they may not have been aware of the specific rules regarding epilepsy and driving (believe it or not, there are instances where this information isn't passed on). Should this patient fail to do as advised, the next step would be to **inform the DVLA** yourself, but it remains good practice to let the patient know why you would be obligated to do this first. To do nothing puts both the patient and members of the public in danger, whilst for you to **inform the police** is an overreaction. To **confiscate the patient's car keys** is inappropriate.

Q220 Elder Abuse

Answer 4 – **Psychological**. This lady has several incontrovertible manifestations of neglectful poor physical care despite living in a setting where appropriate care could and should have been given. **Any or all of the other types of abuse** suggested could have taken place but the evidence for neglect is immediately apparent.

Q221 Acute and Chronic Pain Management

Answer 4 – **Reduce the dose of morphine sulphate gradually**. This option is the most appropriate because the patient is already on a high dose of opioids, which is associated with significant risks, including tolerance, dependence, opioid-induced hyperalgesia, and other side effects. Gradually reducing the dose helps minimise these risks while allowing the patient to potentially benefit from other pain management strategies, such as non-opioid medications and non-pharmacological treatments (e.g. physical therapy, CBT). Tapering off opioids should be done carefully and under medical supervision to manage withdrawal symptoms and ensure patient safety. Why not the other options? **Add in gabapentin**: while gabapentin can be effective for certain types of neuropathic pain, it should not be added without first addressing the high dose of opioids the patient is already taking. Gabapentin can cause sedation and dizziness, which could be compounded by the high-dose opioids, increasing the risk of adverse effects. It might be considered after opioid reduction. **Add in pregabalin**: similar to gabapentin, pregabalin is useful for neuropathic pain but comes with the risk of sedation and dizziness, especially in combination with opioids. Adding pregabalin without addressing the high-dose opioid use first is not advisable.

Increase dose of morphine sulphate to 100 mg twice daily: this option is not appropriate because the patient's pain is not being effectively managed by the current high dose of opioids. Increasing the dose further would likely worsen the risks associated with opioid use, such as tolerance, dependence and opioid-induced hyperalgesia, without providing long-term relief. **Use morphine sulphate liquid for breakthrough pain**: while breakthrough pain management is important, adding more morphine could lead to increased overall opioid consumption, exacerbating the risks associated with high-dose opioid therapy. Addressing the underlying issue with a high dose of opioids should take precedence over simply adding more opioids for breakthrough pain. In summary, the best option is to gradually reduce the dose of morphine to lower the risks associated with long-term high-dose opioid use, while exploring other non-opioid pain management strategies in conjunction with the pain clinic and physiotherapist.

Q222 End of Life Care / Symptoms of Terminal Illness

Answer 4 – **60 mg**, He is taking 60 mg orally twice daily = 120 mg. The equivalent subcutaneously is half the oral dose: 120/2 = 60 mg.

Q223 Falls

Answer 4 – **Drug-induced orthostatic hypotension**. Drug-induced orthostatic hypotension is the most likely cause of the patient's recurrent falls. Evaluation and adjustment of her medications may be necessary to address this issue and improve her safety and quality of life. Orthostatic hypotension is a sudden drop in BP upon standing from a sitting or lying position, leading to dizziness and potentially causing falls. Several factors in the medical history suggest that drug-induced orthostatic hypotension may be the cause of her falls. She experiences falls while walking or changing positions, along with occasional dizziness during these episodes. This is characteristic of orthostatic hypotension. Age: she is elderly, and orthostatic hypotension is more common in older adults. Anti-hypertensive medication: losartan is an angiotensin receptor blocker used to treat hypertension. It is known to cause orthostatic hypotension as an adverse effect, especially in the elderly. NSAID use: ibuprofen, used in this case for joint pain in osteoarthritis, can cause upper gastrointestinal ulcers. Bleeding from an ulcer could further contribute to orthostatic hypotension and increase the risk of falls. The other answer choices are less likely in this scenario:

Age-related gait disturbance: while age-related changes in gait can contribute to falls in the elderly, the mention of dizziness during these episodes suggests a vascular cause, such as orthostatic hypotension. **Cardiovascular syncope**: there is no history of loss of consciousness, chest pain or palpitations, which makes cardiovascular syncope less likely. **Cognitive impairment** can contribute to falls; however, it is not the primary cause in this case. There is no specific information in the history linking her cognitive impairment to her falls. **Osteoarthritis-related joint instability**: while osteoarthritis can cause joint pain and mobility issues, it is less likely to lead to falls in the absence of other factors such as dizziness on standing. In this case, the falls are not directly attributed to joint instability.

Q224 Frailty

Answer 5 – **Presenting with a fall**. Frailty syndromes refer to how a person with frailty may present to healthcare services. The five frailty criteria are falls (hence answer 5 is correct), immobility, delirium, incontinence and the consequences of polypharmacy. The frailty syndromes are not defined by any specific medical diagnoses, such as a **history of prostate cancer** or **history of macular degeneration**, or **BMI** threshold. Although frailty is associated with older persons, **age** per se does not indicate frailty.

Q225 Loin Pain

Answer 4 – **CT kidney, ureter and bladder**. A CT kidney, ureter and bladder (KUB) is the gold-standard investigation to diagnose a ureteric calculi, the most likely diagnosis, and therefore answer 1 is correct. A **CT abdomen and pelvis with contrast** may be indicated if you suspect a bowel obstruction or perforation in the acute abdomen, but less effective at imaging ureteric calculi. A **CT abdomen and pelvis without contrast** is similar to a CT KUB as they are both non-contrast scans; however, given the suspected diagnosis of ureteric calculi, a CT KUB is preferred. A **CT abdominal angiogram** is an assessment of the blood vessels within the abdomen, and would be the most appropriate investigation for a suspected leaking AAA, which is less likely in a 43 year old man with no pulsatile mass and pain that settles with diclofenac. A **US abdomen** would not be particularly useful at investigating for the most likely differentials in this case.

Q226 Misplaced Nasogastric Tube

Answer 3 – **Perform a chest X-ray.** A chest X-ray is needed to confirm the course of the tube and tip position. **Remove the tube immediately as his coughing suggests placement in the respiratory tract**: while the coughing may suggest respiratory tract placement, particularly if it persists, it commonly happens on insertion and does not necessarily mean misplacement. **Remove the tube immediately as the pH suggests placement in the lung**: pH 5.8 is not low enough to confirm placement by pH testing criteria, but again does not necessarily mean misplacement. **Document the tube is safe to use**

as the large volume of green fluid is clearly gastric: although the large volume aspirate is reassuring and makes gastric placement likely, it is not reliable enough to confirm placement, and only the pH testing or X-ray criteria should be used to confirm correct placement. **Flush 40 ml of air down the tube and listen for air flow over the stomach**: this describes the 'whoosh' test which, again, is neither safe nor reliable and should no longer be used.

Q227 Poisoning

Answer 2 – **4 hours after paracetamol ingestion**. Paracetamol levels should be taken at 4 hours after ingestion or as soon as possible thereafter. Delays can lead to delay in care decisions, whilst levels taken prior to 4 hours are prone to misinterpretation.

Q228 Wellbeing Checks

Answer D – **Mental, physical and social health assessment**. Good wellbeing goes beyond physical and mental health. It is a combination of physical, mental, emotional and social factors that enable one to function, to cope with challenges and to lead a meaningful life. Therefore, it goes beyond the absence of an illness/disease, disability or substance addiction. Assessing someone's wellbeing requires a thorough history-taking, and physical and social health assessment.

Q229 Post-surgical Care and Complications

Answer 4 – **Grade IV**. The patient has had complications which fulfil Grade IV of the Clavien–Dindo grade of complications, i.e. 'Life threatening complication (including CNS complications) requiring ICU management'. **Grade I** involves minor complications not requiring intervention (e.g. nausea managed conservatively). **Grade II** includes complications requiring pharmacological treatment (e.g. antibiotics for infection without surgery). **Grade III** involves surgical, endoscopic or radiological intervention, but without ICU admission (e.g. percutaneous drainage of an abscess). **Grade V** is death, which has not occurred in this case.

Q230 Struggling to Cope at Home

Answer 2 – **Collateral history from a family member**. This clinical scenario is not uncommon in the community. Full appraisal, including a good history and examination, is required. A collateral history from a family member may aid in diagnosis and/or planning, allowing a person-centred approach to care. This may facilitate care at home, including for those with mild confusion (so at this stage **her confusion precludes management at home** is not correct). Whilst a **chest X-ray** might be required in certain situations – such as persistent or recurrent chest infection, finger clubbing or persistent cervical lymphadenopathy – the information in this clinical scenario does not suggest a chest X-ray is necessary, at this stage. **Urea and electrolyte bloods**: blood tests, while useful in patients where the clinical picture is unclear and those not responding to treatment, are not always necessary in patient management. **Sputum culture** will take too long to be of any use in this decision.

Q231 Incidental Findings

Answer 1 – **Arrange urgent outpatient CT scan with clinic follow-up**. In the worst-case scenario, the ultrasound has uncovered a potential cancer which must be addressed rapidly. However, since the finding is incidental and the patient asymptomatic, this should be managed on an urgent outpatient basis. Ensuring that both the investigations and follow-up are booked is essential, as is explaining the situation to the patient and informing their GP via the discharge summary. Advising the patient to contact after a certain timeframe if they have not received any follow-up is also excellent practice. **Other options** either do not ensure the required follow-up or cause significant inconvenience / premature alarm.

Q232 Somatisation / Medically Unexplained Physical Symptoms

Answer 2 – **Agree that her pain is real, provide explanations and explore non-drug options**. The history of pervasive pain for 2 years with no localisation, normal examination and cutaneous hypersensitivity strongly suggests a psychosomatic or psychophysiologic condition. **Suggest a step-wise increase in her analgesics**: there is practically no evidence that analgesics, and in particular opiates, are effective in such conditions and they very often cause harm and dependency. **Refer to neurology**: it is tempting to 'refer on' but there is no suggestion here of any underlying neurological condition and the risk is of unnecessary investigation – and more importantly not addressing the real problem. **Arrange a whole-body scan to find the source of her pain**: 232 patients will often ask for more investigations, including scans to find a 'cause' for distressing symptoms. However, any investigation has to be justified in terms of likely benefit and possible risks. In this case, scanning the whole body will almost certainly not be useful diagnostically and may well throw up false positive or incidental findings that may generate yet more investigation. Psychosomatic or psychophysiologic pain is perceived by the body and brain in just the same way as somatic causes of pain. The absolute start of helping a distressed patient is to acknowledge that pain and suffering are 'real' and a result of complex interactions between brain and body. Having acknowledged explicitly that the symptoms described are real and genuine, it is often possible to discuss the interactions between brain and body in terms of commonly understood phenomena, such as tears when upset, blushing when embarrassed and pulse racing when scared. The idea of central sensitisation where the response can continue beyond the initial stimulus can be explored. It is important to reassure that many people recover and that gently progressive exercise, cognitive behavioural techniques and positive relationships have the best evidence base. If there is past or present trauma in a patient's life, a trauma-focused approach can unlock a way forward. Try asking 'what has happened to you?' rather than 'what is wrong with you?' **Advise her that it is all in her head and to get on with life** is not appropriate.

Haematology

8

Q233 Anaemia

Answer 3 – **Iron deficiency anaemia**. Whilst a vegan diet can be rich in iron, it is less easy to extract and absorb the iron. The full blood count given here is highly suggestive of iron restriction with the hypochromic anaemia. You would generally expect **acute myeloid leukaemia** to alter the white cell and platelet count. The **anaemia of chronic disease** can cause hypochromia with a normal MCV but this is less likely than iron loss in a young menstruating woman. **Vitamin B12 deficiency** can be seen in the vegan diet if supplements are not taken, but it is still less common than iron deficiency. **PNH** is an important but rare cause of iron deficiency which can be associated with haematuria and thromboses. It causes an intravascular haemolysis where iron is lost in the urine. Just like acute leukaemia, additional cytopenias are commonly seen.

Q234 Anaphylaxis

Answer 2 – **Epinephrine 0.5 mg intramuscularly**. The history suggests that the patient suddenly became unwell following the administration of an antibiotic. Antibiotics are very commonly associated with anaphylaxis. The symptoms and signs are of are of poor perfusion (agitation, tachycardia and hypotension) as well as bronchospasm. Top of your differential should be anaphylaxis because of sudden onset of cardiorespiratory collapse. The immediate treatment is epinephrine 0.5 mg IM. Epinephrine will halt the mast cell degradation as well as treat the symptoms. **Epinephrine 1 mg intravenously**: intravenous epinephrine should never be given. **Salbutamol** will relieve the bronchospasm only, and **hydrocortisone** and **chlorpheniramine** will attenuate the immune response and reduce a secondary response.

Q235 Pallor

Answer 1 – **Autoimmune haemolytic anaemia**. The patient's recent onset of pallor, shortness of breath, anaemia (Hb 72 g/L), reticulocytosis, elevated bilirubin and positive direct antiglobulin (Coombs) test is highly suggestive of autoimmune haemolytic anaemia (AIHA). The blood film findings of microspherocytes and polychromasia further support this diagnosis, indicating intravascular or extravascular haemolysis. **Glucose-6-phosphate dehydrogenase (G6PD) deficiency** typically presents with acute haemolysis after oxidative stress (e.g. infections, fava beans, drugs) and Heinz bodies on blood film, but it does not cause a positive Coombs test. **Hereditary spherocytosis** can also show spherocytes, but it is a congenital disorder with negative Coombs test and a family history. **Pyruvate kinase deficiency** leads to chronic haemolysis, but it is rare and presents from childhood with negative Coombs test. **Sickle cell anaemia** primarily presents with sickle-shaped cells and vaso-occlusive symptoms, which are not seen in this case.

Q236 Disseminated Intravascular Coagulation

Answer 1 – **Disseminated Intravascular Coagulation**. **Liver disease**, **warfarin overdose** or **vitamin K deficiency** would be a differential diagnosis for prolonged PT and APTT, but the low platelet count and fibrinogen, combined with a history of a known precipitating condition of DIC (severe infection) make this much more likely. Even if the patient has been receiving LMWH as an inpatient, this should not affect the PT or the platelets. **Thrombocytopenia** causes a low platelet count but the PT and APTT should be normal.

Q237 Haemochromatosis

Answer 2 – **25%**. Both parents have one 'normal' (β) gene and one autosomal recessive gene (β0). The child will inherit one gene from each parent. This question is asking what the risk is of the child inheriting two copies of the β0 gene from their parents. The chances of the child receiving two copies of the β0 gene and inheriting the illness is also 25%. The chance of them being a carrier (β/β0) is 50% and the chance of not having any β0 genes (β/β) is 25%. Since the parents both have one 'normal' gene and one affected gene, there are four possible outcomes for the child, as shown in the table below. There is a 1 in 4 chance of inheriting the 'normal' gene from both parents (25%). There is a 2 in 4 chance of inheriting one 'normal' gene and one affected gene (50%). There is a 1 in 4 chance of inheriting two affected genes (25%) and therefore developing beta thalassaemia. Therefore 25% is the correct answer, and **all other options** are incorrect.

Inheritance pattern with both parents being a carrier of beta thalassaemia minor

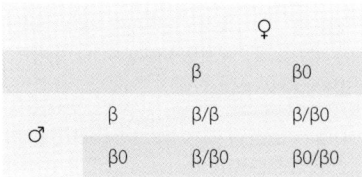

		♀	
		β	β0
♂	β	β/β	β/β0
	β0	β/β0	β0/β0

Q238 Haemophilia

Answer 3 – **Mild haemophilia A**. **Severe haemophilia** will have a factor level VIII of < 1 u/dL and present in infancy. **Acquired haemophilia** usually presents in much older patients with extensive spontaneous haemorrhage. The normal platelet count, factor IX level and von Willebrand antigen and activity levels exclude **all other options**.

Q239 Lymphoma

Answer 3 – **Stage IIIB**. Stage III is disease on both sides of the diaphragm but without extranodal involvement. The weight loss and night sweats are B symptoms. **Stage IB** is disease localised to one lymph node or a regional group of lymph nodes on one side of the diaphragm, with B symptoms. **Stage IIA** is disease localised to one or two regional groups of lymph nodes, with no symptoms (A).

Stage IVA is widespread disease on both sides of the diaphragm, with or without lymph node involvement, with no symptoms (A). **Stage IVB** is widespread disease on both sides of the diaphragm, with or without lymph node involvement, with B symptoms.

Q240 Leukaemia

Answer 2 – **Acute myeloid leukaemia**. The presence of blasts in the blood film suggests an acute rather than a **chronic lymphocytic leukaemia**. Acute myeloid leukaemia is more common than **acute lymphoblastic leukaemia** in adults, making it the most likely diagnosis. **Richter's syndrome** is a high-grade transformation of CLL which usually presents as rapidly enlarging lymphadenopathy.

Q241 Multiple Myeloma

Answer 4 – **Multiple myeloma**. This is a case of light chain myeloma. The renal impairment with the presence of urinary Bence–Jones proteins and a highly elevated lambda light chain in serum, in combination with hypercalcaemia, is essentially diagnostic. The abdominal and bone pain are likely related to the hypercalcaemia. **Bronchogenic carcinoma** can cause hypercalcaemia but that doesn't fit with the rest of the clinical picture. **Diabetic nephropathy** would not explain the hypercalcaemia or the light chains. **MGUS** does not cause CRAB features, at least two of which are present here. **Primary hyperparathyroidism** is ruled out by the suppressed parathyroid hormone.

Q242 Lymphadenopathy

Answer 2 – **EBV IgM serology**. The triad of a short history of pharyngitis, cervical lymphadenopathy and fever in a young patient are highly suggestive of infectious mononucleosis. There are various tests for acute EBV infection (Paul Bunnell, monospot) but all rely on the detection of anti-EBV antibodies and these can be tested for directly by looking for the presence of an IgM antibody rather than IgG, implying acute infection. **CT scan of neck, thorax, abdomen and pelvis** is unnecessary as there is no suspicion of malignancy or deep abscess. **Full blood count** may show atypical lymphocytosis, but it is not diagnostic. **Lymph node biopsy** is not required, as this presentation is consistent with viral lymphadenopathy rather than lymphoma. **Ultrasound scan of neck** is not necessary unless there is a suspicion of abscess or mass, which is not the case here.

Q243 Myeloproliferative Disorders

Answer 2 – **Essential thrombocythaemia**. **Acute infection** and **iron deficiency** can both cause a thrombocytosis, but there are no clinical features to suggest either. The normal CRP makes infection unlikely. Although the normal ferritin does not rule out iron deficiency, it doesn't confirm it either. The presence of the JAK2 mutation means that there is a clonal myeloproliferative disorder so the only question remaining is which one? The rest of the full blood count is normal meaning that this is not **polycythaemia vera**, and there are no clinical features (constitutional symptoms, splenomegaly) to suggest **MF**, which makes ET the most likely diagnosis.

Q244 Pancytopenia

Answer 1 – **Acute leukaemia**. The leucoerythroblastic picture indicates bone marrow infiltration which makes **folate deficiency** unlikely. The other answers are all causes of marrow infiltration, but the presence of circulating blasts indicates an acute leukaemia. Although **myelofibrosis** is associated with circulating blasts, they are not the dominant feature and myelofibrosis would be associated with splenomegaly. In a patient of this age, AML is the most common type of acute leukaemia but further testing is required to definitively distinguish AML from ALL. **Chronic lymphocytic leukaemia** is unlikely, as it typically presents with lymphocytosis rather than pancytopenia and does not usually feature circulating blasts. **Metastatic malignancy** can cause bone marrow infiltration, but it is less likely to present with circulating blasts.

Q245 Patient on Anti-platelet Therapy

Answer 3 – **Aspirin and ticagrelor or prasugrel**. For patients undergoing percutaneous coronary intervention (PCI) for acute coronary syndrome (ACS), dual antiplatelet therapy (DAPT) with aspirin plus a potent $P2Y_{12}$ inhibitor (ticagrelor or prasugrel) is the guideline-recommended regimen to reduce thrombotic complications. **All other options** undertreat the patient.

Q246 Polycythaemia

Answer 1 – **Chronic obstructive pulmonary disease**. There is clear evidence of a secondary cause of polycythaemia due to chronic respiratory illness from both the history and examination findings. The absence of the JAK2 mutation in the presence of a secondary cause is enough to confirm the diagnosis. **EPO-secreting tumour** (e.g. renal cell carcinoma) would typically cause polycythaemia with no respiratory symptoms, and additional imaging would be needed to confirm. **Gaisbock's syndrome** (stress polycythaemia) is seen in hypertensive, stressed or dehydrated individuals but does not usually present with lung disease. **Polycythaemia vera** is a primary bone marrow disorder, but the absence of JAK2 mutation makes it unlikely. **Relative polycythaemia** occurs when plasma volume is reduced (e.g. dehydration) but does not account for the patient's underlying respiratory disease.

Q247 Haemoglobinopathies

Answer 4 – **Non-paternity**. Haemophilia A is an X-linked recessive condition, meaning males who inherit the defective gene on their single X chromosome are affected, while females with one defective gene are typically carriers. If her father truly had haemophilia A, she would have inherited his affected X chromosome and would therefore be a carrier. The fact that genetic testing shows she is not a carrier suggests she did not inherit the X chromosome from her father. This points strongly to non-paternity (the individual identified as her biological father is not her biological father). **Cross-over at meiosis**: while cross-over (genetic recombination) during meiosis can shuffle genes between homologous chromosomes, it cannot 'erase' the presence of a defective gene on the X chromosome. This does not explain why she is not a carrier. **Cross-over at mitosis**: cross-over does not occur during mitosis, as it is not part of normal somatic cell division. This option is irrelevant here. **Non-maternity**: there is no evidence to suggest she is not the biological child of her mother, and this is far less likely than non-paternity. **She has an XY karyotype**: if she had an XY karyotype, she would be biologically male and not capable of being tested as a potential carrier of an X-linked condition.

Q248 Patient on Anti-coagulant Therapy

Answer 1 – **Amiodarone**. Amiodarone is a cytochrome P450 inhibitor, therefore increases the anti-coagulant effect of warfarin. It has a half-life of 58 days, so effects may not be seen for many weeks. Other agents used for rhythm control, such as sotalol and **flecanide**, have no effect on CYP450 enzymes. Flecanide would be contraindicated in this patient due to her impaired LV function. **Bisoprolol** is a beta-blocker that affects heart rate but does not significantly impact warfarin metabolism. **Digoxin** affects cardiac contractility but does not interfere with INR. **Diltiazem** is a calcium channel blocker that can interact with some drugs but does not notably raise INR.

Q249 Sickle Cell Disease

Answer 5 – **Splenic sequestration crisis**. The tender left upper quadrant mass is likely to represent the painful splenomegaly of splenic sequestration crisis. **Acute chest syndrome** presents with fever, hypoxia and respiratory symptoms but does not cause splenomegaly or severe anaemia. **Acute cholecystitis** can occur in sickle cell patients due to pigment gallstones, but it causes right upper quadrant pain and fever, not left-sided mass. **Mesenteric adenitis** is a viral illness causing generalised abdominal pain without anaemia or splenic enlargement. **Parvovirus B19 infection** can cause an aplastic crisis in sickle cell disease, but it is characterised by low reticulocyte count, whereas this patient has reticulocytosis, suggesting active bone marrow compensation

Q250 Transfusion Reactions

Answer 5 – **Stop the transfusion**. It is really important to firstly stop the blood transfusion and keep it for inspection. You can then go on to manage the clinical situation. It is also important to **inform the blood bank that the patient is having a transfusion reaction** once you have control of the clinical situation. **All other options** are incorrect.

Q251 Bruising and Purpura

Answer 5 – **von Willebrand's disease**. The family and personal history suggest an inherited bleeding disorder. **Haemophilia A** and **haemophilia B** are X-linked and would be associated with a prolonged APTT. Von Willebrand's disease can be associated with a prolonged or normal APTT (especially if mild) and would give a platelet pattern of bruising (bruising, menorrhagia) with increased haemorrhage risk on haemostatic challenge, e.g. surgery. **Disseminated intravascular coagulation** typically presents with abnormal coagulation parameters (e.g. prolonged PT, APTT, low fibrinogen) and thrombocytopenia, which are absent here. **Immune thrombocytopenia** would cause isolated thrombocytopenia, but this patient has a normal platelet count.

Q252 Neck Lump

Answer 3 – **Persistent thyroglossal duct**. This can cause a thyroglossal cyst. The history of a midline neck lump presenting in a young patient, which moves on tongue protrusion is consistent with a thyroglossal cyst. **Fascial weakness between the cricopharyngeus and thyropharyngeus muscle** causes a pharyngeal pouch which is not a midline lump. A **second branchial cleft which has failed to obliterate** causes a branchial cleft cyst which presents as a lump anterior to the sternocleidomastoid and doesn't move with tongue protrusion. **Incomplete embryonic epithelial growth at lines of fusion** causes a dermoid cyst which is likely to be subcutaneous and not move with tongue protrusion. **Proliferation of a clone of malignant B cells** is the cause of lymphoma and would present with an enlarged lymph node; these are not usually in the midline.

Q253 Allergies / Allergic Disorder

Answer 1 – **Administer 0.5 mg intramuscular (IM) adrenaline (1:1000).** Suspected anaphylaxis is a medical emergency and, after ensuring the precipitant has been removed and an urgent medical emergency call is made, prompt administration of IM adrenaline should be the next priority. This is the key life-saving intervention in anaphylaxis – however, it is also important to stabilise the patient using oxygen and fluid resuscitation. The patient should also be laid flat with legs elevated to support their BP. Additional adrenaline at a dose of 0.5 mg IM (1:1000) may be indicated after 5 minutes if there has been a suboptimal response to the first round of treatment. **All other options** are inappropriate at this stage.

Infectious Disease

9

Q254 Candidiasis

Answer 1 – **Candida albicans**. The clinical description of creamy white plaques on the surface of the tongue extending to the oropharynx is entirely typical of infection of the oral mucosa with Candida albicans. Anti-fungal treatment and oral hygiene measures will be required to successfully treat. **Corynebacterium diphtheriae** is the causative organism of diphtheria infection. This is a very unusual infection in clinical practice in the UK, where diphtheria vaccination is comprehensive. It is more likely to be seen in migrant populations from countries where vaccination rates are suboptimal. Diphtheria infection is associated with a grey-white exudative membrane in the oropharynx which may give rise to airway obstruction. **Epstein–Barr Virus** (EBV) is the most common cause of infectious mononucleosis. It causes pharyngeal erythema and/or an exudative pustular tonsillitis. It does not typically cause white plaques on the tongue. **Porphyromonas gingivalis** is a gram-negative bacterium typically found in the oral cavity and is associated with periodontal disease. **Streptococcus mitis** is an alpha-haemolytic streptococcus which colonises the oral cavity. It may give rise to invasive disease, such as endocarditis.

Q255 Herpes Simplex Virus

Answer 2 – **Oral aciclovir. Topical aciclovir** will be ineffective. More lesions continue to appear and the patient is in significant pain, so oral aciclovir should reduce the severity and duration of the outbreak. Oral antibiotics, such as **doxycycline**, do not appear to be required, as there is no significant crusting or swelling. **No treatment required** is incorrect, as early anti-viral therapy can shorten the episode and reduce viral shedding. **Topical fucidin cream** is an antibiotic, which would be ineffective as this is a viral infection.

Q256 Hospital Acquired Infections

Answer 2 – **Blood cultures x 2**. The patient is presenting with symptoms of sepsis: fever, tachycardia, hypotension, diarrhoea and new confusion. These symptoms suggest a systemic infection that could be life-threatening. Blood cultures are critical in identifying the causative organism and guiding appropriate antibiotic therapy.

While an **abdominal CT scan** could help identify an abdominal source of infection, it is not the first line of action in a patient showing signs of sepsis. Blood cultures are more urgent to identify bacteraemia. **Lumbar puncture** is usually indicated if there are signs of meningitis, which this patient does not exhibit. New confusion alone without other signs such as neck stiffness or photophobia doesn't directly point to meningitis in the context of his other symptoms. **Prepare for theatre for exploration of wound** – while wound infection could be a source of sepsis, surgical exploration is not the immediate next step unless there is clear evidence of wound dehiscence or abscess that necessitates drainage. Initial step is still blood cultures to guide therapy.

A s**putum sample** could be useful if there is a suspicion of pneumonia, but it doesn't address the urgent need to identify bacteraemia in a septic patient. Blood cultures provide more immediate and broader information.

Q257 Fever

Answer 5 – **Review the patient's previous microbiology results and discuss with the microbiologist.** The recent traumatic catheter change should raise concerns for potential prostatitis but also give an indication that changing the catheter may be difficult and require urology input. The patient most likely has his catheter changed regularly either in the urology department or by a practice nurse. These notes should be reviewed before attempting the catheter change in ED. **Change the urethral catheter and send the tip to the laboratory for culture**: changing the catheter without antibiotic cover could cause dissemination of bacteria and lead to the patient becoming more unwell. Sending the tip is unlikely to add much if a urine sample has already been sent to the laboratory. **Giving antipyretics such as intravenous paracetamol and seeking to optimise his blood glucose** should certainly form part of the management plan but is not the most important management step. **Deferring antibiotic administration until cultures return** in a frail older patient with clear evidence of an acute fever would not be advised. If you can do so in a timely manner, aim to take blood cultures prior to the first dose of antibiotics. In a patient with chronic disease, multiple healthcare contacts, and who lives in residential care with a long-term urinary catheter, the likelihood of colonisation and infection with multi-drug resistant bacteria is high. Antibiotic treatment guided by previous laboratory results is favoured rather than **commencing empirical intravenous antibiotics based on the hospital antibiotic guidance**. Always discuss treatment of multi-drug resistant infections with your local microbiologist.

Q258 Human Immunodeficiency Virus

Answer 1 – **High-dose trimethoprim/sulfamethoxazole**. The patient's presentation and findings are highly suggestive of Pneumocystis pneumonia (PCP), a common opportunistic infection in patients with advanced HIV/AIDS, particularly when the CD4 count is below 200 cells/mm³. The treatment is trimethoprim and sulfamethoxazole. **Immediately start Truvada plus dolutegravir**: these are retrovirals crucial for long-term management, and should be started/restarted after treating the acute infection. **Intravenous co-amoxiclav and clarithromycin** are not first-line treatment. **Meropenem and gentamicin** are not appropriate for PCP. **Oral aciclovir** is used for herpes virus but has no efficacy against PCP.

Q259 Lyme Disease

Answer 3 – **Start oral antibiotics immediately**. The clinical picture gives a high suspicion for Lyme disease. Pointers are fever, rash, arthritis, eye involvement. Management should be for early treatment as delaying it can lead to more severe disease. Oral antibiotics are effective in most situations. There is no need to **admit for intravenous antibiotics**. **Oral steroids** are not indicated and may delay recovery. **Waiting for the microbiology report** delays treatment and is not recommended in cases with high clinical suspicion. **Reassuring and reviewing later** risks disease progression and chronic Lyme arthritis.

Q260 Night Sweats

Answer 3 – **Collect three early morning sputum samples and refer to a respiratory physician urgently**. Productive cough, low-grade fever, night sweats and weight loss should raise the suspicion of tuberculosis.

Immigration from a high-prevalence tuberculosis area is a significant risk factor. As the patient has a productive cough, sputum samples should be collected and sent for TB microscopy and culture. Multiple samples are taken to ensure the tuberculosis organism is successfully cultured. He should be referred to the local respiratory clinic where anti-tuberculous treatment can be initiated. Tuberculosis is a notifiable infectious disease. **A TB Gold QuantiFERON test** confirms previous exposure to tuberculosis but does not differentiate latent from active disease. It is not affected by any previous history of BCG vaccination. Many people coming from endemic tuberculous areas in the world have latent tuberculosis from prior exposure earlier in life and so will have a positive TB Gold QuantiFERON test. Culture of clinical samples is key in confirming both the infection and sensitivities to guide anti-tuberculous therapy. **Check a vitamin D level**: vitamin D deficiency is common in immigrant populations in the UK. It is often seen in association with reactivation of latent tuberculosis but does not in itself cause the range of symptoms described. **Give 1-week course of amoxicillin and follow-up on completion of treatment**: this is an appropriate treatment for community-acquired pneumonia. However, the chronicity of the symptoms would suggest this is unlikely to be bacterial pneumonia. **Refer to the emergency department for urgent chest X-ray**: whilst a CXR would be desirable, arranging this via the emergency department would not be appropriate for several reasons. The symptoms described are chronic. The patient is not acutely unwell. He does not have pleuritic chest pain or sudden-onset breathlessness or any other acute symptoms. Furthermore, adequate control of transmission of any chronic infection, such as tuberculosis, might be difficult to achieve in a busy emergency department.

Q261 Malaria

Answer 4 – **Microscopy of thick and thin smears**. Microscopic examination of thick and thin smears remains the gold-standard investigation for diagnosing malaria. Thick films consist of several layers of red cells which allow a larger number of cells to be examined for the presence of parasites. Low levels of parasitaemia can be more readily detected. Thin films on the other hand consist of a single layer of cells. Thin films are better suited to identifying the morphology and species of the involved parasite. **Blood cultures** are useful for bacterial infections but do not diagnose malaria. **CT thorax, abdomen, pelvis** is unnecessary, as malaria is diagnosed via blood smear, not imaging. **Full blood count** may show anaemia and thrombocytopenia, which are common in malaria, but it is not diagnostic. **Throat swab** is irrelevant, as malaria is a vector-borne parasitic disease, not a respiratory infection.

Q262 Notifiable Diseases

Answer 4 – **Report the case the same day. Mumps is a notifiable disease**. A suspected case of a notifiable disease should be reported immediately. **Undertake testing for mumps and report it if the results come back as positive**: there is no need to wait for confirmation of the infection. It is good practice to let the patient/parents/carers know this is going to be done, although you do not need to seek their permission to do so. **Do nothing unless a second case presents**: even a single case needs to be reported so a picture can be built up of cases in the community. **Admit to paediatrics and expect them to notify if appropriate**: there are no features requiring admission to hospital.

Q263 Surgical Site Infection

Answer 5 – **Swab the exudate, mark the area, change the dressing, commence antibiotics according to local protocol and discuss imaging with senior members of the team**. This man is likely to have a developing collection around his surgical site. He is tender, but not peritonitic, and his bowels are moving post-operatively. His wound is erythematous, tender and discharging. He has some early signs of worsening infection – tachycardia, tachypnoea – but is otherwise reasonably well. He needs antibiotics according to local protocols, swabbing of the wound, and is likely to need imaging to determine the size and extent of the collection. The need for surgical debridement of the wound in theatre is reserved for major life-threatening wound complications, e.g. necrotising fasciitis and complete wound dehiscence. **Order an urgent CT scan and await the results**: bloods and scans are important but they are not the first-line measures. Equally, **drawing around the area of erythema** and **asking the nursing team to change the wound dressing and monitor the observations** are important steps in the follow-up of progress of wound infection and are not the first-line steps alone in the management plan. **Immediate IV fluid resuscitation and emergency laparotomy** is unnecessary at this stage, as there are no signs of sepsis or peritonitis.

Q264 Necrotising Fasciitis

Answer 5 – **Surgical debridement and intravenous antibiotics**. The patient's symptoms, including fever, general malaise, rapidly spreading erythema and swelling in the leg, are highly suggestive of necrotising fasciitis, a severe and rapidly progressing soft tissue infection. This condition is a medical emergency and requires immediate and aggressive treatment. Surgical debridement is essential to remove necrotic tissue, halt the spread of infection, and reduce the bacterial load. Without surgical intervention, the infection can quickly lead to systemic sepsis, multi-organ failure and death. Intravenous antibiotics are necessary to address the underlying infection, but antibiotics alone are insufficient because they cannot adequately penetrate the necrotic tissue. The combination of surgical debridement and intravenous antibiotics provides the best chance of survival and recovery. **Cryotherapy** is inappropriate and ineffective for this condition. **Fluid resuscitation** might be necessary to manage sepsis, but it is supportive care and not the definitive treatment. **Intravenous antibiotics** alone are not sufficient without debridement.

Oral antibiotics are inappropriate for such a severe, rapidly progressing infection.

Thus, surgical debridement and intravenous antibiotics is the correct and most appropriate management plan for this condition.

Q265 Toxic Shock Syndrome

Answer 5 – **Erythroderma**. The earliest dermatological manifestation is usually erythroderma, a diffuse, red, macular rash which resembles a painless sunburn. **Desquamation of palms and soles** tends to occur 1–2 weeks after the onset of illness, and so will not aid your initial diagnosis. **Dry gangrene** may occur following a prolonged period of impaired perfusion, and so would not help your initial diagnosis. **Erythema multiforme** is not associated with toxic shock syndrome. **Erythema toxicum** is a condition associated with neonates.

Q266 Travel Health Advice

Answer 5 – **Awareness, Bite prevention, Chemoprophylaxis, Diagnosis**. This question assesses knowledge around malaria prevention according to WHO guidelines. Answer 5 is the only answer to contain the four aspects of malaria prevention. **Covering up** is incorporated within **bite prevention** so is not correct. **Bite avoidance** and **avoidance** are impossible in some circumstances so are also false. **Drugs** would be too vague a directive, so again is incorrect. Thus, the only answer with specific directives is answer 5.

Q267 Tuberculosis

Answer 3 – **When he has been taking his medication for 3 weeks**. This is because, after 2–3 weeks of appropriate TB treatment, patients are no longer contagious and can safely go out in public. It is important to note that patients should continue taking their medication for the full duration of the treatment course to ensure complete resolution of the infection. **Immediately, if he is wearing a face mask**: although wearing a face covering or mask can help reduce the spread of TB, it is not enough to prevent transmission. **When his symptoms have improved and he is no longer coughing**: these are important indicators of treatment efficacy, but, again, they do not necessarily indicate that the patient is no longer contagious. Likewise, a normal chest X-ray is a good sign, but it also does not necessarily mean that the patient is no longer contagious. **When he has completed 6 months of anti-TB therapy**: completing the full course of antibiotics is necessary to ensure that the TB infection is fully treated; however, patients stop being contagious after 3 weeks of treatment, so a full 6 months of isolation is not necessary.

Q268 Varicella Zoster

Answer 4 – **No test required**. Varicella is usually a clinical diagnosis from the characteristic rash and patient history. This case is a typical presentation for varicella/chickenpox. **PCR testing for varicella zoster virus** can detect current infections and is useful for atypical or severe cases. **IgM antibodies** and **IgG antibodies** can be used to determine recent or previous infection and immunity. The **full blood count** is not indicated in this case.

Q269 Covid-19

Answer 3 – **Consider contacting ITU as a matter of urgency**. The patient is presenting with moderate to severe Covid-19 infection. Despite 15 L of O_2 he is only saturating at 94%. There are also signs that he is tiring and therefore intubation may be required. This patient should certainly not be **given reassurance and advice and discharged home for 10 days of isolation. Admission to hospital for observations only** is not likely to change the progression of disease. O_2 **therapy, intravenous fluids, antibiotics, dexamethasone and remdesivir** may all be indicated later on but should not be given without input from a senior clinician. The patient is young (55) and at risk of deteriorating rapidly. Informing ITU early is the most suitable action to take. **Giving the patient the Covid vaccine** is a preventative measure that enables an immune response should the patient be infected with Covid-19 at a later date.

Mental Health

10

Q270 Abnormal Eating or Exercising Behaviour

Answer 4 – **Hypokalaemia**. The patient has signs suggestive of self-induced vomiting (scratches on knuckles), low BMI and restricted diet. Her ECG is showing signs of hypokalaemia which is common in severe purging. **Hypernatraemia**: sodium would be expected to be low as well, due to malnutrition or laxative abuse. **Low growth hormone**: stress hormones such as the growth hormone would be raised due to starvation. **High LH and FSH**: amenorrhea with low LH and FSH is common in severe eating disorders. **High blood sugar**: her blood sugar could be normal or low.

Q271 Anxiety Disorder – Post-Traumatic Stress Disorder

Answer 4 – **Post-traumatic stress disorder** (PTSD). The patient feels anxious and on edge since giving birth, which suggests significant psychological distress. She had a frightening and traumatic labour, requiring an emergency caesarean section for fetal distress, which is a known risk factor for postnatal PTSD. She experiences re-experiencing symptoms, such as flashbacks ('going back') and intense fear. Emotional numbing and difficulty bonding with the baby are common in PTSD.

Hyperarousal symptoms (being 'on edge') and avoidance of reminders of the trauma are also characteristic of PTSD. **Acute stress disorder** (ASD) is similar to PTSD but occurs within 4 weeks of the traumatic event. Since her symptoms have persisted for 8 weeks, PTSD is the correct diagnosis. **Agoraphobia** involves fear of public spaces and social avoidance behaviours, which is not the main issue here. **Generalised anxiety disorder** (GAD) involves excessive, persistent worry about multiple aspects of life, but it does not involve re-experiencing trauma, flashbacks or emotional numbing. Her symptoms are directly linked to her traumatic birth experience, making PTSD the more accurate diagnosis. **Severe depressive disorder**: while depression can cause guilt, shame and bonding difficulties, it does not feature re-experiencing of trauma, flashbacks or hyperarousal. She has symptoms specifically related to a traumatic experience, which is characteristic of PTSD rather than depression.

Q272 Anxiety Disorder: Generalised, Phobias, Obsessive Compulsive Disorder

Answer 2 – **Intensive CBT combined with SSRI**. The correct answer is intensive CBT, which should be combined with SSRI (which she is on already). The patient presents with OCD. The vital part of the question is in rating the severity of her symptoms and functional impairment. She is having significant problems at work and with family which would suggest a severe functional impairment. As such, a combined approach of SSRI and CBT would be appropriate and she will probably need a referral to secondary care. **Low-level CBT with Exposure and response prevention**: while exposure and response prevention would be an integral part of the CBT in OCD, low level would be inappropriate given the degree of functional impairment. The patient requires active intervention rather than a 'watch and wait approach'. **Diazepam** would be inappropriate as it would not treat the underlying illness and could easily lead to dependence. **Propranolol** can reduce anxiety symptoms, but again would not treat the underlying illness.

Q273 Bipolar Affective Disorder

Answer 5 – **Sodium valproate**. Antipsychotics such as **aripiprazole** or **quetiapine** can be used to treat bipolar depression under the care of a psychiatrist. **Lamotrigine** is an anti-epileptic that can be used to treat bipolar depression. A short course of **diazepam** may be indicated if symptoms of anxiety are high. Sodium valproate can be prescribed as a mood stabiliser; however, it should not be used in women of childbearing age. It greatly increases the risk of neuro-developmental disorders and neural tube defects. Its use in women of childbearing age is tightly regulated and should only be considered as a last resort, and only with effective contraception in place – e.g. an implant or IUS – and under specialist supervision of a psychiatrist.

Q274 Depression

Answer 2 – **Individual guided self-help based on cognitive behavioural therapy (CBT)**. The man has symptoms in keeping with a mild depressive disorder. According to NICE, the first-line interventions for mild to moderate depression are: individual guided self-help based on cognitive behavioural therapy (CBT); computerised CBT; a structured group physical activity programme. In the first instance, treatment should be provided in primary care, hence **referral to secondary care services** is not indicated. **Commence an** SSRI: it is not recommended to routinely use antidepressant medications for people with subthreshold or mild depressive symptoms. **Reassurance** is unlikely to be appropriate, and **psychodynamic psychotherapy** is not a first-line intervention.

Q275 Low Mood / Affective Problems

Answer 5 – **Severe depression with psychosis**. This man presents with symptoms of depression, e.g. low mood, low energy, flat affect. It is severe enough to have caused mood-congruent nihilistic delusions that his bowel is leaking. Individuals with **schizophrenia** are more likely to present with persecutory delusions that others are trying to harm them or are controlling them, or to have persecutory auditory hallucinations. **Delusional disorder** presents with a single systematised delusional belief system in the absence of major mood abnormalities. This is the first psychiatric presentation, therefore a diagnosis of **bipolar disorder** would not be made at this point. If he had a manic/hypomanic episode in the future, then the diagnosis would probably become bipolar disorder. **Schizoaffective disorder** requires both mood and schizophrenia-like symptoms, but this patient's delusion is mood-congruent rather than suggestive of schizophrenia.

Q276 Eating Disorders

Answer 1 – **Admit to the medical wards for monitoring and weight restoration**. This patient is physiologically compromised and at high risk of death. She has a low BMI and haemodynamic instability. She requires urgent admission to a medical ward for blood and ECG monitoring whilst weight restoration is undertaken. This would usually be under the gastroenterology team with liaison psychiatry support. All other options are inappropriate due to the degree of physiological compromise and risk of death. This patient is very unwell; community treatment may be an option once stabilised.

This would be with the **Eating Disorders Service**, not primarily a **GP** or **self-help services**. **Refer to acute psychiatry team for admission to eating disorder unit**: an admission to an eating disorder unit may be indicated, but stabilisation and weight restoration take precedence.

Q277 Suicidal Thoughts

Answer 5 – Previous impulsive suicide attempt. **Married status**: marriage tends to act as a protective factor. **Female gender** is associated with less risk of completed suicide when compared to the male gender. Moderate **alcohol intake** has no clear increase in risk. The link between **being menopausal** and suicide risk is not currently clear from research, but associations are emerging. Previous suicide attempt has the greatest influence upon her suicide risk.

Q278 Personality Disorder

Answer 3 – Intensive community support for crisis management. **Dialectal behaviour therapy** has an evidence base for the treatment of Emotionally Unstable Personality Disorder. It is not appropriate to start therapy during a severe crisis, but when the crisis has passed and the patient is better able to engage. **Diazepam 10 mg twice daily for 3 weeks** is inappropriate as benzodiazepines can increase impulsivity and worsen emotional dysregulation. **Intensive community support for crisis management** may be useful in the short term but does not provide the long-term skills-based therapy needed for EUPD. **Quetiapine as a mood stabiliser** is not first-line for personality disorders, as medication has limited efficacy in treating the core features of EUPD. **Voluntary inpatient psychiatric admission** is unnecessary as the patient is amenable to working with liaison psychiatry, and inpatient care is usually reserved for imminent risk of suicide or self-harm that cannot be managed in the community.

Q279 Elation / Elated Mood

Answer 2 – Bloods and a urine dip and drug screen. In the first instance, you would want some basic investigations to rule out common physical causes for this behaviour, such as hyperthyroidism or illicit drug intoxication, specifically with stimulants. This will be accompanied with a full history and physical examination. **CT scan head**: this may be part of the plan later if a neurological cause for these symptoms is suspected, but a full history, physical examination and routine bloods should be undertaken first to ascertain if imaging is indicated. **Call security as he has spoken inappropriately to a member of staff:** whilst it is important to maintain a safe environment for patients and staff, the question does not make it clear that the patient has done anything more than ask for the staff member's phone number. If the nurse were to feel threatened in any way, then calling security may become necessary. Calling security prematurely may escalate the situation. **Contact the psychiatric liaison team:** you may require advice from the team or for them to assess at a later stage, but at this point you are still at the information-gathering stage and it is not clear if the underlying cause is medical or psychiatric. Should you require more information about how to handle the situation, they may be a valuable resource for you. **Arrange MHA assessment**: detention is not indicated at this time as physical causes for this presentation have not been excluded. If they had an organic cause for their presentation, managing this should take precedence rather than immediate detention under the MHA. He is also so far willing to be in the emergency department, thus not requiring detention.

Q280 Schizophrenia

Answer 5 – **Switch haloperidol to a depot formulation**. The patient's presentation is fairly typical for an individual living in the community with schizophrenia. Many patients with schizophrenia have ongoing symptoms despite adequate treatment with antipsychotic medication. Adherence to medication can be challenging. Haloperidol comes as a depot, so trialling this instead of tablet medication may improve adherence, but it may not result in lessening of symptoms. **A trial of clozapine** should be considered as he has treatment-resistant illness and it can be particularly efficacious for those who have had a suboptimal response to other antipsychotics. **A blister pack** may help improve adherence to medication, but the preferable medication would be clozapine, not haloperidol. **Increasing the frequency of visits from the CPN** may provide extra support but probably won't alter his presentation a great deal. There is currently no indication for **admission to hospital**, especially under the MHA, as risks are low and community management is safe and viable. With community management, it is likely that his presentation will settle and he can remain living in the community.

Q281 Somatisation

Answer 5 – **Somatic symptom disorder**. The most likely diagnosis in this case is Somatisation Disorder. The patient's presentation is characterised by the presence of multiple physical symptoms across different organ systems, occurring over an extended period, and causing significant distress and impairment. The absence of any medical explanation for her symptoms, along with her frequent healthcare visits, suggests a pattern consistent with Somatisation Disorder. Additionally, the patient's preoccupation with her physical health and frustration about the lack of a definitive medical diagnosis align with this diagnosis. **Factitious disorder** involves intentional symptom fabrication for psychological gain (e.g. assuming the 'sick role'), which is not evident here. **Functional neurological symptom disorder** (conversion disorder) presents with neurological symptoms (e.g. weakness, paralysis, sensory loss) that are inconsistent with medical conditions, whereas this patient has symptoms across multiple systems. **Generalised anxiety disorder** involves excessive worry about multiple life aspects, not just physical health. **Illness anxiety disorder** (formerly hypochondriasis) is characterised by excessive worry about having a serious illness despite minimal or no physical symptoms, whereas this patient has multiple distressing physical symptoms.

Q282 Substance Misuse / Use Disorder

Answer 5 – **Therapeutic trial of intravenous naloxone**. This woman has signs consistent with opiate toxicity. The treatment would be naloxone, which should initially be administered as a trial dose, which can be administered more quickly and the response assessed. If it has helped, this confirms the diagnosis and an infusion of naloxone should then be set up. **Bolus of intravenous fluids** might also be helpful, but in an ABCDE assessment the respiratory issue would be addressed first, as the most life-threatening. **Artificial ventilation** would not be required if the patient responds adequately to naloxone, and neither **intravenous lorazepam** nor **intravenous infusion of adrenaline** is indicated in this situation.

Q283 Self-Harm

Answer 1 – **Conduct a mental capacity assessment**. The patient is in an urgent and potentially life-threatening situation. She is not behaving in a way that is normally expected and her actions could cause harm. There is enough information in the vignette to question whether her personality disorder could be impairing her decision-making capacity. The most appropriate step is to assess her capacity to consent to treatment under the MCA. If she lacks capacity, treatment should be guided in her best interests under the frame-work of the MCA. **Discharge the patient as requested**: this is incorrect, given the risks involved, and the patient, and her capacity to consent to treatment, should be considered in the first instance. **Refer for MHA assessment** is incorrect: the MCA is more appropriate for considering her capacity to consent to treatment, in this urgent situation. The MHA is for treatment of mental disorders. Whilst theoretically the patient could be detained to the general hospital and the overdose treated under the MHA, it would be a convoluted care pathway, waste precious time and is not a primary function of the MHA. **Treating her against her wishes as she could die from the overdose** is incorrect: to provide treatment for any individual, they need to have capacity to consent. If they have capacity, treatment cannot be enforced. If they lack capacity, they should be treated under a suitable legal framework, e.g. MCA or MHA. **Watch and wait** is incorrect: whilst much can be gained from giving time and space, this is an urgent situation and requires quick decision-making and consideration of appropriate legal frameworks. The patient may develop liver failure, risking death, if too much time elapses.

Q284 Acute Stress Reaction

Answer 3 – **Nurse 1:1 in a quiet area**. This patient presents with an acute stress reaction following a traumatic assault. Individuals will often benefit from being nursed in a quieter environment on a 1:1 basis. It can be very traumatic for people to be restrained, which can maintain the current trauma, complicate the current trauma or retrigger past traumas. Therefore, reassuring the patient, giving space and grounding is the first principle of management. It is probable that, with appropriate intervention in ED, she will not require a **MHA assessment** or hospital admission. An organic explanation is unlikely, given the scenario. The benefits of **taking MSU and bloods for delirium markers** or imaging, such as **CT head scan** under restraint is outweighed by the harm done of obtaining them under restraint. A benzodiazepine such as **oral lorazepam** or diazepam could be helpful to reduce arousal or distress, but only once the patient is being nursed in a less stimulating environment.

Q285 Addiction

Answer 2 – **Advise him to self-refer to the local substance misuse service and to keep drinking alcohol in the meantime**. This ensures immediate withdrawal symptoms are postponed. Self-referral empowers the patient and shows commitment to overcoming their addiction. **Admit him to a medical ward for a reducing regimen of benzodiazepines**: this is not an indication on its own for admission to a medical bed. **Phone the community drug worker to arrange an inpatient detox** is not wrong, but likely to take time to arrange and fails to address the immediate danger posed by acute alcohol withdrawal. **Prescribe him acamprosate and advise follow-up by his GP**: this fails to address the alcohol withdrawal. **Provide a prescription for a reducing regimen of chlordiazepoxide with GP follow-up**: this would only be appropriate through a community drug and alcohol service, rehab unit or inpatient ward, not from the emergency department to a patient being discharged back into the community.

Q286 Behaviour/Personality Change

Answer 2 – **Investigate which medications have been changed**. There are many potential diagnoses. For example, delirium caused by steroids as part of her COPD treatment, hyponatraemia from an increase in furosemide. She has risk factors for having an infection (diabetes) and for developing delirium (age, cardiac disease). An organic diagnosis is most likely, so **undertaking a full MHA assessment** and **referral to the psychiatry liaison team** are inappropriate as physical healthcare takes precedence. **Restraining the patient to administer medications and fluids as indicated** is incorrect. An MCA has not taken place and there is currently no biochemical or clinical indication for treating the patient with intravenous fluids. The patient is clearly acutely unwell, so **allowing her to self-discharge** is inappropriate. A capacity assessment should be considered if the patient wished to self-discharge. to decide whether they have the ability to make this decision. Investigating which medications have been changed is a good objective way to find out more information – think of it like detective work.

Q287 Fixed Abnormal Beliefs

Answer 4 – **Psychosis**. This diagnosis fits the scenario best. The individual has a fixed, false belief (delusion) that he's being followed and monitored by the police, despite evidence to the contrary (no cameras found, no odd behaviours observed by others). This belief is causing distress and interfering with his functioning, as seen by his withdrawal from hobbies and friendships. **Bipolar disorder**: while bipolar disorder can involve delusions during manic or depressive episodes, the symptoms described in the scenario don't align with the classic presentation of bipolar disorder. There's no mention of mood swings between manic and depressive states. **Mania** involves elevated mood, increased energy, and impulsivity, which are not prominent features in this case. While the individual may show some irritability, it's not the primary symptom. **Panic disorder** involves recurrent panic attacks, often accompanied by a fear of future attacks or a change in behaviour to avoid situations that may trigger panic. There's no indication of panic attacks or avoidance behaviours in the scenario. **Severe depression with psychosis**: while psychosis can occur in severe depression, the key features of depression, such as pervasive low mood, anhedonia (loss of interest in previously enjoyed activities) and withdrawal, are present in this case. However, the primary symptom driving the distress and functional impairment seems to be the delusional belief, rather than the depressive symptoms. Therefore, psychosis is a more appropriate diagnosis.

Q288 Pressure of Speech

Answer 3 – **Mania**. This is a classic presentation of mania. She has pressured speech, increased energy, disinhibition and grandiose delusions. **Bipolar disorder** requires both manic and depressive episodes. There is no history of depression in this patient. **Delusional disorder**: while grandiose delusions are present, the overall pattern of behaviour, including increased energy and rapid speech, is more indicative of a manic episode rather than delusional disorder.

While **personality disorder** can involve erratic behaviour, the sudden onset and specific symptoms described in the scenario (such as pressure of speech and grandiosity) are more consistent with a manic episode rather than a personality disorder. **Schizophrenia** involves a range of symptoms, including hallucinations, delusions, disorganised speech and negative symptoms. While delusions are present, the absence of other hallmark symptoms of schizophrenia suggests it is not the most appropriate diagnosis in this case.

Q289 Threats to Harm Others

Answer 4 – **Physical health screening**. Before proceeding with psychiatric management, it is essential to rule out organic causes of psychosis, such as substance-induced psychosis, metabolic imbalances, infections or neurological disorders. The patient's daily cannabis use increases the likelihood of substance-induced psychosis, which requires a thorough physical health screen, including blood tests, toxicology and neurological assessment. **Admitting under medics** is not the most appropriate next step, as medical admission alone would not address the underlying psychiatric symptoms. **Completing a mental capacity assessment** is premature, as his presentation suggests psychosis rather than an isolated capacity issue. **Discharging into the community with psychiatric follow-up** is unsafe, given his active threats and lack of insight. **Referring for Mental Health Act assessment** may be necessary, but first, an organic cause must be excluded before assuming a primary psychiatric disorder.

Neurology

11

Q290 Brain Abscess

Answer 5 – **Staphylococcus aureus**. This is the most likely causative organism in this scenario and is particularly common in patients with a history of intravenous drug abuse. It is commonly implicated in cutaneous infections and, in a patient who is likely immunocompromised (diabetes), the risk of a cutaneous infection progressing to a systemic infection (including a brain abscess) is high. **E. coli** brain abscesses are rare, and **HSV** does not usually present with brain abscesses – rather, as an encephalitis. **SARA-CoV-2**: whilst Covid is now a common viral infection, there are no reported cases of the virus being the direct causative organism for brain abscesses. **Mycobacterium tuberculosis** can cause tuberculomas or meningitis, but this would present more chronically.

Q291 Brain Metastases

Answer 5 – **Small cell lung metastasis**. Considering the history, the most likely diagnosis is a malignant neoplastic process as he has systemic symptoms (weight loss, haemoptysis). **Meningiomas** are (usually) benign dural-based extra-axial tumours arising from the meninges; vermian lesions are on the other hand intra-axial. This could be a **primary brain tumour** but is most likely a metastasis, as these are more common. Any solitary cerebellar lesion in an elderly patient is a metastasis until proven otherwise. **Primary central nervous system lymphoma** – lymphomas affecting the cerebellum are not very common and neither are **prostatic metastases** to the brain. The commonest primary cancer metastasizing to the brain is lung cancer, followed by breast cancer. In an elderly man with a solitary cerebellar lesion, who has a long smoking history and who presents with haemoptysis, the most likely diagnosis is lung cancer with cerebellar metastasis.

Q292 Abnormal Involuntary Movements

Answer 1 – **Drug-induced myoclonus**. The patient exhibits brief, shock-like jerks of the whole body (myoclonus) during admission, which settled over a few days. Given his history of acute kidney injury and use of a morphine patch, opioid-induced myoclonus is the most likely cause. Morphine and other opioids can accumulate in renal impairment, leading to neurotoxic effects such as myoclonus. **Drug-induced tremor** typically presents as rhythmic, oscillatory movements rather than sudden, jerky myoclonic movements. **Epileptic seizures** would present with loss of consciousness, tonic–clonic activity or postictal confusion, which are not described here. **Functional movement disorder** is less likely, as opioid-induced myoclonus is a well-recognised physiological cause. **Hemiballismus** presents as unilateral, violent flinging movements, rather than generalised myoclonus.

Q293 Chronic Fatigue Syndrome

Answer 3 – **Pain clinic referral**. **Initiate opiate medication:** there is no evidence that opioids help the pain and other symptoms in CFS patients. The long-term use of opioids in chronic pain patients can lead to multiple side effects like tolerance, dependence, and opioid-induced hyperalgesia – i.e. having more opioids increases the pain further – constipation, and suppression of immunity and hypothalamus–pituitary axis **Oral steroids for 3 weeks** or **steroid injection into trigger points:** the assessment by the rheumatologist suggests there is no inflammation. So, there is no role for steroids. Moreover, steroids can result in multiple side effects like GI irritation, mood changes, insomnia, venous thromboembolism, increased infection risks and weight gain. **Regular anti-inflammatory medication** can lead to severe gastric irritation, renal damage, and cardiac, bleeding and respiratory complications. Psychology-based programmes can help to cope with the symptoms.

Q294 Dementias

Answer 3 – **Dementia with Lewy bodies**. The correct diagnosis for this 61 year old man is dementia with Lewy bodies (DLB). The evidence supporting this diagnosis includes progressive cognitive decline (i.e. inability to concentrate on TV programmes), presence of psychiatric symptoms (i.e. talking to objects and people not present, restlessness, short temper and anger outbursts), parkinsonism (i.e. slow walking, reduced arm swing on the left, shuffling gait) and smaller handwriting. All these are characteristic symptoms of DLB.

Alzheimer's disease is less likely because it primarily presents with memory loss and the MRI would typically show hippocampal and temporal lobe atrophy, which was not observed here. **Creutzfeldt–Jakob disease** often presents with rapidly progressing dementia, myoclonus and characteristic changes on EEG, none of which are reported. **Frontotemporal dementia** is characterised by personality changes and executive dysfunction but typically lacks the parkinsonism seen here. **Vascular dementia** often presents after a stroke or series of mini-strokes, and MRI typically shows evidence of cerebrovascular disease, such as white matter changes or lacunar infarcts, which was not observed in this case.

Q295 Encephalitis

Answer 1 – **Aciclovir**. The history of acute behavioural change, pyrexia and seizure is highly suspicious for viral (HSV-1) encephalitis, strongly supported by results of cerebrospinal fluid analysis. The most important initial management is with intravenous aciclovir at a dose of 10 mg/kg every 8 hours. Whilst **benzylpenicillin**, **ceftriaxone** or **dexamethasone** might be considered for the treatment of bacterial meningitis, the lack of meningism or photosensitivity makes this less likely, whilst cerebrospinal fluid analysis would be expected to show prominent neutrophilia in this instance (note: TB meningitis typically causes lymphocytic CSF with very high protein – however, presentation is usually subacute). **Phenytoin** is a first-line treatment for status epilepticus but would not be indicated after a single seizure with full recovery.

Q296 Epilepsy

Answer 4 – **It can help define an epilepsy syndrome**. The clinical history is suggestive of juvenile myoclonic epilepsy (combination of myoclonic, absence and tonic–clonic seizures), which is associated with specific changes on interictal EEG and is known to respond favourably to certain medications. An EEG does not **confirm**, or **rule out a diagnosis of epilepsy**: this is based on the clinical assessment of seizures, and in this case two unprovoked tonic–clonic seizures over a month is sufficient to diagnose epilepsy. Where there is clinical doubt, a prolonged EEG to capture an event may give support for or against epilepsy. **It can demonstrate that the collapse was actually a syncope**: the diagnosis of syncope would be made on the clinical history. **It can determine whether she is allowed to drive**: she will not be allowed to drive following a seizure regardless of what the EEG shows, although in some cases the duration of the driving ban may be influenced by the results of investigations including MRI and EEG.

Q297 Fits/Seizures

Answer 2 – **ECG**. The history is convincing for a generalised seizure. The recommended investigations are blood glucose, electrolytes and an ECG. These will identify possible triggers for a seizure (e.g. hypoglycaemia, hyponatraemia) and screen for cardiac conduction defects (which may be associated with seizures or be a cause of syncope, a common alternative diagnosis for collapses) that need urgent management. **Serum prolactin** is not a reliable discriminator between seizures and other causes of collapse. A **CT head** or an **MRI head** could be considered if there is evidence of a structural cause for the seizure (e.g. significant trauma, focal neurological deficit); otherwise, neuroimaging will be considered after specialist assessment. A **lumbar puncture** would only typically be indicated if there are signs of meningoencephalitis as the cause of a seizure.

Q298 Essential Tremor

Answer 4 – **Recommend lifestyle modifications**. This is looking at treatment for essential tremor. All of the options are useful in some circumstances, so it is really a question of what you would try first. Recommend lifestyle modification is the first, followed by **propranolol** +/− **referral to physiotherapy**. If that fails, then **primidone**. If the essential tremor does not respond to medical therapy, then **initiating deep brain stimulation** is a final option.

Q299 Extradural Haemorrhage

Answer 2 – **Arrange an urgent CT head**. This patient could be suffering from the delayed appearance of a post-traumatic extradural haematoma. Clinical pointers include the history of direct trauma to the head, headaches and an altered level of consciousness. An extradural haematoma typically occurs in a patient who has sustained direct trauma to the head, resulting in a skull fracture. The fracture typically tears the middle meningeal artery resulting in the accumulation, over several hours, of an extradural haematoma. **Admit for neuro-observation and review again in 4 hours**: if the patient is observed, deterioration is expected and this could result in death or a poorer prognosis for recovery. **Call the neurosurgeons immediately to review him for theatre**: if the neurosurgeons are contacted, they will state that a CT brain scan is required. Other investigations suggested (**CXR, ECG, routine bloods**) will not provide a diagnosis. **Discharging home with head injury advice** with this clinical history exposes the patient to harm.

Q300 Migraine

Answer 3 – **Headaches last 5 days at a time**. Migraines, according to the consensus definition of the International Classification of Headache Disorders (ICHD), last up to 72 hours. Headache episodes lasting 5 days at a time contradict this, and therefore this patient's headache does not meet criteria for migraine. Headaches **always preceded by visual disturbance** may indicate an aura, which is a potential feature of migraines. **Aggravation by routine physical activity**, **presence of nausea/vomiting during the headache**, and **pulsating quality** are all features of migraines specified by the ICHD.

Q301 Motor Neurone Disease

Answer 1 – **Amyotrophic Lateral Sclerosis** (ALS). This is the most common form of motor neurone disease, and is most likely in this case, due to mixed upper motor neurone signs (brisk reflexes) and lower motor neurone signs (atrophy with fasciculation). In a typical age group with the classical history of relentless progression from limb to limb, ALS is the most likely diagnosis. **Primary lateral sclerosis** would not typically have lower motor neurone signs, and **progressive muscular atrophy** would not have upper motor neurone signs. **Spinal muscular atrophy** is a disease that normally afflicts children and adolescents and is therefore not the most likely form of MND in this patient. **Kennedy disease** typically affects lower motor neurones of men of between 30 and 60 years old; a pathognomonic sign is peri-oral fasciculation due to bulbar involvement.

Q302 Confusion

Answer 4 – **Perform a set of observations and assess the patient clinically**. This allows you to assess and potentially treat the underlying cause of the confusion. This patient is presenting with an acute delirium following surgical procedure. All the options are appropriate – but it is what you do first which is being asked here.

Call family members to ask about the patient's baseline cognitive function: the patient becomes more confused, indicating the problem. The relatives' report is not necessary at this stage (although would be useful later, once the patient is treated). **Organise a chest X-ray, a set of confusion screen blood and urine tests**: this would be the next option after examining the patient. **Organising CT head scan** would again be a good option – but later. **Prescribing lorazepam** should not be done unless the patient is posing a potential risk to either himself or others.

Q303 Multiple Sclerosis

Answer 3 – **Primary progressive multiple sclerosis**. According to McDonald criteria, primary progressive multiple sclerosis can be diagnosed in patients with disability progression *from the start* in those with no better explanation for the clinical presentation (the ancillary testing in this patient was negative) in the context of:

- 1 year of disability progression (retrospectively or prospectively determined) independent of clinical relapse

plus two of the following:

- *one or more* T2-hyperintense lesions characteristic of multiple sclerosis in one or more of the following brain regions: periventricular, cortical or juxtacortical, or infratentorial
- *two or more* T2-hyperintense lesions in the spinal cord
- presence of CSF-specific oligoclonal bands

So it is possible to make a diagnosis at this stage. The absence of attacks in advance of the history of progressive symptoms would not be consistent with **secondary progressive multiple sclerosis**. The absence of episodic attacks is not consistent with **relapsing multiple sclerosis**. The history and presentation were not consistent with **clinically isolated syndrome**.

Q304 Muscular Dystrophies

Answer 1 – **Creatine kinase**. The boy's presentation is characteristic of Duchenne muscular dystrophy and an urgent creatine kinase could confirm this as the likely diagnosis on the same day. A **genetic test for Duchenne muscular dystrophy** would give an accurate diagnosis but the results would take longer. None of the other tests are indicated in this case. A **muscle biopsy** would only be requested if there was no clear diagnosis. There is no indication of syndromic features which may prompt **karyotype analysis**.

Q305 Parkinson's Disease

Answer 5 – **Parkinson's disease**. The presentation is very typical for Parkinson's disease, having many of the classic signs and symptoms – notably, slowing down (bradykinesia); difficulty using a knife and fork; change in facial expression; constipation and anosmia (loss of sense of smell); reduced arm swing on one side; paucity of facial expression; progressively reduced amplitude of finger tapping; rigidity detected during examination; and resting tremor.

Alzheimer's disease causes cognitive decline; **essential tremor**: typically the tremor is with action; **motor neurone disease**, muscle disease and wasting without tremor and bradykinesia; **multiple sclerosis** gives more varied neurological symptoms.

Q306 Peripheral Nerve Injuries/Palsies

Answer 4 – **Traumatic common peroneal nerve injury**. **Diabetic neuropathy** classically produces bilateral distal sensory loss rather than a focal sensorimotor deficit. **Injury to the lateral cutaneous nerve of the thigh** produces sensory loss in the distribution of the nerve in the lateral aspect of the thigh. The sural nerve is a sensory nerve which supplies sensation to the posterolateral leg and ankle, and therefore **traumatic sural nerve injury** would not cause a foot drop. A **prolapsed intervertebral disc** causing an L4/5 radiculopathy can be responsible for a foot drop. However, given the recent history of a fracture of the fibula, a common peroneal nerve injury is the most likely cause of the symptoms.

Q307 Head Injury

Answer 3 – **Extradural haematoma** (EDH). The symptoms are classic for EDH – initial transient loss of consciousness followed by a lucid interval and then a rapid deterioration in Glasgow Coma Score, on a background history of trauma. The biconvex lens shape on CT head occurs because the bleed is in the space outside the dura and dura attaches to the inside of the skull at the skull sutures. This is also why EDH doesn't cross the midline. **Acute subdural haematoma** would appear as a crescent-shaped bleed that can go up to the midline on one side. **Chronic subdural haematoma** occurs in elderly patients or patients on blood thinners with history of falls. Usually, history is of gradual-onset symptoms. **Traumatic subarachnoid**

haemorrhage would again be unlikely to present with the history above. The blood would be in the grooves of the brain / on the brain surface. **Intracerebral haemorrhage** appears as localised bleeding within brain tissue rather than an extradural (epidural) location.

Q308 Radiculopathies

Answer 1 – **Arrange an emergency whole spine MRI**. This lady has features consistent with 'incomplete' compression of the cauda equina nerves. She does not yet have a full house of bilateral sciatica, lumbar nerve root weakness and overflow incontinence. However, the urinary hesitancy and bilateral numbness are symptoms of concern. Examination identified features consistent with a central disc prolapse afflicting bilateral nerve roots. The features of cauda equina compression must be recognised early: an emergency MRI is required. This is normally best obtained via referral to the local emergency department with onward referral to a spinal surgeon if the clinical suspicion is confirmed. **All other options** include delays in management that will enable the cauda equina syndrome to become more severe, with less prospect of recovery.

Q309 Raised Intracranial Pressure

Answer 1 – **CT head scan**. A CT head is a relatively quick and accessible investigation modality available in most UK hospitals. This usually takes 5–10 minutes and will reveal space-occupying lesions, hydrocephalus or cerebral oedema. **Fundal photography** is a specialist assessment for papilloedema, and is inappropriate in the context of a patient who is clearly obtunded. Fundoscopy will not reveal the cause of the raised ICP. **Lumbar puncture** is potentially dangerous as it could result in cerebellar tonsillar herniation (coning) and brainstem/midbrain compression causing irreversible neurological injury/death. Like a CT head, **MRI** will show the cause of the raised ICP but in even better detail. However, it is not readily accessible and a typical scan can take up to 45–60 mins. There is no role for **transcranial doppler** (TCD) ultrasound in this patient. It gives no information on raised ICP or the cause.

Q310 Spinal Cord Injury

Answer 3 – **Referral to the Regional Spinal Cord Injury Centre**. **Ventilation to avoid hypoxia** – a thoracic injury is not normally associated with hypoxia; ventilation is commonly required for a cervical spine injury. **Spinal angiography** is invasive and could exacerbate any neurological deficit. There is no evidence that **administration of hypertonic saline** is useful. This treatment may cause volume depletion and exacerbate spinal ischaemia. There is no evidence to strongly support the use of steroids such as **methylprednisolone** after spinal cord trauma. Early involvement of the Regional Spinal Cord Injury Centre is recommended.

Q311 Spinal Fracture

Answer 3 – **Pan CT**. Pan-CT (or trauma CT) scan evaluates multiple systems (e.g. chest, pelvis, long bones, spine, head) and is appropriate given the history. Any spinal fractures will be identified. Most osteoporotic thoracolumbar fractures are stable. **X-ray of the spine**: X-rays lack sensitivity; a **bone scan** or **whole body MRI** would not be relevant in the acute situation – more complex to perform and lack sensitivity for all possible injuries. An **LP** is utilised if the history is consistent with a causative spontaneous subarachnoid haemorrhage and the CT head scan is normal.

Q312 Tremor

Answer 4 – **Idiopathic Parkinson's disease**. Parkinson's disease is characterised by an insidious onset of symptoms. There is often evidence of non-motor symptoms that can be elicited in the history prior to the motor symptoms' start. The triad of resting tremor, bradykinesia and rigidity should always raise suspicion for Parkinson's disease. **Essential tremor** is associated with action tremors. **Paraneoplastic cerebellar degeneration** presents as a rapidly progressive pan-cerebellar syndrome. **Autonomic neuropathy** and **hereditary spastic paraparesis** do not have tremors as a symptom.

Q313 Stroke

Answer 4 – **Haemorrhagic transformation**. The sudden change in presentation could result from any of the listed options – however, observed seizure activity would be most associated with haemorrhagic transformation. **Allergic reaction to alteplase** is rare and would typically present with anaphylaxis or angioedema, not seizures and decreased consciousness. **Aspiration pneumonia** can occur in stroke patients but would present with fever, respiratory distress and consolidation on imaging, not sudden neurological decline and seizures. **Concomitant myocardial infarction** is unlikely as the primary cause of the sudden deterioration; there is no chest pain or

ECG changes reported. **Venous thromboembolism** (e.g. pulmonary embolism) could cause hypoxia and collapse, but it does not explain the seizure and worsening neurological status.

Q314 Subarachnoid Haemorrhage

Answer 2 – **CT scan of the head**. The history is consistent with a subarachnoid haemorrhage. A CT head scan has a very high specificity and sensitivity for the detection of subarachnoid haemorrhage and is the first-choice investigation. The distribution of blood can be very helpful at identifying the most likely source of a haemorrhage. If a CT head scan is reported as not showing blood, the Society of British Neurological Surgeons recommends that a **lumbar puncture** is performed. This should be delayed until 12 hours after the ictus to allow the breakdown of red blood cells which results in xanthochromic CSF. An **MRI of the head** is less sensitive than a CT scan for subarachnoid haemorrhage, although specific vessel wall sequences are emerging that can help establish which aneurysm has ruptured in some cases where a patient has multiple aneurysms and there is uncertainty about the culprit aneurysm. A **CT angiogram** is very useful once a plain CT head scan has confirmed a subarachnoid haemorrhage: the CT angiogram frequently identifies the causative lesion and anatomical information helps with the planning of endovascular or surgical treatment. A **full blood count** does not contribute to the diagnosis of a subarachnoid haemorrhage, though is an appropriate investigation in this situation.

Q315 Tension Headache

Answer 1 – **Amitriptyline 10 mg once nightly**. Amitriptyline is the only recommended preventive (prophylactic) pharmacological treatment for tension-type headache, with aspirin and paracetamol both recommended for acute episodes by BASH. **Regular paracetamol** and **regular aspirin** without cessation put this patient at risk of medication-overuse headache, and would not be appropriate preventive management. Neither **triptans** nor **oramorph as required for acute attacks** are recommended for use in tension-type headache.

Q316 Transient Ischaemic Attacks

Answer 2 – **Aspirin**. The NICE guidelines currently recommend giving 300 mg of aspirin for a suspected TIA. The patient was not in AF, and therefore a **warfarin loading dose** and **dabigatran** are not appropriate. **Alteplase** is a fibrinolytic given for thrombolysis which can be given in an acute ischaemic stroke confirmed on cerebral vascular imaging (CT/MRI angiography). **Atorvastatin** can be useful in managing cholesterol as a risk factor in the long term, which this patient will likely need, but is not the best immediate management from the options given.

Q317 Visual Hallucinations

Answer 3 – **MRI brain**. The presentation is suspicious of posterior circulation stroke leading to cortical blindness and Anton's syndrome. Brain imaging is warranted. **Electroencephalogram (EEG)** is used for seizure activity or encephalopathy, but the presentation is more suggestive of a vascular event. **Lumbar puncture** is used for infectious or inflammatory conditions (e.g. meningitis, encephalitis, autoimmune disorders), but there is no fever or signs of infection. **Psychiatry review** is unnecessary at this stage, as delirium due to an acute neurological event should be ruled out first. **Referral to the Parkinson's team** may be helpful later, but this presentation is not typical for Parkinson's-related confusion (e.g. dopamine agonist toxicity, Lewy body dementia) – it is more suggestive of a stroke.

Q318 Trigeminal Neuralgia

Answer 5 – **Trigeminal neuralgia**. The history provided is typical of trigeminal neuralgia. Spontaneous **subarachnoid haemorrhage** normally presents with a sudden onset of severe headache, rather than repeated daily episodes. **Dental abscess** and **maxillary sinusitis** normally cause continuous facial, maxillary or mandibular pain. **Brainstem gliomas** typically present with painless cranial nerve and sometimes corticospinal deficits.

Q319 Wernicke's Encephalopathy

Answer 2 – **AIDS**. Wernicke's encephalopathy is a neurological disorder caused by a deficiency of thiamine (vitamin B1). It is commonly associated with chronic alcoholism, probably due to poor nutritional intake, but other conditions can also increase the risk. The specific risk factor here, aside from alcohol excess, is AIDS. The reason for this is a combination of malnutrition (poor intake, opportunistic bowel infections reducing absorption – and therefore thiamine intake), inflammation, chronic infection and high metabolic demand (depleting thiamine stores). Other conditions – **age**,

COPD, **type 2 diabetes** and **temperature** only have a minor impact on thiamine availability.

Q320 Subdural Haemorrhage

Answer 2 – **Chronic subdural haematoma**. The gradual, progressive history is typical of a chronic SDH. **Ischaemic stroke** and a spontaneous intracerebral haemorrhage are abrupt in onset. An **acute SDH** is normally associated with trauma. The rare spontaneous acute SDH is of sudden onset. **Extradural haematoma** and traumatic **intracerebral haematoma** present soon after a traumatic brain injury, although both can be associated with a deterioration in condition some hours after trauma.

Q321 Altered Sensation, Numbness and Tingling

Answer 2 – **Guillain–Barre syndrome**. In this particular scenario, note the acute-onset positive symptoms, with involvement of proximal and distal weakness along with a history of likely infectious gastroenteritis prior to this. GBS has an acute onset with rapid progression, and disease manifests completely within 4 weeks. Most patients reach their nadir within 14 days. The triggering event could be an infectious respiratory or gastrointestinal illness 4–6 weeks prior to the onset of symptoms. **ALS**, **PD** and **MG** do not have neuropathic symptoms. Although **MS** can present acutely, this illness has a predominantly UMN pattern examination, unlike GBS which has purely LMN pattern signs.

Q322 Auditory Hallucinations

Answer 3 – **Hearing loss**. The patient is experiencing prolonged auditory hallucinations of music. This is recognised to occur in individuals with hearing loss. There are no clinical features of psychosis to suggest late-onset **schizophrenia**. **Epilepsy** may rarely cause hallucinations, but these would be short-lived. **Parkinson's disease** dementia or Lewy body dementia typically cause visual hallucinations. There is no history of **head injury**.

Q323 Decreased / Loss of Consciousness

Answer 3 – **Perform lying and standing BP**. Postural hypotension is a common cause of falls in older patients and can be readily detected by measurement of lying and standing BP. This is an initial investigation that can easily be conducted at the time of the clinical examination. **Arranging an MRI head** is unnecessary unless there are neurological symptoms suggesting stroke or transient ischaemic attack. **Routine blood tests** may help identify contributing factors (e.g. anaemia, electrolyte imbalances) but are not the first-line test. **Immediate referral to the emergency department** is not required, as she is well between episodes. **Starting anti-epileptic medication** is inappropriate, as there is no history of seizures, postictal confusion or abnormal movements.

Q324 Diplopia

Answer 4 – **Infarction**. The examination is classical for a third nerve palsy. The onset is sudden (making it less likely to be **malignancy** or **abscess**); history of hypertension and diabetes (makes infarction more likely); the pathology is only affecting the third nerve, making **haemorrhage** unlikely. There are no previous episodes of neurological loss so **demyelination** is less likely.

Q325 Bell's Palsy

Answer 5 – **Urgent CT head**. A CT head is required to rule out an acute stroke, given the weakness does not appear to be localised to the facial nerve. **Anti-viral therapy** and a **high-dose corticosteroid** are potential management options in confirmed Bell's palsy, and **MRI brain** would be useful if a neoplasm were suspected. **Chest X-ray** would be indicated if this were a Horner's syndrome – looking for a pancoast tumour.

Q326 Facial Pain

Answer 2 – **Carbamazepine**. The description of paroxysmal shooting pain exacerbated by cold weather and eating is typical of trigeminal neuralgia. Carbamazepine represents the gold-standard first-line drug recommended for long-term treatment. Whilst the benefit of carbamazepine has been validated in multiple randomised controlled trials, treatment may be limited by adverse effects which include drowsiness, dizziness, rash, ataxia, hyponatraemia, hepatotoxicity and the potential for multiple drug interactions. In order to minimise the risk of side effects, it is recommended that carbamazepine is initiated at a low dose (200–400 mg daily in divided doses) and uptitrated at weekly or 2-weekly intervals to a maximum daily dose of 1600 mg. Oxcarbazepine represents an alternative to carbamazepine, and may be associated with fewer side effects. **Amitriptyline** is used for general neuropathic pain but is not the first-line treatment for trigeminal neuralgia. **Duloxetine** is primarily used for diabetic neuropathy and fibromyalgia, not trigeminal neuralgia. **Lidocaine patches** are used for localised postherpetic neuralgia but are ineffective for deep nerve pain like trigeminal neuralgia. **Pregabalin** is used for generalised neuropathic pain but is less effective than carbamazepine for trigeminal neuralgia.

Q327 Facial Weakness

Answer 1 – **Bell's palsy**. The examination features are consistent with a LMN pattern of facial weakness. While a **pontine stroke** and **multiple sclerosis** could affect the facial nerve nucleus in the brainstem and cause an LMN-pattern facial weakness, these would almost always cause other cranial nerve signs as well. A **right MCA territory stroke** would cause a UMN-pattern facial weakness. The unilateral LMN facial weakness with associated hyperacusis and taste impairment is typical for Bell's palsy. **Lyme disease** could be considered if the weakness does not start to improve within 4 weeks (as expected for Bell's palsy) or there was a history of a tick bite or erythema migrans rash.

Q328 Myasthenia Gravis

Answer 2 – **Double vision**. Myasthenia is a neuromuscular junction disorder causing fatigable muscle weakness (i.e. worse with recurrent use of the affected muscles). This commonly affects the eyes in the first instance, leading to diplopia and ptosis, which is worse with prolonged use and at the end of the day. It has no effect in the central nervous system, including the brain, so would not cause **headache** or **confusion**, and does not cause any **hip girdle stiffness**. **Foot drop** would be suggestive of permanent/persistent nerve damage leading to a muscle weakness specific to the area affected.

Q329 Fasciculation

Answer 2 – **Benign fasciculation syndrome**. This patient is clearly generally fit and well, with no change in his motor function for the last 5 years. It is most likely that the fasciculation is occurring because of exercise, but it could also be due to use of a salbutamol inhaler in an asthmatic patient. Lack of neurological findings on examination reinforces this. **Amyotrophic lateral sclerosis** would present with progressive weakness, muscle atrophy and widespread fasciculations, which are absent here. **Chronic inflammatory demyelinating polyneuropathy** causes progressive weakness and sensory changes, not isolated, non-progressive fasciculations. **L5/S1 nerve root lesion** would cause weakness, sensory loss or radicular pain, none of which is present. **Multifocal motor neuropathy** presents with asymmetric weakness and conduction block on nerve conduction studies, which is not described in this case

Q330 Headache

Answer 5 – **Urgent CT head scan.** Reaching maximal intensity within 5 minutes of onset defines this as a thunderclap headache, for which a serious vascular cause such as a subarachnoid haemorrhage needs to be excluded prior to further investigation. **Preventive migraine treatment, reassurance and discharge** and **referral to neurology outpatients** fail to address the potential acute issue at hand. **Lumbar puncture** may well be required following the initial CT head to look for xanthochromia or evidence of neurological infection, but the CT should be done first.

Q331 Diabetic neuropathy

Answer 4 – **Improved glycaemic control**. This will help to control further progression of his diabetic neuropathy by reducing the neuronal damage caused by hyperglycaemia. The other four answers are drug treatments that will control symptoms, but will not prevent progression of the diabetic neuropathy. **Midodrine** can be used for postural hypotension in autonomic neuropathy, and **gabapentin/amitriptyline/duloxetine** can be used for neuropathic pain.

Q332 Limb Weakness

Answer 2 – **Left anterior cerebral artery stroke**. Given the history of hyperacute onset along with vascular risk factors (hypertension and PAF), this points to the clue that this could likely be a vascular event. The signs of right leg weakness along with urinary incontinence indicate a lesion of the paracentral lobule which is supplied by the anterior cerebral artery. **GBS** presents in a subacute manner with ascending or descending weakness and it often causes an asymmetric lower motor neurone lesion (peripheral neuropathy) with all symptoms manifesting within 7–28 days since the index event. **Myasthenia gravis** usually presents with weakness and fatiguability and will predominantly have proximal muscle weakness accompanied by bulbar symptoms. **NPH** has a more chronic history and is unlikely to present with acute weakness. **Todd's paresis** often precedes a history of seizures and on carefully reviewing the history we can clinch the diagnosis.

Q333 Limp

Answer 4 – **MRI lumbosacral plexus**. The patient's symptoms suggest a localised neurological problem, likely affecting the lumbosacral plexus, given the pattern of weakness, sensory deficits and foot drop. The normal MRI of the lumbosacral spine rules out common causes of radiculopathy, such as disc herniation or spinal stenosis, leading to the suspicion of a plexus-level pathology. An MRI lumbosacral plexus is the most appropriate next investigation as it can help identify structural abnormalities, such as tumours, inflammation or other lesions affecting the plexus, which are not visible on the standard spine MRI. Other options, such as **HbA1c and bloods** for systemic causes, **Lumbar puncture, antibody panel +/– nerve biopsy** for potential inflammatory or infectious causes, **MRI brain and whole spine** and **ultrasound of the course of the sciatic, tibial and peroneal nerves**, are less immediately relevant or are secondary considerations based on the clinical presentation and initial imaging results.

Q334 Memory Loss

Answer 5 – **Vascular dementia**. This is a very typical presentation of memory loss.

The most likely cause is vascular dementia – risk factors being the same as those for cerebrovascular disease: smoking, hypertension, obesity, underlying claudication and probable undermedicated AF. With these points, this type of dementia becomes more likely than **Alzheimer's disease**. **Delirium** is of acute onset of less than 1 week. **Dementia with Lewy bodies** usually has a Parkinsonian-type gait. **Pick's disease** usually occurs in younger individuals and is associated with personality changes (loss of inhibition).

Q335 Meningitis

Answer 5 – **Streptococcus pneumoniae**. This is the most common cause in infants, young children and adults. **Neisseria meningitidis** affects mainly teenagers and young adults. **Haemophilus influenzae** type B was once a leading cause, but new Hib vaccines have reduced this. **Listeria monocytogenes** can be found in unpasteurised dairy products, and pregnant women, newborns and the immunocompromised appear particularly susceptible. Listeria can cross the blood–brain barrier. **E. coli** is less common but can still cause meningitis.

Q336 Neuromuscular Weakness

Answer 4 – **Myasthenia gravis**. This is the correct answer as it is the only one of the five pathologies which is associated with anti-acetylcholine receptor antibodies positivity and presents with the pattern of weakness described in the question's text and at a later stage in life, but without myalgia. **Congenital myopathy** usually manifests early in life and is not associated with the antibodies. **Inflammatory myopathy** is often associated with myalgia and would not have positive anti-acetylcholine receptor antibodies. **Motor neurone disease** and **peripheral neuropathy** do not come with positive antibodies either. The clinical picture (particularly bulbar signs such as dysphagia or unilateral ptosis) would also not be in keeping with a peripheral neuropathy. It is also unlikely for motor neurone disease to clinically present as described (unilateral ptosis, symptoms worse in the evening, strictly proximal limb weakness).

Q337 Spinal cord compression

Answer 5 – **Sustained clonus**. This is the only upper motor neurone sign. **All other options** are lower motor neurone signs. The other upper motor neurone signs include hypertonia, brisk reflexes and up-going plantars.

Q338 Ptosis

Answer 3 – **Oculomotor**. The oculomotor nerve (cranial nerve III) is responsible for controlling most of the eye's movements, including constriction of the pupil and maintaining an open eyelid. The cause of ptosis (drooping of the upper eyelid) is 3rd nerve lesion. **Abducens** (VI) controls only the lateral rectus muscle (abduction of the eye). **Facial** (VII) controls muscles of facial expression, not eye movements. **Optic** (II) is responsible for vision, not eye movements. **Trochlear** (IV) controls the superior oblique muscle (intorsion and depression of the eye when adducted).

Q339 Sleep Problems

Answer 4 – **Obstructive sleep apnoea**. Obstructive sleep apnoea is the best answer as the patient has risk factors (COPD and obesity). There is also a history of snoring, excessive daytime sleeping and fatigue. It is unlikely to be a **circadian rhythm sleep–wake disorder** as the patient doesn't work night shifts, which can affect the sleep cycle. **Insomnia** involves difficulty falling or staying asleep, but this patient's primary issue is daytime sleepiness despite sleeping at night. **Narcolepsy** is characterised by sudden sleep attacks, cataplexy, sleep paralysis and hallucinations, none of which is present. **Restless leg syndrome** causes uncomfortable leg sensations at rest, relieved by movement, rather than loud snoring and daytime sleepiness.

Q340 Unsteadiness

Answer 5 – **Right cerebellar hemisphere**. Right-sided clumsiness and intention tremor suggest dysfunction of the right cerebellar hemisphere, which controls coordination and fine motor movements on the same side (ipsilateral control).

Unsteadiness on walking is consistent with cerebellar involvement, particularly affecting balance and coordination. Headaches at night and morning vomiting suggest raised intracranial pressure (ICP), which can occur with a posterior fossa lesion.

Bilateral papilloedema further supports increased ICP, commonly seen in posterior fossa masses affecting cerebrospinal fluid outflow. **Cervical spine**: pathology here would cause spinal cord symptoms such as weakness, sensory loss or reflex changes, but not intention tremor or papilloedema. **Foramen magnum** could cause compression of the brainstem, leading to cranial nerve dysfunction, but would not localise as specifically to the right cerebellar hemisphere. **Left internal capsule** would cause contralateral weakness and sensory deficits, not cerebellar signs such as tremor or unsteadiness. **Pituitary fossa**: a pituitary lesion would primarily cause visual field defects (e.g. bitemporal hemianopia) or endocrine disturbances, neither of which are present here.

Q341 Cervical Cancer

Answer 3 – **Stage 2**. This patient has previously tested positive for HPV which can cause cervical cancer. Due to the lesion extending from the cervix to the upper third of the vagina, this would be classed as stage 2. **Stage 0** is carcinoma *in situ*, limited to the cervical epithelium without invasion. **Stage 1** is confined to the cervix only, without vaginal or pelvic spread. **Stage 3** involves extension to the lower third of the vagina or pelvic wall or causes hydronephrosis. **Stage 4** indicates distant metastasis or extension to the bladder, rectum or beyond the pelvis.

Q342 Atrophic Vaginitis

Answer 1 – **Atrophic vaginitis**. The patient meets the criteria for being classified as at high risk of bladder or **uterine prolapse** due to her age, weight, and multiple pregnancies. As a result of physical examination, prolapse is not detected. **Pelvic inflammatory disease** is ruled out because, although the patient has a few signs and symptoms, she has no vaginal discharge or fever. The same argument can also be made for **bacterial vaginitis**. **Endometrial cancer** usually presents with abnormal bleeding, which is not reported. The diagnosis of atrophic vaginitis is appropriate because the patient is post-menopausal, with low oestrogen reserves causing decrease in vaginal secretions and thinning of the endothelium, and predisposing women to mechanical weaknesses. The earliest signs are usually burning or dyspareunia which can be exacerbated by a superimposed infection, such as a UTI.

Q343 Bacterial Vaginosis

Answer 3 – **Metronidazole**. Fishy-smelling discharge is very suggestive of bacterial vaginosis (treated with metronidazole). **Azithromycin** is for chlamydia. Chlamydia usually gives a strong-smelling yellow discharge with other symptoms. There are no painful blisters suggestive of herpes (excluding **aciclovir**). **No treatment now but await swab findings**: you would treat before swabs are taken. Only **refer to the sexual health clinic** if history is suggestive of sexually transmitted disease. Note: the phrase 'having the same partner for x years' usually (but not always) points to a non-sexually transmitted disease.

Q344 Cervical Screening (HPV)

Answer 2 – **Perform a smear as she is a year overdue**. The patient is due her smear test. As she is HPV negative, she no longer needs smear tests – screening continues regardless of an HPV negative result. **Reassure her that her next test is not due for another year due to her age**: NHS screening intervals change to 5 years for women *over* 50 years of age. **Rearrange smear after 2 weeks of topical oestrogen therapy**: this is not appropriate as, from clinical examination, smear should be easy to take. **Urgent referral to gynaecology as her periods are intermittently heavy**: clinical examination and history do not support a referral.

Q345 Cord Prolapse

Answer 4 – **Pull the emergency buzzer**. Additional help is urgently needed as transfer and preparations must be made for an immediate caesarean section. Pulling the emergency buzzer is the fastest way to summon help. **Bleep the anaesthetist**: the first person to arrive would be asked to put out an Obstetric Emergency 2222 bleep, which will in turn summon the members of the team who are not within earshot of the buzzer, including the anaesthetist. The midwife who diagnosed the cord prolapse should give the patient a brief explanation of what has happened and instruct her on how to adopt the all-fours knees-to-chest position on her bed, while awaiting enough assistance to make the transfer to obstetric theatres. **Checking the woman's observations** and **starting a CTG** are not relevant at this point as they will delay transfer to theatre, where they can be checked. **Insert a cannula**: a cannula will be required in theatre so if there is a competent clinician available and it will not delay transfer, it could be sited, after the necessary calls have been put out.

Q346 Abnormal Cervical Smear Result

Answer 4 – **Repeat smear in 12 months.** HPV positivity without abnormal cytology is managed with repeat cervical screening in 12 months, as most HPV infections clear spontaneously within a year. If HPV persists for 2 consecutive years, **referral to the colposcopy clinic** for further assessment is warranted to detect potential cervical changes. Otherwise, referral is only indicated if there are abnormal cells. Since no abnormal cells were found, colposcopy is not necessary at this stage. **Immunisation with HPV vaccine** is most effective when given before exposure to the virus (typically before sexual activity, around ages 11–14). While beneficial for future protection, it does not clear an existing infection. **No additional action necessary**: this is incorrect, as HPV positivity requires monitoring due to its association with cervical cancer. **Treatment with anti-virals**: there is no anti-viral treatment for HPV; the immune system usually clears the infection naturally.

Q347 Diabetes in Pregnancy (Gestational and Pre-existing)

Answer 4 – **Give advice regarding diet and exercise changes and review again in 1–2 weeks**. This is correct because her fasting blood glucose was less than 7.0 mml/L and her ultrasound is normal. This means a trial of diet and exercise changes first, and a re-review in 1–2 weeks. If her fasting blood glucose had been more than 7.0 mmol/L, or her ultrasound had demonstrated complications associated with diabetes such as macrosomia or polyhydramnios, immediate treatment with **metformin and insulin** would be advised. **Repeat the OGTT to confirm the result**: the OGTT does not get repeated, and **weight loss** is generally not advised in pregnancy (rather, avoidance of gaining excess weight is advised). **Commencing insulin only** is premature without first attempting dietary and lifestyle modifications.

Q348 Ectopic Pregnancy

Answer 2 – **Ectopic pregnancy**. This patient has an ectopic pregnancy. This is supported by the fact that her last period was several weeks ago, and she has a positive pregnancy test. It is further supported by vaginal bleeding, which may be spotting in some cases. **Appendicitis** can cause right lower quadrant pain but would not explain the positive pregnancy test or vaginal bleeding. **Normal menses** is unlikely given the missed period and positive pregnancy test. **Ovarian cyst** can cause lower quadrant pain but typically does not cause vaginal bleeding or a positive pregnancy test. **Urinary tract infection** may cause abdominal pain but would also present with dysuria, frequency, and no positive pregnancy test.

Q349 Endometriosis

Answer 1 – **Diagnostic laparoscopy +/– excision of endometriosis**. The patient may need a fertility work-up including a **hysterosalpingogram** in due course, but it is important to treat any endometriosis first. This should also help her pain. An **MRI** would not be used as first-line here, and **GnRH agonists** are contraindicated as she wants to conceive. **Referral to the fertility team for IVF** may be appropriate if surgical treatment fails, but addressing endometriosis surgically can improve natural conception rates.

Q350 Fibroids

Answer 5 – **Uterine fibroids**. The most likely answer in this scenario is uterine fibroids, although consideration needs to be given to all the other conditions. A physical examination should have ruled out **cervical cancer**. She has regular periods, so **pregnancy** is unlikely. A bulky uterus is more in keeping with uterine fibroids than **ovarian cancer**. **Overactive bladder** may also be implicated, but more likely her urinary symptoms and heavy periods are being caused by pressure on the bladder from the enlarged uterus.

Q351 Hyperemesis

Answer 3 – **Molar pregnancy.** Severe, worsening nausea and vomiting at 11 weeks of gestation, especially when accompanied by new-onset hypertension, raises concern for molar pregnancy (hydatidiform mole), a form of gestational trophoblastic disease. Molar pregnancies are associated with higher levels of human chorionic gonadotropin (hCG), which can lead to excessive nausea and vomiting (similar to hyperemesis gravidarum) as well as early-onset hypertension. While **anxiety** can cause transient increases in BP, it is unlikely to cause persistent hypertension at such high levels (160/110 mmHg), especially in pregnancy. **Hyperemesis gravidarum** involves severe nausea and vomiting in early pregnancy but is not typically associated with hypertension. The severe nausea in this case may be due to elevated hCG levels from a molar pregnancy. **Multiple pregnancy** can cause elevated hCG levels and increase nausea and vomiting, but they typically cause uterine enlargement. The fact that the fundus is not palpable at 11 weeks makes this diagnosis less likely. **Preeclampsia** generally occurs after 20 weeks of gestation, so it is unlikely at 11 weeks. Additionally, pre-eclampsia is usually associated with proteinuria, which is not mentioned here.

Q352 Human Papilloma Virus Infection

Answer 2 – **Perform a smear test.** The patient has not yet had a smear despite meeting screening criteria. **Full set of bloods including CA125** – the patient history does not contain any information to suggest that she has ovarian cancer. The history does not support **prescribing antibiotics** – swabs are normal, and antibiotics are not indicated for routine coil fit. Clinical examination, history and swab results do not support a need to **refer to sexual health clinic.** An ectropion without unusual features or symptoms does not require **urgent referral to colposcopy.**

Q353 Obesity and Pregnancy

Answer 3 – **Insulin resistance**. Gestational diabetes typically develops because of insulin resistance, especially during the second and third trimesters of pregnancy. Here's why insulin resistance is the key mechanism: pregnancy hormones (such as human placental lactogen, progesterone and cortisol) cause the body to become more resistant to insulin – this is a normal part of pregnancy that allows more glucose to be available for the growing fetus; in women with predisposing factors (such as obesity – a BMI of 35 kg/m^2 in this case), this insulin resistance can become excessive, leading to gestational diabetes because the pancreas is unable to produce enough insulin to overcome this resistance. **Increased excretion of insulin** is not a recognised mechanism for gestational diabetes. **Increased metabolism of insulin** is not relevant to gestational diabetes pathophysiology. **Lack of production of insulin** suggests type 1 diabetes, which is not the case here. **Overproduction of insulin** occurs as a compensatory response to insulin resistance, not as a primary cause of gestational diabetes.

Q354 Menopause

Answer 4 – **Sequential combined HRT**. The patient is perimenopausal (as menopause is defined in retrospect – 1 year of no periods) and experiencing menopausal symptoms – hot flushes. She has hot flushes due to oestrogen deficiency and having periods. HRT will help in treatment by providing required oestrogen. Sequential combined HRT is preferred: combined as she has a uterus, and sequential as she is still having periods. **Continuous combined HRT** is not the correct treatment as this is given when women do not have periods and have a uterus. **Oestrogen only HRT (oral tablets** or **patches or gel)** cannot be correct as oestrogen only treatment is given when the patient does not have a uterus – otherwise, it will stimulate the endometrium and predispose towards cancer.

Tibolone has oestrogen, progesterone and androgenic properties but cannot be given in peri-menopause as it causes chaotic bleeding.

Q355 Ovarian Cancer

Answer 1 – **Bloods (FBC, urea and electrolytes, liver function tests, CA125)**. It is important to initially arrange some blood tests which can guide you towards further investigations including imaging and endoscopy. In this scenario, ovarian cancer is a possible diagnosis, often presenting with unspecific symptoms such as those of bloating, feeling of indigestion and frequent urination. It is important to consider this diagnosis in any woman, especially in the post-menopausal cohort, and to arrange a serum CA125 as first-line investigation. **Transabdominal and transvaginal ultrasound** is the next-line investigation for assessing ovarian and pelvic pathology, helping to identify ovarian masses, cysts or ascites, and if there is a strong suspicion this should be organised before blood results come back. **CT scan of thorax, abdomen and pelvis** is not a first-line test for suspected ovarian cancer; it is used once a mass is identified to assess for metastasis. **Colonoscopy** is more appropriate for lower gastrointestinal symptoms (e.g. rectal bleeding, change in bowel habits). **Gastroscopy** is indicated for upper gastrointestinal symptoms (e.g. dysphagia, reflux) but not for bloating and urinary symptoms.

Q356 Placenta Praevia

Answer 1 – **Admit to the maternity department for assessment and ongoing management**. This patient needs to be seen in the maternity unit to assess the cause of bleeding, need for admission and ongoing management. A speculum examination is safe in bleeding in pregnancy, as it will not go through the cervix. **A manual vaginal examination** could result in a finger going through the cervix and causing further damage or bleeding. **Reassure the patient and** discharge them: all bleeding in pregnancy is abnormal and should be assessed and investigated. Also, you do not know the patient's rhesus status and whether they require anti-D prophylaxis. **Requesting an ultrasound** is not necessary – we are aware of the placental positioning, and so the immediate need is for clinical assessment in the maternity unit. There is no need to **start intravenous fluids**, as this patient has now stopped bleeding, and is haemodynamically stable.

Q357 Postpartum Haemorrhage

Answer 4 – **Theatre for an examination under anaesthesia and removal of placenta**. This lady is bleeding from a combination of atony and tissue retention. Surgical removal is required. The placenta remains *in situ* and needs removing. If there is ongoing atony after this has been removed, **a compression balloon** may be required subsequently. At this stage, the patient does not require a **blood transfusion**, and it is not definitive treatment. This patient has a history of pre-eclampsia, so **ergometrine** should be avoided. Whilst **tranexamic acid** should be administered, it is not going to treat the underlying cause.

Q358 Pre-eclampsia, Gestational Hypertension

Answer 3 – **Labetolol**. **Atenolol** is associated with growth restriction and **enalapril** increases the risks of congenital abnormalities, and so both of these antihypertensives are generally avoided. **Nifedipine** is used if labetolol is not suitable, and **methyldopa** is used if both labetolol and nifedipine are not suitable. Nifedipine, labetolol and methyldopa are all considered suitable for use during pregnancy; however, methyldopa and nifedipine are not specifically licensed for use in pregnancy.

Q359 Vulval/Vaginal Lump

Answer 4 – **Marsupialisation**. Treatment is marsupialisation, where abscess is incised and cut edges of cyst wall are stitched with vulval skin using interrupted stitches such that the cavity of the cyst is marsupialised. These cysts are lined with cuboidal epithelium which secretes mucoid material to keep the vulva moist. Ducts of these glands are lined with transitional epithelium and obstruction of these ducts causes Bartholin's cysts to appear. Antibiotics are given in initial stages, in case infection has caused ducts to block but in advanced cases, drainage is to be done. **Antibiotics** are given at an initial stage but not after formation of an abscess, and antibiotics cannot penetrate into pus contained in a cyst. **Cystectomy** is also not correct as it is often not possible to dissect the cyst wall from vulval tissue, and this can cause scarring. **Incision and drainage** is not done as the cyst wall closes again after temporary relief and the abscess forms again. There is no indication to **refer to sexual health clinic**.

Q360 Vasa Praevia

Answer 1 – **Category 1 (immediate) caesarean section**. The CTG is likely to reflect fetal anaemia and hypoxia. Any delay will increase the mortality. The caesarean section needs to be conducted as fast as possible and is classified as a category 1 caesarean section as there is immediate threat to the life of the baby. **Category 2 (urgent) caesarean section** is for non-life-threatening emergencies. **All other options** are too slow.

Q361 Venous Thromboembolism in Pregnancy and Puerperium

Answer 2 – **Discussion with the woman concerning a ventilation/perfusion scan or CT pulmonary angiogram**. She is demonstrating symptoms consistent with a PE and has multiple risk factors in addition to pregnancy. **Check her D-dimer and calculate her Wells score**: at present, D-Dimer and Wells are not validated or reliable for use in pregnancy, therefore they should not be used to determine the need for further investigation. She is also showing no signs of deep vein thrombosis, so venous dopplers are inappropriate. Just as in a non-pregnant patient, starting treatment prior to any investigations carries a low risk of complication when compared to the risk of the embolus evolving whilst awaiting imaging. However, she is not showing signs of a massive life-threatening embolus, therefore **starting thrombolysis** is not indicated. In this case, her CXR is normal so either a V/Q or CT pulmonary angiogram would be an appropriate first-line option, depending on what is available in your unit and after discussion with the mother. **Repeating chest X-ray in 4 hours** is unnecessary given the normal initial result and high clinical suspicion of PE. **Requesting bilateral compression duplex ultrasound** is useful for deep vein thrombosis (DVT) but is not first-line if there are no leg symptoms or signs.

Q362 Amenorrhoea

Answer 5 – **Urgent referral to a gynaecologist**. Menopause is a clinical diagnosis, and the history is certainly suggestive. However, the age of the patient is outside the currently accepted range and warrants a secondary care referral for consideration of less benign causes. **Asking her to make an appointment at the sexual health clinic** is inappropriate, as her symptoms are hormonal and not suggestive of a sexually transmitted infection or sexual health issue. **Referral for transvaginal ultrasound** could help assess for endometrial or ovarian pathology, but it is not a substitute for a comprehensive gynaecological evaluation. **Routine referral to endocrinology** may be useful for complex endocrine causes, but a gynaecologist is more appropriate as a first step given the gynaeco-logical nature of her symptoms. **Starting treatment for hormone replacement therapy** is premature without further investigation to exclude other causes of her symptoms.

Q363 Bleeding Antepartum

Answer 1 – **Placental abruption**. All of the listed conditions can cause antepartum bleeding. Out of these, only **uterine rupture** and placental abruption are likely to cause severe abdominal pain. Two major risk factors for placental abruption are present in this case – cocaine use and hypertensive disease of pregnancy. Lastly, a tense or 'woody' uterus is very suggestive of placental abruption. **Placental praevia** usually presents with painless, bright red vaginal bleeding and a soft, non-tender uterus, which does not fit this presentation. **Preterm premature rupture of membranes** (PPROM) presents with sudden gush of fluid without severe pain or a tense uterus. **Vasa praevia** causes painless vaginal bleeding when fetal vessels rupture during membrane rupture, which is inconsistent with the severe pain and tense uterus described here.

Q364 Endometrial Cancer

Answer 2 – **Multiparity**. **Obesity** and increasing age (patient's **age 65**) are the two major risk factors for developing endometrial cancer. It predominantly effects post-menopausal women, with peak inci-dence between 75 and 79 years old in the UK. Therefore, **time elapsed since menopause** can be eliminated from the answer list, although this may be relevant if they have taken unopposed oestro-gen as part of HRT, but there is no mention of this in the question stem. A high total number of ovulatory cycles, as in early menarche and late menopause, also increases risk, but this is different from time elapsed since menopause.

Type 2 diabetes and hypertension are also associated with increased risk of developing endometrial cancer, and so are not protective. Having children and breastfeeding are both protective factors against endometrial cancer and therefore multiparity is the correct answer.

Q365 Bleeding Postpartum

Answer 5 – **Uterine atony**. All of the options listed are reasonable for postpartum bleeding. Uterine atony is the most common cause of postpartum haemorrhage, with as many as 70% of cases attributed to this. The large uterus on examination suggests that the uterine tone is not adequate. After delivery of the neonate, the uterus should contract to about the size of a grapefruit.

Q366 Complications of Labour

Answer 1 – **Amniotic fluid embolism** (AFE). This is a rare but life-threatening obstetric emergency that can occur during labour, delivery or immediately postpartum. It is characterised by the sudden entry of amniotic fluid, fetal cells or other debris into the maternal circulation, triggering an allergic-like reaction that can lead to severe cardiopulmonary collapse. Key features supporting this diagnosis are: timing – the sudden onset of breathlessness, wheezing and rapid progression to circulatory collapse shortly after a procedure (artificial rupture of membranes) strongly suggests an acute embolic event; asthma history – while the patient has a history of asthma, the acute onset of severe symptoms during a delivery procedure is more consistent with AFE than a primary asthma attack; risk factors – being a multiparous woman and undergoing induction of labour increases the risk of AFE. **Anaphylaxis** could present with wheezing and circulatory collapse, but there is no clear exposure to an allergen in this scenario. The timeline and context (labour) are more suggestive of amniotic fluid embolism. **Asthma attack with tension pneumothorax**: although the patient has a history of asthma, tension pneumothorax typically presents with unilateral decreased breath sounds and a more gradual decline in respiratory status. The sudden collapse after a procedure during labour is not typical of a spontaneous asthma attack or pneumothorax. While possible, **myocardial infarction** is less likely in this context due to the abrupt onset of respiratory symptoms and circulatory collapse, which align more closely with AFE. **Pulmonary embolism** is a consideration, especially given the patient's risk factors (BMI, smoking), but the timing with labour induction and the rapid progression from respiratory symptoms to collapse point more towards AFE as the cause.

Q367 Labour

Answer 4 – **Cervical dilatation to 10 cm to delivery of the fetal head**. The second stage of labour begins when the cervix is fully dilated at 10 cm and ends with the delivery of the fetal head. It includes the pushing phase and ends with the birth of the baby. **Cervical dilatation to 4 cm and delivery of the placenta** describes part of the first stage of labour and the third stage (placental delivery). **Cervical dilatation to 4 cm to delivery of the fetal head** describes part of the first stage, not the second. **Cervical dilatation to 10 cm and delivery of the placenta** includes both the second and third stages of labour. **Uterine contractions occurring regularly for 1 hour or more** is part of early labour but does not define the second stage.

Q368 Menopausal Problems

Answer 4 – **Transdermal oestrogen with progesterone**. This is a case of peri-menopause and this patient will greatly benefit from HRT, in particular until the age of natural menopause and beyond. She has a uterus so she must have progesterone as well as oestrogen to prevent endometrial hyperplasia. Transdermal oestrogen is safer than **oral** because it does not have the thromboembolic risk. **Vaginal oestrogen** is very low risk but is only used to treat genitourinary syndrome of the menopause. She is still having periods so would need sequential rather than continuous combined HRT. As she is not menopausal, if she was to become sexually active she would need contraception. A good option would be the IUS as this covers both HRT and contraception. **None, HRT is contraindicated** is incorrect because transdermal HRT is not contraindicated in women with a history of **DVT**.

Q369 Pregnancy Risk Assessment

Answer 1 – **Carbon monoxide breath test**. This is correct as carbon monoxide is a poisonous gas contained in cigarette smoke. Measuring levels in the body can be a good assessment of the patient's exposure to cigarette smoke. A raised carbon monoxide level of 4 parts per million (4 ppm) or above is a sign that further investigation or support is needed. **Nicotine level testing** is incorrect as nicotine testing is not available on the NHS. Cotinine (the first metabolite in the breakdown of nicotine) can be detected, but is only available privately.

Oxygen saturations are used to check oxygen levels in the blood and cannot detect a patient's exposure to cigarette smoke. **Peak expiratory flow rate** is a screening test for asthma. A test for **serum tar level** does not exist.

Q370 Menstrual Problems

Answer 5 – **Tranexamic acid**. The patient has heavy, painful periods (menorrhagia and dysmenorrhea) and is not responding to simple analgesics. **Tranexamic acid** is a first-line treatment for heavy menstrual bleeding in women who do not wish to conceive immediately and is particularly suitable here given her use of a progesterone implant and migraine with aura (which contraindicates the combined oral contraceptive pill). **Providing a prescription for codeine** might help with pain but does not address heavy bleeding and can lead to dependence and constipation. **Reassuring her without treatment** is inappropriate given her significant symptoms. **Endometrial ablation** is reserved for refractory cases in women who do not wish to conceive at all. **Starting the combined oral contraceptive pill** is contraindicated due to her history of migraine with aura, which increases the risk of stroke with combined hormonal contraceptives.

Q371 Mental Health Problems in Pregnancy or Postpartum

Answer 5 – **Sodium valproate**. Sodium valproate is contraindicated in pregnancy. Sodium valproate should be avoided in women of reproductive age unless all other options are ineffective / not tolerated. In 2019 the Medicines and Healthcare Products Regulation Authority (MHRA) released this information regarding sodium valproate use in pregnancy:

10% of babies exposed to any dose of valproate in pregnancy are born with a congenital malformation

30–40% have a developmental delay – (talking/walking later), lower intellectual abilities and poor language skills (speaking/understanding)

Babies who are exposed to valproate *in utero* have a threefold risk of autism and it may also be linked to ADHD.

The other medications may be used carefully in pregnancy.

Q372 Pelvic Mass

Answer 3 – **Serum CA125**. This woman presents with non-specific symptoms and risk factors for ovarian cancer and a normal examination. **Serum CEA** is not useful here as this is a marker for non-ovarian cancers. She has no bowel symptoms, so **colonoscopy** is not indicated in this scenario. A **CT scan of thorax, abdomen and pelvis** risks excessive radiation exposure and would not be a first-line investigation. The first line investigation here would be a CA125; if this is above 35, an **ultrasound scan of pelvis** and referral as indicated by ultrasound findings would be the next steps.

Q373 Normal Pregnancy and Antenatal Care

Answer 5 – **Refer to a consultant obstetrician for an individualised management plan**. This the correct answer because this patient has a BMI of over 30, which poses some increased risks in pregnancy. An individualised care plan will need to be made by an obstetrician which includes offering a dietitian referral and organising serial growth scans, as a symphysis–fundal height measurement may not be accurate. **Advise her to lose weight to reduce her BMI towards the normal range**: it is not advisable to lose weight in pregnancy (rather, avoidance of excess weight gain is advised). **Advise her to increase her exercise to at least 1 hour every day of the week**: the UK Chief Medical Officer's advice for exercise in pregnancy is to aim for 150 minutes of moderate-intensity activity every week, with muscle-strengthening activities twice per week. **Discuss her increased risk of back pain in pregnancy**: she may be at increased risk of musculoskeletal pain during pregnancy due to carrying excess weight, but this is not the next best step here. **Continuing with routine low-risk care** is unsafe given her high-risk status.

Q374 Pelvic Pain

Answer 4 – **Ruptured ectopic pregnancy**. A ruptured ectopic pregnancy is likely because she has a missed menstrual period. The vaginal bleeding should not be mistaken for a menstrual period when her normal cycle is 29 days (also making **endometriosis** unlikely as she is mid-cycle). She has an increased risk of developing an ectopic pregnancy due to a history of PID. The positive urinary hCG confirms that it is likely to be an ectopic pregnancy. Whilst she is the correct age to be at risk of STIs, and therefore **PID**, the vignette implies that she has had one sexual partner in the last year. In addition, she is afebrile, and the character of pain is different from what you would expect with PID. Whilst she has a history of PID, a **tubo-ovarian abscess** is unlikely as it resolved a year ago. Whilst **ovarian torsion** presents as sharp unilateral pain, it is associated with nausea and does not explain why she is hypotensive.

Q375 Intrauterine Death

Answer 3 – **Intrapartum asphyxia**. The last recorded fetal heart rate was 165/min, which is elevated and suggests fetal distress. The fact that fetal monitoring was done by intermittent auscultation (rather than continuous monitoring) could mean that a critical event, such as asphyxia, went undetected in the final minutes of labour. The baby was delivered at 42 weeks, which carries a higher risk of complications such as fetal asphyxia or placental insufficiency due to the prolonged pregnancy. The absence of obvious congenital anomalies or dysmorphic features suggests that a chromosomal abnormality or major structural abnormality is less likely. While **chromosomal abnormality** can cause stillbirth, there is no mention of dysmorphic features or other abnormalities that would point to this cause. Additionally, chromosomal issues usually lead to early pregnancy loss or stillbirths with lower birth weights. The serology for toxoplasmosis and cytomegalovirus is negative, ruling out these common **congenital infections**. There's no indication of other signs of infection in either the mother or baby. There is no mention of **maternal autoimmune disease**, such as antiphospholipid syndrome or lupus, which could lead to stillbirth due to placental problems. Her glucose tolerance test and infection screens were normal. **Placental abruption** typically presents with significant maternal symptoms (e.g. abdominal pain, bleeding) and can lead to sudden fetal distress. There is no mention of maternal bleeding or abdominal pain in this case, making abruption less likely.

Q376 Reduced / Change in Fetal Movements

Answer 4 – **Refer for review by the maternity department via their triage service**. The patient should be reviewed by the maternity services and a plan put in place by them. **Arranging an ultrasound scan** is incorrect as this presentation requires same-day assessment and review to determine fetal wellbeing. **Asking patient to go home and concentrate on their movements for an hour before coming in** could result in false reassurance and a diminishing of concerns and delay necessary care. The fetus may require delivery and certainly needs a review of their overall wellbeing. Fetal movements should have developed a pattern by now, and so **reassuring her that this is normal** is incorrect. **Sending the patient to the emergency department for review** is incorrect as the ED is not the place for pregnancy assessments – they do not have the equipment or the expertise in obstetrics to assess these patients. Maternity services all have emergency department-type arrangements (triage / day assessment depending upon unit) and these should be utilised for pregnancy problems.

Q377 Small or Large for Gestational Age

Answer 5 – **Ultrasound scan to check the fetal size**. This is a screening test and an ultrasound is more accurate at estimating fetal size. **Arrange caesarian section at 36 weeks** is premature without further assessment of fetal growth and wellbeing. **Arranging a glucose tolerance test** can be useful if the ultrasound suggests fetal macrosomia, but it should not precede a scan. **No action is required** is inappropriate given the decreased fetal movements and large fundal height. **Requesting a senior clinician to repeat the examination** might help, but an ultrasound provides more definitive information about fetal size and health.

Q378 Placental Abruption

Answer 1 – **Category 1 caesarean section**. There is an immediate threat to the life of the fetus and mother. The woman has a partially detached placenta and concealed haemorrhage, which is a medical emergency. Urgent (**category 2 caesarean section**) is for situations where there isn't immediate risk of loss of life – but still urgent (i.e. needs to be done in 30–60 minutes' time). Anything slower (i.e. **all other options**) is not appropriate.

Q379 Vaginal Prolapse

Answer 3 – **Ring pessary**. The patient's symptoms, including the sensation of a mass 'coming down her vagina' and the need to apply digital pressure on the posterior vaginal wall to empty her rectum, strongly suggest pelvic organ prolapse, specifically a rectocele (posterior vaginal wall prolapse). She also reports stress incontinence, which is common with prolapse, especially after multiple vaginal deliveries. A ring pessary is a conservative, non-surgical option that can provide mechanical support to the pelvic organs, helping to relieve the symptoms of prolapse. It is often the first-line treatment in women who have not yet tried conservative measures or who wish to avoid surgery. While **vaginal mesh** was historically used for surgical repair of prolapse, concerns about complications such as infection, erosion and pain have led to restrictions on its use. Mesh is generally reserved for surgical management after failure of other treatments, not as a first-line option. **Radical hysterectomy** is a major surgery usually reserved for the treatment of cancer, particularly cervical or uterine malignancies. There is no indication of cancer in this case, and it would not address the prolapse symptoms. An **oestrogen pessary** is used to manage symptoms of vaginal atrophy, particularly in post-menopausal women. The patient is still menstruating and her symptoms are related to prolapse, not atrophy, so an oestrogen pessary is not appropriate here. **Vaginal hysterectomy and repair** may be considered for more severe or persistent cases of uterine prolapse, or when conservative measures fail. However, this patient appears to have a rectocele, and a ring pessary should be tried first before considering surgery.

Q380 Vulval Itching/Lesion

Answer 5 – **Vulval intraepithelial neoplasia**. This is vulval intrae-pithelial neoplasia (VIN), a pre-cancerous lesion requiring follow-up and treatment to prevent it from developing into vulval cancer. Risk factors include smoking, previous LLETZ (suggesting previous HPV infection) and the description of the lesions. She should be referred to a vulval clinic for ongoing management. **All other options** are incorrect.

Q381 Breast Lump

Answer 5 – **Request an urgent (2-week-wait) appointment**. A firm lump in the breast of a breastfeeding woman should be evaluated thoroughly to rule out potential serious conditions such as breast cancer. While most breast lumps in breastfeeding women are benign (e.g. due to blocked milk ducts or lactational changes), any new, persistent breast lump should be taken seriously and warrants further investigation. Urgent (2-week wait) referral is standard practice for breast lumps, especially in women over 30, to promptly assess for malignancy through imaging (e.g. ultrasound, mammogram) and possibly biopsy if needed. **Advise her to stop the carbamazepine and review in one month**: there's no mention of the patient taking carbamazepine, nor is it relevant to the management of a breast lump.

Prescribe antibiotics and review: while antibiotics may be appropriate if the patient had signs of infection or mastitis (e.g. fever, redness, warmth), the current presentation (firm lump, no fever or other signs of infection) does not suggest infection, so this is not the best option. **Reassure and review in 1 month**: delaying evaluation of a breast lump is not recommended, as any suspicious breast lump should be investigated promptly to exclude malignancy. **Refer to breastfeeding advisory nurse**: while a breastfeeding nurse can assist with lactational issues, the presence of a firm breast lump warrants more urgent assessment to rule out more serious conditions such as breast cancer.

Q382 Breast Abscess / Mastitis

Answer 1 – **Continue to feed from both breasts**. The woman likely has lactational mastitis, which is a localised inflammation of the breast tissue commonly occurring in breastfeeding women. The symptoms include a painful, red and tender area on the breast, as seen in this case. Here's why continuing to breastfeed from both breasts is the best course of action: frequent feeding helps to keep milk flowing, which can prevent milk stasis (milk build-up), one of the causes of mastitis. There's no harm to the baby from breastfeeding while the mother has mastitis. The infection is in the breast tissue, not the milk, so continuing to breastfeed is safe for the baby. **Only feeding from the affected breast** is not advised because feeding from both breasts maintains regular milk flow and prevents issues like milk stasis in the non-affected breast. Continuing to alternate between breasts helps keep both functioning properly. **Only feed from the non-affected breast**: stopping feeding from the affected breast can lead to worsening of mastitis due to milk stasis, increasing the risk of abscess formation and prolonging the condition. The affected breast needs to be drained to resolve the infection. **Stopping breastfeeding for 24 hours** would increase the risk of milk stasis and worsening of the condition. Breastfeeding should be continued even during mastitis. **Stopping breastfeeding until symptoms resolve** is not advised, for the same reasons. Stopping breastfeeding would increase the risk of complications and prolong the duration of mastitis. Therefore, continuing to breastfeed from both breasts is the most appropriate advice to help resolve the condition.

Q383 Breast Cysts

Answer 3 – **Breast ultrasound**. This is the correct answer, as it is the least invasive and will allow you to confirm whether the lump is fluid filled – in which case, it is a breast cyst – or solid, in which case you will have to investigate further due to suspicion of cancer. Even though **biopsy of the lump** is important to rule out cancer, but it wouldn't be the appropriate next step as the diagnosis in this case is most likely breast cyst. **BRCA-1 genetic profiling**: there are no systemic symptoms such as weight loss, so unlikely to be cancer. **CT chest, abdomen and pelvis** and **FBC** are less likely to show anything abnormal.

Q384 Fibroadenoma

Answer 3 – **Fibroadenoma**. Based on the patient's age, the most likely diagnosis is fibroadenoma. Fibroadenomas have been reported in up to 9% of the female population. They are most common in young women aged between 21 and 25 years old. Fewer than 5% occur in women over 50 years of age. Their cause is unknown. **Breast cancer** is less likely in this age group and typically presents as a hard, irregular and immobile mass. **Breast cyst** can cause palpable lumps, but they are more common in older premenopausal women and often fluctuate with the menstrual cycle. **Intraductal papilloma** presents with nipple discharge rather than a distinct lump. **Lipoma** is a soft, compressible and non-tender mass and is less common in the breast compared to fibroadenomas in young women.

Q385 Breast Cancer

Answer 2 – **An infiltrative border**. Malignant tumours have acquired mutations that allow them to divide rapidly and move through surrounding tissue, disrupting the normal structure (and therefore function) of the tissue. This 'disruption' can be visualised as an infiltrating border in ultrasound, sectioned and stained core biopsies and mammogram images. The presence of **adipose tissue** is normal and does not signify malignancy. **Oedema** can be present if a tumour restricts the drainage of fluid, and is indicated in inflammatory breast cancer, metastasis from an extra-mammary malignancy, or mastitis and normal changes during the menstrual cycle. **Fluid-filled cysts** are benign. Complex breast cysts can have a mix of fluid and solid components, and may indicate breast cancer in up to 20% of cases.

Micro-calcifications can be associated with malignancies such as DCIS.

Q386 Difficulty with Breastfeeding

Answer 1 – **Continue to breastfeed or express both sides**. Mastitis is not a contraindication to breastfeeding. Continuing to breastfeed or express from both breasts helps to prevent milk stasis, which can worsen the infection and increase the risk of abscess formation. Flucloxacillin is safe in breastfeeding, so the baby is not at risk from the antibiotic. Draining the affected breast (via breastfeeding or expressing) can help clear the infection more quickly. There is no risk to the baby, as breast milk itself does not carry harmful bacteria in this context. Milk needs to be drained from both breasts to maintain supply and prevent further complications, so the patient should not **continue to breastfeed or express on the affected side, letting the normal side rest. Continue to breastfeed or express only on the normal side, letting the affected side rest** is incorrect. Avoiding feeding from the affected breast can lead to worsening engorgement and abscess formation. **Stop breastfeeding altogether** is incorrect. Stopping abruptly can lead to engorgement, worsening infection, and reduced milk supply. **Stop breastfeeding while taking antibiotics, then try to restart** is incorrect. Flucloxacillin is safe for breastfeeding, so there is no need to stop. Interrupting breastfeeding can lead to reduced supply and increased discomfort.

Q387 Breast Tenderness/Pain

Answer 1 – **No further action needed**. The patient has breast pain without any palpable lumps or abnormal findings on examination. In the absence of concerning features (e.g. lumps, skin changes, nipple discharge or significant family history of breast cancer), breast pain (mastalgia) is often benign and can be managed conservatively: simple analgesics (e.g. paracetamol or ibuprofen) are typically first-line treatments for managing breast pain; follow-up ensures that, if symptoms persist or worsen, further investigation can be conducted at a later stage. **Prescribing the combined oral contraceptive** can worsen mastalgia due to hormonal fluctuations and is not indicated. **Requesting a mammogram** is unnecessary without a palpable lump or other red flags. A **routine outpatient appointment** is not needed if the symptoms are well controlled and there are no alarming features. An **urgent (2-week-wait) outpatient appointment** is reserved for suspicious findings such as a new lump, nipple discharge or skin changes, none of which are present.

Q388 Nipple Discharge

Answer 2 – **Complete a breast and ophthalmic examination**. It is important to complete a thorough examination to help include/exclude certain differentials before moving on to investigations. It would be sensible to **arrange an MRI head** after any investigations including blood tests, as this diagnosis is pointing towards a pituitary adenoma/prolactinoma. The visual loss in her peripheries is known as bitemporal hemianopia and this is there is compression at the optic chiasm. The white discharge is usually referred to as milky discharge, seen in prolactinomas. You would also expect menstrual cycle disturbances as LH and FSH release would be affected. **Referral to the 2-week-wait breast clinic** for a mammogram and fine-needle aspiration is not the answer as there is no suggestion of a breast lump. It is unlikely to be a migraine as she is experiencing nipple discharge which would be unexplained by a migraine. **Prescribing cabergoline/bromocriptine** (dopamine agonists) is appropriate for prolactinoma but should follow imaging confirmation. **Reassuring** without investigation is inappropriate given the concerning symptoms.

Ophthalmology

13

Q389 Benign Eyelid Disorders

Answer 2 – **Excision biopsy**. The risk factor for developing tumours of the skin include: (1) white race; (2) long exposure to sunlight; and (3) previous history of tumour elsewhere in the body. A farmer by the nature of his job is constantly exposed to sunlight and if he had a previous history of tumour removal elsewhere in the body, he is more likely to get a tumour again. This patient has a lesion which is raised, and he also mentions that this may have got bigger, and with a history of bleeding, this raises the possibility of a malignancy. The next line of management would be to excise the tumour completely and arrange a histological examination. **Prescribing topical anti-biotic cream** is not correct as this is not likely to be of infective origin. **Reassurance and review in 6 months** would lead to increase in the size and potential spread of the tumour. **Taking a scraping from the surface looking for fungal hyphae** is not an option as this is unlikely to be a fungal infection. **Crushing the lesion with forceps and applying cryopexy** may lead to haematogenous spread, although cryotherapy may kill the tumour cells. A histology specimen is definitive in establishing the exact nature of the tumour and also will establish whether the tumour has been completely removed.

Q390 Blepharitis

Answer 4 – **Meibomian gland**. Blepharitis is associated with dys-function of the meibomian gland which is found in the tarsal plate of the eyelid. **Lacrimal gland** is incorrect as that produces tears, and damage to that can cause dry eyes and not blepharitis. The **gland of Moll** is present in the lid and it produces sweat. It can get blocked leading to the formation of a cyst of Moll, but is not associated with blepharitis. The **parotid gland** produces saliva, and inflammation of this gland causes parotitis, so that is incorrect in this scenario. The **accessory lacrimal gland of Krause** is involved in producing basal tear secretion, and damage to this structure produces dry eye syndrome not blepharitis.

Q391 Squint

Answer 3 – **Patch one eye**. A 65 year old poorly controlled diabetic patient presents with binocular diplopia which he is able to overcome by closing one eye. This is most likely a left-sided 6th nerve paralysis. The underlying pathology is due to microangiopathy of the vasa nervorum of the 6th nerve and is usually self-limiting. If there is no papilloedema, then the immediate management would be to treat his diplopia. This can be treated by patching one eye, hence option 3 is the correct answer. Glasses by themselves cannot correct double vision if it is binocular and muscle related, so **asking optician to review prescription for glasses** is not correct. Although blood sugar control is important, this is not the immediate management but treating the symptom of double vision, and ruling out intracranial pathology is important, so **referral to GP for improved diabetic control** is not correct either. Urgent MRI is not needed as, in the absence of papilloedema, the underlying problem is purely a 6th nerve paralysis, due to microangiopathy, so **urgent MR scan of head** is not correct. A baseline Hess charting is useful but is not the immediate management, so **Hess screening to measure the deviation** is not correct.

Q392 Cataracts

Answer 1 – **Advise surgery as soon as possible for the cataracts**. There is no known effective treatment option for cataract other than surgery. This involves removing the cataract and replacing it with an artificial plastic intraocular lens. The patient's visual acuity has dropped to 6/18 in both eyes, and a vision of 6/12 is needed in the good eye to drive legally in the UK. Hence, improving his visual acuity is important so that he can drive legally to earn his livelihood. **Stopping the steroid cream** is incorrect as this will not reverse the cataract, and neither will it improve his vision. Moreover, steroids may be necessary for him to control his dermatitis. **Advise that he takes vitamins A and E** – there is no evidence that vitamins A and E, or **prescribing regular aspirin**, will reverse the cataract or improve the vision. **Review in 6 months' time to check cataract maturity** – waiting for 6 months will cause further worsening of his vision, so this is incorrect. He needs cataract surgery as soon as possible to restore his sight to driving standards.

Q393 Central Retinal Arterial Occlusion

Answer 4 – **Ocular massage to the right eye**. The cholesterol embolus with retinal ischaemia is the reason for his sudden painless loss of vision. The aim of the treatment is to dislodge the cholesterol embolus from the branch retinal artery to the peripheral retinal circulation and save the macula from damage. There is a window of opportunity of less than 4 hours to treat retinal artery occlusion before irreversible damage sets in in the retina. The cholesterol embolus can be dislodged by reducing the intraocular pressure. This can be achieved by administering IV acetazolamide and also by ocular massage. This is not an inflammatory disease, so **high-dose IV corticosteroids** are not useful. **Immediate CT head** is incorrect as the patient needs immediate treatment and neuroimaging is not required, as the diagnosis and pathology are obvious. Although artery occlusion can be caused by both embolus and inflammation, embolus in this case is obvious, so **urgent temporal artery biopsy** is not correct. Although the prognosis for visual recovery may be guarded, treating the patient can salvage some vision and should be initiated, hence **No treatment needed for this patient** is incorrect.

Q394 Diabetic Eye Disease

Answer 5 – **Vitreous haemorrhage**. Patients with type 1 diabetes mellitus who are poorly controlled are at high risk for developing neovascularisation in the retina due to proliferative diabetic retinopathy. This can cause bleeding resulting in vitreous haemorrhage. Mild vitreous haemorrhage can cause symptoms of either a floater or a cobweb, as this patient reported initially. Subsequently, a massive haemorrhage led to a global blurring of vision. Poorly controlled diabetic patients can develop acute **cataract** rarely, with sudden loss of vision, but this will produce some blurring initially but no cobwebs, and hence this option is not correct. **Diabetic macular oedema** can be associated with type 1 diabetes mellitus but causes either distortion of vision or blurred vision and never acute loss of vision. Acute angle closure glaucoma can cause sudden loss of vision, but this is not the case with **open angle glaucoma**, which is associated with gradual loss of vision. Inflammatory **optic neuritis** is not associated with diabetes mellitus, but there is an association with ischaemic optic neuropathy. However, optic neuritis can cause sudden loss of vision, but is not preceded by cobwebs, and so is not correct in this case.

Q395 Conjunctivitis

Answer 2 – **Topical chloramphenicol eye drops with oral doxycycline**. Chlamydial infection of the eye cannot be completely eradicated by topical antibiotics alone. Concurrent systemic antibiotic is needed to eradicate the infection, or else it tends to recur. Topical chloramphenicol with a course of oral doxycycline or erythromycin will eradicate the infection, and hence is the correct answer. **Topical beta-blocker eye drops** are used for treating glaucoma in the eye, hence these are incorrect. **Topical fusidic sodium eye ointment** is not effective against chlamydia, so this is incorrect. Topical steroids, will make the eye white and may give some symptomatic relief but will not treat the chlamydial infection, neither will oral penicillin. Hence **topical prednisolone eye drops with oral penicillin** is incorrect. **Topical quinolone antibiotic drops** are again not an effective treatment option for chlamydial infection as mentioned.

Q396 Infective Keratitis

Answer 5 – **Take corneal scrape for gram stain and bacterial culture sensitivity**. The clinical diagnosis is suggestive of a severe infective keratitis. Although mild keratitis can be treated empirically, for severe infection it is important to take a corneal scrape for gram stain and bacterial culture and sensitivity. Starting treatment with a broad-spectrum antibiotic is the norm as it usually works against a wide range of bacteria. A bacterium resistant to an antibiotic can cause progressive and irreversible damage to the cornea. Identifying the offending bacteria and sensitivity to commonly used antibiotics is important so that the appropriate antibiotic is substituted should the current antibiotic not be effective. Since this is a severe infection, antibiotics are crucial and **prescribing topical tear supplements** will not help with treating the infection, so this is incorrect. Although **starting broad-spectrum topical antibiotics** is correct, that should follow the corneal scraping and not precede it. Topical antibiotics have greater availability at the site of the corneal infection, whereas oral antibiotics do not, hence **starting oral antibiotics** is incorrect. Steroids suppress the immunity and allow the bacteria to replicate and this can cause rapid destruction of the cornea, hence **starting topical steroids** is incorrect.

Q397 Facial/Periorbital Swelling

Answer 2 – **Normal eye movements**. A history of sore throat and runny nose implies possible paranasal sinus involvement. Due to the proximity of the sinus to the orbital cavity and the peri-orbital tissue, the lid is swollen in both preseptal and orbital cellulitis. The swelling of the orbital tissue in orbital cellulitis leads to proptosis and chemosis. Since the extraocular muscles are inflamed in orbital cellulitis, this restricts the movement of extraocular muscles, which can lead to diplopia and pain in eye movements. Restriction of extraocular muscle movement with diplopia is one of the cardinal signs of orbital cellulitis. Vision may or may not be affected in the initial stage of orbital cellulitis but is not a feature in preseptal cellulitis. In the suggested answers, **proptosis** is a classical sign of orbital cellulitis. As explained above, the involvement of extraocular muscles leads to **pain on eye movements** and **diplopia**, or double vision. **Reduced vision** is also a feature of orbital cellulitis, whereas the optic nerve is not involved, and hence the vision is not affected, in preseptal cellulitis. Normal eye movements are a feature of preseptal cellulitis, as the extraocular muscles are not involved. Hence the correct response is normal eye movements.

Q398 Iritis

Answer 3 – **Iritis**. This man has a red and sore right eye with photophobia, which can sometimes be a non-specific symptom for many ocular conditions. The symptoms have to be interpreted in relation to other local or systemic associations. The absence of discharge in this case makes it unlikely to be bacterial conjunctivitis. There is usually severe watering of the eye and associated nasal discharge with sore throat in **viral conjunctivitis**, so this is unlikely. In **bacterial keratitis** the pain is pretty constant, exacerbated while blinking, with associated lacrimation. The absence of these rules this out. **Endophthalmitis** is usually seen following intraocular surgery/ trauma and the pain is very severe, not relieved by painkillers. The vision is also drastically reduced, hence this is unlikely. In **ocular migraine**, there is pain on one side of the head, sometimes associated with nausea, vomiting and intolerance to light, with variable degree of blurring of vision. The eye itself is not sore. The symptoms mentioned here are more ocular than cranial pathology, which rules this out. The patient has sore red eye with photophobia. There is known systemic association of iritis with ankylosing spondylitis. With a chronic back pain and a suspected diagnosis of ankylosing spondylitis, coupled with typical symptoms of iritis, this is the most likely diagnosis.

Q399 Chronic Glaucoma

Answer 4 – **Latanoprost eye drops**. Topical eye drops are the first line of treatment for primary open angle glaucoma. Latanoprost, a prostaglandin analogue, is the preferred drug of choice. **Goniotomy** is the treatment of choice for congenital glaucoma, and hence is incorrect for this patient. **Cyclocryopexy** is a destructive procedure aimed at damaging the ciliary body, hence reducing the production of aqueous humour formation and intraocular pressure. This treatment modality has become obsolete now due to the morbidity associated with it. Also, this was used as a modality for intractable glaucoma, and is incorrect in this scenario. **Peripheral iridotomy** is the treatment for narrow angle glaucoma, not for open angle glaucoma, and hence is incorrect. **Drainage tube** surgery is reserved for complicated glaucoma and is not the treatment of choice for uncomplicated primary open angle glaucoma, so this too is incorrect.

Q400 Macular Degeneration

Answer 4 – **Late and wet active AMD**. This 79 year old woman has presented to the emergency department with acute-onset symptoms of central vision loss and distortion of images. She was already diagnosed with dry AMD suggesting she had **early AMD**, so this is incorrect. In **late and dry AMD**, the vision is severely affected but is gradual in onset, hence this is incorrect. The end stage of wet AMD is **late and wet inactive AMD** and one of the types is **disciform scar**, hence both of these are incorrect. Wet active AMD presents acutely with blurring of central vision or distortion of vision or both. Inability to do crossword puzzles suggests this patient has loss of visual acuity for near vision, and distortion in her vision led her to miss the kerb with a near accident. Hence option C is the correct answer.

Q401 Optic Neuritis

Answer 3 – **Establish the diagnosis by examining the affected eye**. The diagnosis of multiple sclerosis can follow after an attack of optic neuritis in 20% of patients, whereas 75% of patients diagnosed with multiple sclerosis will develop at least one episode of optic neuritis during their lifetime. In this patient diagnosed previously with multiple sclerosis, although there is a high risk of developing optic neuritis, this should not be assumed. There may be many reasons for ocular discomfort with blurred vision. The diagnosis of optic neuritis should be confirmed by clinical examination, hence this is the correct response. Arranging investigation without comprehensive eye examination is a wrong clinical approach, hence **arranging an urgent CT scan of the brain** is a wrong response. Moreover, once the systemic diagnosis of MS has been made and optic neuritis is suspected, CT scan will not give additional information. **Immediate lumbar puncture to look for CSF proteins** without clinical examination and a provisional diagnosis is a wrong approach to a disease, and hence is incorrect. Lumbar puncture is an invasive procedure with associated risk and should not be ordered without weighing the pros and cons and the benefit it would provide in arriving at a clinical diagnosis. **Reassure patient and order next-day electrodiagnostic test:** patients presenting with symptoms should not be reassured and sent home without a working diagnosis and providing symptomatic relief. Clinical diagnosis can be reached in most instances by comprehensive examination, and rarely will there be a need for electrodiagnostic testing. Next-day electrodiagnostic test is not needed. If the patient has infection and has not been assessed properly, intravenous methylprednisolone can have serious side effects, hence **treating urgently with bolus of IV methylprednisolone** is incorrect. Investigations and treatment should always follow comprehensive clinical examination.

Q402 Retinal Detachment

Answer 1 – **Within 24 hours**. Acute rhegmatogenous retinal detachment not involving the fovea is a surgical emergency. Retinal detachment can involve any quadrant of the retina. Inferior retinal detachment is less likely to progress quickly, whereas superior retinal detachment is more likely to progress quickly to involve the fovea (centre of macula) due to the effect of gravity. If the retinal reattachment surgery is performed after the fovea is detached, then the visual acuity recovery may not be optimal, hence the urgency to operate. The timing of surgical intervention is critical and even if the fovea is detached, if the surgery is performed within 24 hours, then the chance of visual recovery is good, compared to operating after 24 hours or later. The visual acuity recovery gets poorer as the time advances, hence **all other options** are incorrect. As explained above, timing is critical for optimal visual recovery.

Q403 Scleritis

Answer 2 – **Diffuse scleritis**. Patients with diffuse scleritis often present with pain in the eye radiating to the forehead, brow and jaw. The eye is tender to touch and awakens the patient at night. The pain is not completely relieved by analgesics. Nearly half the patients with scleritis have an autoimmune disorder. The typical symptom of pain and the localised redness with a possible suspected autoimmune disorder makes the diagnosis of diffuse scleritis the most likely one. An attack of **acute angle closure glaucoma** does not occur at night and neither does it wake up the patient. This usually occurs at dusk when the ambient light is low, in predisposed patients with narrow angles. The pain is so severe that the patient cannot tolerate the pain for 3 days without seeking medical help. The ocular findings in acute angle closure glaucoma, with its redness in the eye being diffuse not localised, mean this is unlikely to be the diagnosis. The pain of migraine is usually one-sided, associated with nausea, intolerance to light and vomiting. There may be some pain in the eye but it is unlikely to be painful with localised redness in the eye, so **typical migraine** is incorrect. **Orbital pseudotumour** is rare and is usually associated with some proptosis, chemosis of conjunctiva, and double vision with painful eye movement. There is no localised redness in the sclera; all these features make this unlikely here. **Superior limbic keratoconjunctivitis** is a rare condition and is seen in patients having thyroid ophthalmopathy, or dry eye syndrome. There is redness in the upper bulbar conjunctiva and the superior limbus of the cornea with formation of filaments. This stains with fluorescein and rose Bengal dye. Patients usually complain of a foreign body sensation, excessive blinking, photophobia, burning and pain. The constellation of symptoms and the disease association makes this unlikely.

Q404 Foreign Body in Eye

Answer 2 – **CT scan orbits**. In the past, X-ray was commonly used for imaging the eyeball for detection of an intraocular foreign body, but it is limited in sensitivity and can detect only 40% of IOFB so is not an ideal imaging modality, so **X-rays of the globe in two positions of gaze** is incorrect. Even if the foreign body is 0.5–0.6 mm in size, a CT scan can detect these in 100% cases, so currently it is the best method of imaging and detecting a metallic intraocular foreign body, so CT scan orbits is the correct answer. The magnetic force in MRI can cause movement of the metallic foreign body and damage ocular structures so this is contraindicated with a suspected metallic foreign body, hence **MRI of orbits** is incorrect. Although sensitive in detecting IOFB, ultrasound is not useful in penetrating ocular injury due to the risk of extrusion of intraocular contents by the pressure of the ultrasound probe, hence **bedside rapid assessment by ultrasound of the globe and orbit** is incorrect. PET scans are used for functional imaging of tissues and organs of the body, particularly for cancer, and not for detecting foreign bodies, hence **PET scan of the orbit** is incorrect.

Q405 Thyroid Eye Disease

Answer 2 – **Detailed ocular assessment to rule out compression of the optic nerve**. A prominent eyeball (exophthalmos) noticed by the family but not by the patient herself is probably of gradual onset and, coupled with systemic symptoms of palpitation and weight loss, is suggestive of thyroid-related eye problem. The common cause of unilateral and bilateral proptosis is thyroid eye disease. This is more common in females compared to males. Exophthalmos can potentially lead to compression of the optic nerve and blindness, hence assessing the patient for this condition is critical. Moreover, the patient has presented with visual symptoms, so this is the correct answer. This is not orbital cellulitis and hence prescribing **broad-spectrum antibiotics** is not correct. She does need assessment and treatment by a physician for her palpitations and weight loss, but not immediately. This can wait till the comprehensive ocular examination is carried out, hence **referral to the cardiologist** is not correct. She needs blood tests for her thyroid functions rather than for **routine blood tests**. In mild forms of thyroid eye disease, topical lubricants are what is needed, but prescribing **topical lubricants and reassuring** the patient without doing comprehensive ocular examination is incorrect.

Q406 Uveitis

Answer 1 – **anterior uveitis**. In 50% of cases, the aetiology of uveitis is unknown. The presence of an underlying systemic disease can be identified in the rest. It can involve the joints, skin or gastrointestinal tract. This patient complains of back pain and could have underlying undiagnosed ankylosing spondylitis. HLAB27 arthropathies like the above are commonly associated with anterior uveitis, which this patient is likely to have. Hence this is the correct response. **Intermediate uveitis** and **posterior uveitis** are typically associated with painless blur, floaters or photopsia. The unilaterality and lack of discharge make the much more common **conjunctivitis** less likely. The commoner form of **episcleritis** presents with irritation, photophobia and localised redness. Pain is not a feature of this condition.

Q407 Acute Change in or Loss of Vision

Answer 5 – **Urgent blood test consisting of CRP, FBC and plasma viscosity**. An 82 year old white lady presents to the emergency department with visual impairment in the right eye, with the visual acuity dropping to 6/36. She has loss of weight, and reduced appetite. She also complains of pain in her jaw and scalp, while eating and combing her hair respectively. This constellation of symptoms and swelling of the optic disc is highly suggestive of GCA (giant cell arteritis). This is a vasculitis of the medium- and large-sized blood vessels. This is a blinding condition and untreated will affect the other eye with disastrous outcome. Treatment with steroid is sight-saving for the unaffected eye. This needs to be started immediately, after confirming the diagnosis with inflammatory markers in the blood consisting of CRP and viscosity. Hence, among the given options, urgent blood test is the correct one. Delaying the treatment by **reassuring her and requesting a routine blood test** will inevitably result in blindness. The symptoms and the optic disc swelling are suggestive of GCA, and glasses will not improve her vision, hence **referral to the optician for corrective lenses** is incorrect. The optic disc swelling due to GCA is not embolic in nature from blocked carotid arteries, hence a **carotid duplex scan** is incorrect. This condition is a medical emergency. Sending the patient home without investigating and treating her will result in irreversible blindness, hence **reassurance and review in outpatients in 2 weeks** is incorrect.

Q408 Periorbital and Orbital Cellulitis

Answer 4 – **Intravenous antibiotics**. The patient has presented with a proptosis of his right eye with painful and restricted eye movements. This is suggestive of orbital cellulitis/abscess. He is also pyrexial and unwell which might indicate septicaemia. The next step in the management involves securing an IV line immediately and giving broad-spectrum antibiotics. With the IV access line, blood is drawn for aerobic and anaerobic bacterial cultures and full blood count. Imaging of the orbit and brain is needed after giving IV antibiotics to look for localised areas of pus which need drainage and for the source of pus, usually from infected sinuses. **CT scan of brain**

and orbits is not the correct answer. Being an infective condition, the patient needs high-dose antibiotics and not steroids as they suppress the immune system and worsen the infection, hence **IV steroids** is incorrect. The patient does need **ENT review** but this is not the immediate step in the management once diagnosis is made. Blood samples are needed for blood cultures and full blood count, and not for testing immunodeficiency, hence **blood sample to exclude immunodeficiency** is incorrect.

Q409 Eye Pain/Discomfort

Answer 5 – **Traumatic corneal abrasion**. The patient presents with severe pain after gardening without using protective goggles. He is tearing and has photophobia, and the pain is not relieved by taking acetaminophen. Gardening without protective goggles can cause injury to the eye from flying objects like grit, wood, leaves, etc. This can lead to corneal abrasion due to rubbing caused by irritation. Corneal abrasion causes severe pain, watering and photophobia. Hence, this is the correct response. **Acute mucopurulent conjunctivitis** does not produce severe pain, and the hallmark of this condition is mucopurulent discharge, which is not a symptom in this patient. **Ruptured hordeolum externum** (stye) produces discomfort and may be accompanied by mild discharge, but severe pain and photophobia are not a feature of this condition, so this diagnosis is not correct. **Necrotising scleritis** is rare and is usually associated with an autoimmune disease. Severe dull pain is a feature of this condition but it is not associated with photophobia and tearing. This is unlikely to be exacerbated by gardening, which is a presentation in this case, so necrotising scleritis would not be correct. **Traumatic carotico-cavernous fistula** is brought about by significant head trauma accompanied by exophthalmos. This is not a feature in this clinical presentation, so this diagnosis is not correct.

Q410 Eye Trauma

Answer 4 – **Irrigate her eyes with saline checking the pH of the conjunctival sac periodically**. Industrial accident due to splash of caustic soda is a chemical injury by an alkali. Alkali injury is an ophthalmic emergency and potentially has a blinding sequela. The first step is to minimise the contact of the alkali with the ocular surface tissue. The eye should be irrigated with copious saline or water, and the pH checked periodically to ensure 7 (neutral). The irrigation should include the conjunctival fornices as some may be impacted under the lid. The chemical was stored in a metallic container, but the patient was not injured by it, so there is unlikely to be a metallic foreign body in the eye, so **exploration of the eyeball in theatre to rule out a globe rupture** is incorrect. Also, a fluid splash is unlikely to cause globe rupture. Although the patient will benefit from analgesia, **intramuscular analgesia and discharging her with topical lubricants** is not the proper treatment. Similarly, prescribing **immediate, intense steroids to counter the inflammation** is incorrect as the immediate treatment is irrigation of the eye, due to the explanation given above. **Urgent CT scan** is not required unless there is suspicion of intraocular foreign bodies or orbital fractures, which is not suggested by the history.

Q411 Flashes and Floaters in Visual Fields

Answer 5 – **Urgent ophthalmology referral.** Flashes (photopsia) and floaters are classic warning signs of posterior vitreous detachment (PVD) or retinal detachment, both of which require urgent ophthalmological evaluation. Myopia is a major risk factor for retinal detachment, as it increases the likelihood of vitreoretinal traction due to a thinner and more stretched retina. Early detection and treatment (e.g. laser photocoagulation or surgery if detachment is confirmed) can prevent permanent vision loss. **Immediate laser photocoagulation**: laser treatment is only done if a retinal tear or detachment is confirmed. The patient needs urgent assessment first.

Start oral steroids: steroids are not used for flashes and floaters. If this were optic neuritis, steroids could be considered, but the symptoms here are more consistent with retinal pathology. **Perform tonometry to check intraocular pressure**: elevated intraocular pressure (IOP) is relevant for glaucoma, but this patient's symptoms are not typical of acute glaucoma, which usually presents with severe pain, blurred vision, and a fixed, mid-dilated pupil. **Refer for urgent MRI of the brain**: while a neurological cause (e.g. occipital stroke, migraine aura) could be considered, the pattern of symptoms (flashes, floaters, myopia, normal acuity) strongly suggests an ophthalmic cause rather than a central nervous system issue.

Q412 Gradual Change in or Loss of Vision

Answer 3 – **Optometrist assessment.** The 10 year old boy has poor vision seeing the blackboard but can see better when he is sat in the front row. When examined his visual acuity is 6/36 and this improves to almost normal vision of 6/9 with a pin hole. This suggests that the boy has a refractive (focusing) error. Refractive error can be corrected by prescription glasses. In contrast, if the pinhole test does not improve vision, it suggests a pathological disease process of the eye. Hence optometrist assessment is the correct answer. Since he does not have pathological disease of the eye, **urgent ophthalmological review** is incorrect. He does not have headache, which is an important symptom of intracranial pathology, hence does not need MRI/CT scan, so **arrange urgent MRI/CT** is incorrect. Pencil push-ups are helpful if patient has latent squint, but his eye examination is reported as being normal so **advise pencil push-ups** is incorrect. He does not complain of dryness, irritation and watering of the eye – an important symptom of dry eye – hence **tear supplements** is incorrect. Moreover, watering in the evening is suggestive of eye strain and not dry eye. Also, dry eye is extremely rare in the younger age group.

Q413 Loss of Red Reflex

Answer 3 – **Dilated eye examination with ultrasound**. High-impact ocular trauma with contact sports such as rugby is known to cause physical injury, wherein the eye may also be involved. This boy has a risk factor for developing retinal detachment due to trauma, and the risk increases if he has evidence of a connective tissue disorder. Dad has Stickler syndrome, a connective tissue disorder associated with lattice degeneration of the retina (present in 100% of affected patients) and high myopia (present in 80%). These contribute to a lifetime risk of retinal detachments. The child may have inherited Stickler syndrome from his father, as it is autosomal dominant (50% chance). The fact that he has been wearing glasses since early childhood is suggestive of the possibility of his having myopia. Due to this risk, **reassure and discharge** is not correct, as discharging him without a comprehensive eye examination would miss retinal detachment and could lead to potential blindness. Of children with retinoblastoma, 92% present before the age of 6, so **arrange an urgent MR scan** is less likely; moreover, a complete eye examination would reveal retinoblastoma if present. The urgency here is to diagnose acute blinding conditions, and **arranging an urgent geneticist appointment for counselling** is unnecessary at this stage. **Topical steroids and antibiotics**: traumatic uveitis is a possibility, and can be diagnosed by examining the eye, though this would not give rise to an abnormal greyish reflex in the pupillary area. Hence the correct option is dilated eye examination with ultrasound.

Q414 Acute Glaucoma

Answer 4 – **Treat with intravenous acetazolamide 500 mg**. IV acetazolamide is very effective in reducing the intraocular pressure and is the first-line treatment for this condition, although additional adjunctive pressure-lowering eye drops will be needed besides acetazolamide. The clinical feature of cornea oedema with shallow anterior chamber and a raised intraocular pressure of 60 mm Hg points to an attack of acute angle closure glaucoma. This condition is one of the few ophthalmic emergencies. The principle of treatment consists of reducing the intraocular pressure to the normal range of less than 20 mmHg. Topical anti-glaucoma drops such as timolol (0.5%) are not effective in reducing the intraocular pressure to such a level from 60 mmHg. Hence **Treat with topical beta-blocker (timolol 0.5%) eye drops** is incorrect. The vomiting is due to raised intraocular pressure, and hence reducing the intraocular pressure will resolve the vomiting, although sometimes it may need symptomatic relief. Since this is an eye emergency, delaying treatment by **referring the patient to a physician for his vomiting** will lead to irreversible loss of sight, and hence is incorrect. The clinical signs are diagnostic of acute angle closure glaucoma, and the vomiting is due to the raised intraocular pressure and is not due to CNS pathology, so **arranging an urgent CT scan to rule out intracranial lesion** is not required. **Arrange an urgent laser peripheral iridotomy**: laser peripheral iridotomy is difficult to perform in the presence of oedematous cornea and is not effective due to the swollen iris tissue. It is done once the intraocular pressure approaches the normal range and the corneal oedema has resolved. This laser procedure is not a first-line management.

Q415 Red Eye

Answer 3 – **Levofloxacin**. The patient in the vignette has a corneal ulcer secondary to contact lens use. Although her symptoms of pain, redness and photophobia are not exclusive to corneal ulcers, the history of sleeping in the contact lens and the opacity on the cornea is suggestive of a microbial infection. **Ganciclovir gel** is used for herpetic corneal ulcers which have a classical branching pattern. **Hypromellose 0.3%** is a lubricant eye drop used to alleviate symptoms of dry eyes. **Natamycin 5%** eye drops are used for fungal infections, which are common in tropical climates and following ocular injury with vegetal matter. **Prednisolone eye drops** are used in inflammatory eye conditions. The correct answer is to start treatment with intensive broad-spectrum antibiotic eye drops that can be tailored following results of microscopy, culture, and sensitivity of corneal scrapes.

Q416 Visual Field Defects

Answer 4 – **Parietal lobe**. Parietal and temporal lobe lesions cause quadrantic field defects. The superior quadrantic field defects are due to temporal lobe lesions, whereas inferior quadrantic field defects are due to parietal lobe lesions. Hence, parietal lobe is the correct answer. Cataract produces generalised blurring of vision or sometimes double vision but doesn't cause a selective shadow in the inferior field of vision. An automated visual field testing in cataract can produce generalised depression but not homonymous or heteronymous hemianopsia, hence **lens of the eye** is not correct. Retinal dystrophy produces either generalised depression, peripheral constriction or central scotoma on visual field testing, hence **retina** is incorrect. Hemianopia or quadrantanopia are caused by lesions behind the **optic chiasma**. Lesions affecting the optic chiasma produce bitemporal hemianopia, hence optic chiasma is incorrect. Typically, occipital lobe lesions produce homonymous hemianopia with macular sparing, hence **occipital cortex** is incorrect.

Orthopaedics and Trauma

14

Q417 Lower Limb Fractures

Answer 3 – **Hemiarthroplasty**. The patient has a displaced intracapsular neck of femur fracture and therefore needs a replacement rather than fixation. Given her cognitive comorbidities, the appropriate management would be a hemiarthroplasty. **Cannulated screws** are suitable for undisplaced intracapsular fractures but have high failure rates in displaced fractures in elderly patients. **Dynamic hip screw** is used for extracapsular fractures (intertrochanteric fractures), not intracapsular ones. **Intramedullary nail** is used for subtrochanteric or unstable intertrochanteric fractures. **Total hip arthroplasty** is usually recommended for active elderly patients without cognitive impairment and has a higher risk of dislocation in patients with dementia.

Q418 Lower Limb Soft Tissue Injury

Answer 4 – **Vastus lateralis.** 20 cm below the anterior superior iliac spine is lateral and approximately halfway from the hip to the knees. The **femoral artery**, **femoral nerve** and **femoral vein** run medially as does the **vastus medialis**. The only lateral structure mentioned is vastus lateralis.

Q419 Pathological Fracture

Answer 2 – **MRI of the whole spine.** The history is highly suggestive of cord compression (in the history – severe back pain and weakness in both legs, history of prostate cancer; examination – sensory level and weakness; investigations – collapse of T9, bladder scan showing some retention). So he needs an early and accurate evaluation of the spinal cord and surrounding tissues: MRI whole spine. **CT-guided**

biopsy of the T9 vertebra would get histology – it is not the immediate next step; **occupational therapist assessment** may be needed
before discharge – again not immediate; **referral to the spinal
surgery team for spinal stabilisation** may be necessary but MRI is
needed to guide their management; **urinary catheter** may be needed
in a few hours' time, depending on whether the patient goes into
acute retention.

Q420 Upper Limb Fractures

Answer 1 – **Anterior interosseous branch of median nerve**. The
anterior interosseous nerve supplies motor power to the flexor pollicis longus in the thumb and the flexor digitorum profundus in the
index finger, both required to make the 'OK sign'.

Q421 Immobility

Answer 2 – **Obtain corroborative history followed by a detailed
clinical examination**. This lady shows functional decline, confusion
and cognitive impairment. Part of the initial assessment is to assess
how much decline. Before involving other services (such as **contacting the police**, **arranging occupational therapy assessment** or **referring to the dietitians**) or proceeding with specific investigations
(including **routine blood investigations**), it is crucial to gather
a comprehensive history and conduct a detailed clinical examination.
This will help identify immediate medical needs, potential causes of
her current state, and any safeguarding concerns.

Q422 Osteomyelitis

Answer 3 – **Surgical debridement, removal of the intermedullary
nail**. This removes the likely colonised intramuscular nail, and allows
for debridement of infected tissue back to healthy margins. **Above-
knee amputation** is incorrect: the patient is 25 and, although he may
eventually need amputation, limb salvage should always be
attempted or considered before amputation. **Long-term antibiotics
only is** incorrect: foreign bodies such as intramuscular nails should
always be removed in the case of local infection, due to colonisation
and biofilm formation, which means that antibiotics alone will not
remove the infection. **Surgical debridement of discharging tract** is
incorrect, for reasons provided in relation to long-term antibiotics
above.

    Symptom control with analgesia and physiotherapy is incorrect:
this will not treat the issue and leaves the patient at risk of sepsis.

Q423 Septic Arthritis

Answer 1 – **Joint aspiration**. As the patient is not septic, she can wait to have antibiotics until after a joint aspiration is performed. Performing it before antibiotics are commenced gives the best chance of a positive culture. **Reassurance and review in 2 weeks** is incorrect: this presentation should be considered septic arthritis until that can be ruled out. **Routine referral to rheumatology** is incorrect for the same reason. **Start on intravenous antibiotics** is incorrect: this patient does need antibiotics, but this is not the FIRST step that should take place. If the patient were septic and haemo-dynamically unstable, then antibiotics should be given first and joint aspiration attempted later. Patient safety is of utmost importance. **Take to theatre for debridement of joint** is incorrect: the patient may eventually require debridement, but first we have to confirm the diagnosis with a joint aspiration and gram stain.

Q424 Musculoskeletal Deformities

Answer 5 – **Rheumatoid arthritis**. Rheumatoid arthritis generally presents with pain in the morning that eases later in the day and is 2–3 times more likely to affect women rather than men. It is an inflammatory arthropathy and produces a characteristic ulnar devi-ation at the metacarpophalangeal joints as well as swan neck deform-ities of the fingers. **Ankylosing spondylitis** affects men more than women and generally presents with back pain or large joint involve-ment rather than in the hands. **Gout** generally presents with a monoarthropathy, with a hot swollen joint rather than deformity. **Osteoarthritis** pain gets worse through the day, with patients having to stop using the affected limb by the evening in more severe cases. **Psoriatic arthritis** affects the distal interphalangeal joints first, has nail changes (onychodystrophy – nail pitting) and is preceded by a rash with plaques over the extensor surface of joints.

Q425 Compartment Syndrome

Answer 1 – **Assess the neurovascular status of his leg**. Following splitting the plaster cast, the next step is to assess the neurovascular status of his leg and the following step is to inform the senior team for urgent assessment. In this scenario, the first differential diagnosis should be compartment syndrome of the lower leg. Since the patient is complaining of pain out of proportion to his injury despite having adequate analgesia, as per the BOAST guidelines, one should split the plaster cast and assess the distal nerves and the pulses as well as the calf tenderness. The most important examination is to check for pain on passive extension/flexion of toes and ankle. Discussing immediately with senior colleagues and early referral of the patient to trauma and orthopaedic surgeons is essential. **CT scan of his leg** is unnecessary initially, as clinical assessment is the priority for suspected compartment syndrome. **Elevating the limb more** can worsen compartment syndrome by reducing arterial perfusion. **Ice application** is contraindicated as it may cause vasoconstriction and exacerbate ischaemia. **Venous ultrasound** to exclude thrombosis is inappropriate at this stage, as the concern is for arterial compromise and nerve compression, not venous obstruction.

Q426 Bone Pain

Answer 2 – **Femoral MRI and a CT chest, abdomen and pelvis**. This patient has a concerning lesion in her femur with a history of breast cancer. It is likely that this is a metastatic deposit from the breast cancer. However, there is too little information to make this diagnosis. Assuming this is the case, the definitive management may well be **primary stabilisation with an intramedullary nail**. To confirm the diagnosis, local staging with a femoral MRI and distant staging with a CT chest, abdomen and pelvis is the best first initial step in her management. **Radiotherapy followed by excision of the lesion** – any decision about radiotherapy needs to be made with the local oncology team. **Primary excision of the lesion and referral to oncology** is best suited to primary bone tumours, which are rare, and would be performed at a regional bone tumour centre. **Commence bisphosphonates** – bisphosphonates are used in osteoporosis and, considering she already has this diagnosis, she may already be on them.

Q427 Lacerations

Answer 1 – **Abduction of the fingers**. The ulnar nerve supplies sensation to the palmar surface of the little finger and ulnar half of the ring finger. The dorsal sensation of these fingers remains intact, indicating that the superficial branch of the ulnar nerve is spared, which suggests an injury distal to the ulnar nerve's branching point. Abduction of the fingers (spreading them apart) is controlled by the dorsal interossei, which are innervated by the deep branch of the ulnar nerve. An ulnar nerve injury at the wrist affects the deep motor branch, leading to weakness of finger abduction (e.g. inability to spread fingers apart). **Extension of the little finger** is incorrect.

The extensor digiti minimi extends the little finger and is innervated by the radial nerve, which is unaffected here. **Flexion of the distal interphalangeal joint of the little finger** is incorrect. The flexor digitorum profundus (FDP) of the little finger is innervated by the ulnar nerve, but proximal to the wrist. If the lesion were at the wrist, FDP function should remain intact. **Flexion of the interphalangeal joint of the thumb** is incorrect. This movement is controlled by the flexor pollicis longus, which is innervated by the median nerve, not the ulnar nerve. **Palmar abduction of the thumb** is incorrect. Palmar abduction (moving the thumb perpendicular to the palm) is controlled by the abductor pollicis brevis, which is innervated by the median nerve, not the ulnar nerve.

Q428 Soft Tissue Injury

Answer 4 – **Control any bleeding with topical dressings and refer for immediate specialist assessment**. The greatest concern in this case is the suspected tendinous injury, indicated by the lack of ability to adduct the thumb. This injury should be reviewed and assessed by appropriate trained specialist teams (in this case, an orthopaedic hand surgeon or plastic surgeon) for consideration of wound exploration and potential tendinous repair. **Admit for elevation and intravenous antibiotics** – based on the history, there is no immediate indication for intravenous antibiotics. **Close the wound with interrupted sutures and refer for outpatient follow-up** – as there is a suspected tendinous structure injury, the wound should not be immediately closed. **Close with wound closure strips and cover with non-adherent dressings** – wound closure strips would also not be an appropriate method of closure in this case. **X-raying the thumb** may highlight any concurrent bony injury; however, it will not replace the need for specialist assessment. There is acceptance that a number of these options may occur concurrently, but the priority here should be specialist assessment and return/preservation of digit function.

Q429 Trauma

Answer 4 – **Pelvic binder application**. This should be considered using the <C>abc Approach (i.e. catastrophic haemorrhage, airways, breathing, circulation). In principle, when prioritising interventions in trauma, injuries that will kill the patient the quickest should be dealt with first. When resuscitating patients in a large team, the order may be slightly disrupted as simultaneous interventions occur. There is debate about whether the pelvic binder is an intervention that could be considered in the '<C>' or 'c' section. Certainly in this patient, who is shocked with clear signs of pelvic haemorrhage (scrotal haematoma), it would be reasonable to consider the pelvic binder as a device to manage <C>, in which case it comes before all other interventions. If you consider the pelvic binder as part of the 'c' section; in this vignette 'a' and 'b' have been managed and therefore 'c' needs to be managed next. **Antibiotics, reduction and splintage of his fracture**, **cervical spine X-rays** and **urgent neurosurgical opinion do** not address c problems. **Large-bore intravenous access and 1 L of Hartmann's solution** does address 'c'. However, controlling haemorrhage should be prioritised over replacing lost volume (again, in principle – often these occur simultaneously). In addition, this patient requires resuscitation with blood products, not crystalloid. Hence, pelvic binder application is the best option.

Q430 Upper Limb Soft Tissue Injury

Answer 1 – **Distal biceps tendon rupture**. This is the most likely diagnosis. This is because the mechanism of injury (commonly, forced extension with the elbow in partial flexion) is consistent with a rupture of the distal biceps tendon. The swelling in the upper arm (often referred to as a 'Popeye' sign, due to the bunching of the bicep muscle belly) is commonly seen, and is separate from the site of maximal tenderness, which would be around the tendon insertion in the antecubital fossa. An **elbow dislocation**, while it would potentially display some of the features described, would not allow a full range of movement at the elbow. **Lateral epicondylitis** would be more consistent with a chronic inflammatory process, rather than an isolated, acute injury. **Proximal biceps tendon rupture** is commonly seen in more elderly patients, and rarely causes pain distal to the shoulder. And rotator cuff tear such as **teres minor** would also be more likely to cause pain on movement of the shoulder, and would not result in swelling or bruising to the elbow.

Q431 Massive Haemorrhage

Answer 2 – **Initiate the Massive Haemorrhage Protocol and call for a blood transfusion**. In Class III haemorrhagic shock, characterized by a 30–40% blood loss, the primary intervention is to initiate the Massive Haemorrhage Protocol. This protocol involves activating a coordinated response, including senior medical staff, anaesthetic/ ITU team, transfusion lab, porter staff and senior nursing staff. The pre-agreed pack delivered to the clinical site contains red blood cells

(RBC) and fresh frozen plasma (FFP) units, among other components, to address the life-threatening blood loss. The timely initiation of blood transfusion, in accordance with British Society for Haematology guidelines, is crucial for stabilising the patient and improving outcomes in this critical state of shock. **Administering crystalloid solutions** may be used temporarily, but excessive crystalloid in Class III shock can lead to dilutional coagulopathy and hypothermia. **Ordering a CT angiogram** is inappropriate as the patient is haemodynamically unstable and requires immediate resuscitation. **Performing early definitive airway management** is secondary unless there are clear airway or breathing compromises. **Splinting and aligning fractures** is part of secondary management after stabilising the patient's haemodynamic status.

Q432 Back Pain

Answer 1 – **Active rehabilitation**. The most appropriate management is active rehabilitation – physical exercise is the most suitable management in this scenario (back pain, young person, no concerning features). **Add opiate pain relief** is not appropriate due to risk of dependency and side effects; there is no need for **blood test for FBC and PSA** in this context (would be appropriate in a man > 60); **lumbar spine X-ray** is not appropriate – it rarely is for simple back pain. **MRI lumbar spine** is not appropriate with no concerning features.

15

Renal and Urology

Q433 Abnormal Urinalysis

Answer 5 – **Pyelonephritis**. **Diabetic ketoacidosis** is incorrect: glucose would be present in the urine and, although there are ketones in the urine, this would usually be > 1+, and other features include weight loss, abdominal pain and increased thirst. The question clearly states pregnancy test is negative, which excludes an **ectopic pregnancy**. **Glomerulonephritis** would usually present with blood and protein in the urine, alongside a decline in eGFR; flank pain, fever and dysuria are not associated with this condition. **Lower urinary tract infection** is a possibility but the presence of flank pain makes pyelonephritis the most appropriate answer.

Q434 Acute Kidney Injury

Answer 1 – **1 L of 0.9% saline**. The patient's abdominal pain, anuria for 24 hours, hyperkalaemia, elevated urea (28 mmol/L), elevated creatinine (375 μmol/L) and high PCV (0.56%) suggest pre-renal acute kidney injury (AKI) likely due to dehydration and hypovolaemia from poor oral intake and possible sepsis (temperature 39.2 ° C). The next step is aggressive fluid resuscitation with 1 L of 0.9% saline to restore intravascular volume, improve renal perfusion and enhance urine output.

40 mg intravenous furosemide is inappropriate in suspected pre-renal AKI, as diuretics can worsen dehydration. **Infusion of calcium gluconate** is used for severe hyperkalaemia (K+ > 6.5 mmol/L or ECG changes) but is not indicated here; rehydration alone may correct potassium levels. **Intermittent haemodialysis** is premature without a trial of fluid resuscitation and response assessment.

Parenteral nutrition is not a priority in acute management and should be considered only after stabilising renal function and volume status.

Q435 Benign Prostatic Hyperplasia

Answer 2 – **Finasteride**. This is correct and will take about 6 months for symptomatic benefit. **Doxazosin** is an alpha-blocker and therefore contraindicated in postural hypotension. **Stopping fludrocortisone** will have no effect on the patient's BPH. **Tamsulosin** is contraindicated as the patient has postural hypotension. **Transurethral resection of the prostate**: a surgical approach would be recommended if medical therapy is unsuccessful or the patient has renal complications.

Q436 Chronic Kidney Disease

Answer 3 – **Add ramipril 2.5 mg once daily**. This patient requires improved BP control. In the context of proteinuria, a stricter target of < 130/80 would normally be set. While any of the antihypertensives (**indapamide** and increasing **amlodipine**) could be used, ramipril also has anti-proteinuria effect so would be the best choice. **Metformin** should be avoided if the eGFR is < 30 due to accumulation. **Preparation for dialysis** normally starts when the eGFR is < 20 and at this point in the patient journey, active management would be the most appropriate option.

Q437 Urinary Incontinence

Answer 5 – **Weight loss.** The patient is not experiencing urge incontinence because she doesn't report urgency to urinate or frequent urination, therefore **bladder training** is not suitable. The **oestradiol ring** or **topical oestrogen gel** are not correct due to the young age of this patient – they are unlikely to be peri/menopausal. Therefore, the vaginal wall will still be muscular due to high levels of oestrogen in comparison to menopausal women. This patient's age and that they are nulliparous suggest that the sphincters should be functioning well and that they have not been damaged by childbirth. **Pelvic floor exercises** could be used as a secondary treatment. Obesity causes incontinence, as the raised abdominal mass increases the pressure on the pelvic floor. Weight loss will reduce this pressure and her pelvic floor muscles should resume normal function following weight loss.

Q438 Diabetic Nephropathy

Answer 4 – **Sodium-glucose cotransporter-2 (SGLT2) inhibitor**. The patient has microalbuminuria and is already on maximum dose ACE-inhibition, to control the microalbuminuria, and SGLT2-I would be the next step in management, as per NICE guidelines. The patient has adequate glycaemic control therefore **dipeptidyl peptidase intravenous (DPP IV) inhibitor** and **sulpho-nylurea** would not be the next step in management. The patient's BP control is adequate at present **therefore beta-blockers and calcium channel blockers** would not be the most appropriate next management to initiate.

Q439 Epididymitis and Orchitis

Answer 2 – **Escherichia coli**. In older men, E. coli and pseudomonas are more prevalent than STIs and initial treatment should be aimed at these, rather than **the other options**.

Q440 Prostate Cancer

Answer 4 – **Posterior**. Adenocarcinoma of the prostate typically begins in the posterior lobe. On DRE, the prostate could be asymmetrical, hard or large. Sometimes the cancer is too small to palpate. The location of most prostate malignancies leads to urethral compression and symptoms of lower tract obstruction later.

Q441 Testicular Cancer

Answer 4 – **Testicular cancer**. A young, fit and well man presented with a small painless lump. Based on the examination findings, as it is painless and non-tender, it makes **testicular torsion** and **epididymo-orchitis** unlikely. The mass did not feel cystic and did not transilluminate, hence making **hydrocele** unlikely. **Inguino-scrotal hernia** often presents with a soft, reducible mass in the inguinal region or scrotum, not a hard testicular lump.

Q442 Urinary Tract Calculi

Answer 5 – **Urine dipstick**. A urine dipstick would be an appropriate first test to help differentiate between urinary tract infection and urinary calculi. The presence of blood in the absence of nitrites and leukocytes would increase the suspicion of renal colic. **Non-contrast CT KUB** is the gold standard for confirming urolithiasis, but a urine dipstick is a quicker, less invasive and cost-effective first step. **Bloods**

for kidney function help assess the impact of obstruction but do not provide immediate diagnostic information. **Contrast CT KUB** is not recommended initially due to nephrotoxicity risks. **Ultrasound scan abdomen** is useful in pregnancy or when radiation is a concern but is less sensitive for ureteric stones compared to CT.

Q443 Urinary Tract Infection

Answer 2 – **Cystitis**. The patient has no systemic indication of **pyelonephritis**, nor pain indicative of it. She has a long-term partner making **STDs** less likely and her symptoms are more likely to be associated with a lower urinary tract infection along with a normal pelvic exam. She gives no symptoms attributable to **renal calculi** and there are no bloods provided to indicate **AKI**.

Q444 Nephrotic Syndrome

Answer 5 – **Renal vein thrombosis secondary to nephrotic syndrome**. This patient presents with nephrotic syndrome; she is clinically oedematous and hypoalbuminaemic, with significant proteinuria on her urine dip. Renal vein thrombosis is a known complication of nephrotic syndrome; this presents with haematuria, flank pain and AKI. **Renal colic** may present with similar flank pain and haematuria, but would not explain her proteinuria. **Portal vein thrombosis secondary to nephrotic syndrome** would present with deranged liver function tests and right upper quadrant pain. **Acute interstitial nephritis secondary to valsartan** is not often associated with significant proteinuria. The clinical history is not suggestive of infection and CRP is only mildly elevated, hence **AKI secondary to pyelonephritis** is a poor fit.

Q445 Haematuria

Answer 1 – **Immediate 2-week-wait referral to urology**. Visible haematuria without evidence of urinary tract infection in anyone over the age of 45 should receive a '2-week-wait' referral as per NICE guidelines, so **making a non-urgent referral to urology** and **a follow-up appointment following mid-stream urine analysis** are incorrect. Painless, visible haematuria carries the highest risk for cancer and requires referral for further investigation, therefore **reassuring the patient that the symptoms should resolve spontaneously** would be inappropriate. Urine dip was negative for leukocytes and nitrites and so **prescribing antibiotics for presumed urinary tract infection** is not required.

Q446 Oliguria

Answer 2 – **Oliguria due to hypovolaemia**. This patient presents with oliguria due to a combination of prolonged vomiting, bowel surgery with open abdomen and possibly inadequate perioperative fluid administration, leading to dehydration. This diagnosis is suggested by vital signs, examination, low urine output and the results of the renal function tests. **Septic shock** patients present with similar vital signs but also: high temperature (pyrexial), systolic BP below 90 mmHg unresponsive to fluid administration, confusion. This patient has no **asthma exacerbation** as chest is clear without any wheezing. There is no **perioperative fluid overload** as chest is clear with normal SpO_2, absent crackles on chest auscultation and no pulmonary or peripheral oedema. In a **postoperative opioid overdose**, the patient would be confused, drowsy, with slow RR.

Q447 Bladder Cancer

Answer 3 – **Perform bedside urinalysis**. Whilst all answers are correct and would be useful in determining the cause of his symptoms, attention must be paid to the question, which asks for the best next immediate investigation. This should be a bed-side test in the form of urinalysis which will confirm the presence of haematuria and potentially diagnose the most common cause of haematuria: infection. **Refer for 2-week-wait urology referral** would be indicated once infection is ruled out. **Full blood count** may detect anaemia and the presence of raised white cells may suggest infection, but this is unlikely to lead to a definitive diagnosis. **Checking his PSA levels** can be useful if prostate cancer is suspected, but other causes of haematuria should be excluded first. A flexible cystoscopy would be a good investigation for haematuria if infection has been ruled out, but this is an invasive diagnostic procedure and other differentials, in particular infection, should be ruled out first. **Referral for CT urogram** may give further information on the cause of haematuria, particularly if an upper tract or renal cause is suspected, but usually comes after or as part of more invasive diagnostic tests such as a flexible cystoscopy.

Q448 Scrotal/Testicular Pain and/or Lump/Swelling

Answer 2 – **Hydrocele**. The patient's painless, progressive swelling in the right hemiscrotum that is cystic and transilluminant is characteristic of a hydrocele, which is an accumulation of fluid within the tunica vaginalis. **Epididymal cyst** can also be cystic and transilluminant but is usually separate from the testicle and smaller. **Inguinal hernia** often presents as a non-transilluminant, reducible mass that increases with coughing or straining. **Testicular tumour** presents as a non-transilluminant, solid, painless mass. **Varicocele** feels like a 'bag of worms', does not transilluminate, and is usually more prominent on the left side.

Q449 Urinary Symptoms

Answer 3 – **Ask him to complete a symptom score**. Also offer him lifestyle advice and an alpha-blocker. Initial management should include assessment of his symptoms using a validated questionnaire, then later stepwise treatment including medical therapy, before consideration of surgical options. There is no evidence in the history or examination to suggest acute urinary retention. An **anticholinergic medication** would not improve voiding lower urinary tract symptoms. **5-alpha reductase inhibitors** require at least 3 months of use before having an effect. **Bladder outlet surgery** is reserved for severe symptoms or complications and is premature without a symptom score assessment. **Urgent bladder scan** is not indicated as there are no symptoms of acute retention, significant post-void residual volume or sudden onset of symptoms.

Q450 Testicular Torsion

Answer 4 – **Refer to the on-call urologist for operation imminently**. From the history given, the primary concern should be a possible torsion which would require urgent review by the on-call urology doctor. Whilst a **USS of the patient's scrotum** may be considered if the history is uncertain, this is a decision that should be made by the on-call urologist. **Discharge with analgesia and antibiotics and review in the STI clinic**: sending home with analgesia is not appropriate for a possible torsion. A **CT scan of the abdomen and pelvis** would not be able to rule out a testicular torsion. Finally testicular torsion is a urological emergency, if the testicle was twisted a delay in exploration could lead to loss of the testicle, hence **intravenous antibiotics and review by the urology team** would not be appropriate.

16 Respiratory

Q451 Respiratory Failure

Answer 1 – **Apply oxygen to target SpO$_2$ of 88–92%**. This is an acutely unwell patient presenting in type 2 respiratory failure with a compensated respiratory acidosis as highlighted by the raised bicarbonate level which suggests a degree of chronic illness. Whilst this may mean he has an impaired hypercapnic drive to ventilation, he is hypoxic with a low arterial pO$_2$ and oxygen saturations, meaning the initial management with an ABCDE resuscitation approach is to apply oxygen to an appropriate saturation target for this patient. Whilst **contacting the critical care registrar on call** and **starting non-invasive ventilation** may be part of his management, appropriate resuscitation should take place in the first instance. This may well also include **giving an intravenous fluid bolus of 250 ml Hartmann's solution** and **an intravenous antibiotic**; however, oxygen is the priority.

Q452 Respiratory Arrest

Answer 4 – **Open the airway and assess for breathing and a pulse**. All of the options are reasonable steps. When addressing a collapsed patient, there should be a very brief period of assessment to confirm the problem before any intervention is started. Then **calling for help and beginning CPR**, **beginning bag-mask ventilation with a self-inflating bag**, and **administering 400 mcg naloxone intravenously** should follow in order, in keeping with advanced and basic life support algorithms. If cardiac arrest is confirmed, CPR would take priority, but if only respiratory arrest is present, then bag-mask ventilation should be started. **Performing a primary survey to rule out any trauma** would come after immediate life-saving steps.

Q453 Asbestos-Related Lung Disease

Answer 3 – **Mesothelioma**. The patient's symptoms and their insidious onset (developing over a period of months) make **pneumonia** highly unlikely. **Asbestosis** does cause progressive breathlessness, but chest pain and a pleural effusion are not associated symptoms of this condition. This man's lethargy and significant weight loss are concerning for malignancy, making benign conditions such as **benign asbestos-related effusion** less likely. **Pleural plaques** are usually asymptomatic and do not cause effusions. The main differential diagnoses are mesothelioma and lung cancer. His occupational asbestos exposure, combination of symptoms, and otherwise clear lung fields on chest X-ray, make mesothelioma the most likely diagnosis.

Q454 Fibrotic Lung Disease

Answer 5 – **Pulmonary fibrosis**. The most correct answer in this case is pulmonary fibrosis. Several clues in the patient's history and clinical findings point towards this diagnosis:

1. Age – pulmonary fibrosis is more commonly seen in older individuals.
2. Progressively worsening breathlessness – pulmonary fibrosis is characterised by progressive dyspnoea.
3. Dry cough – the presence of a dry cough throughout the day is consistent with pulmonary fibrosis. In contrast, **asthma** symptoms are characteristically variable and the cough is usually productive in **bronchiectasis**.
4. Smoking history – this is a risk factor for developing pulmonary fibrosis.
5. Occupational history – exposure to certain chemicals, dust or fumes can contribute to the development of pulmonary fibrosis.
6. Examination findings – the features described are characteristic findings in pulmonary fibrosis.
7. Radiographic findings – the pattern described is consistent with pulmonary fibrosis.

While the above listed differentials are all possible, the combination of the patient's history, clinical examination findings and radiographic features supports the diagnosis of pulmonary fibrosis. **Chronic obstructive pulmonary disease (COPD)** is associated with smoking history, but presents with wheezing, hyperinflation and productive cough rather than velcro crackles and reticular shadowing. **Lung cancer** can cause cough and shortness of breath, but would more likely present with a mass or nodules on imaging rather than basal reticular shadowing.

Q455 Influenza

Answer 2 – **Direct patient to self-care with support of friends and family and with appropriate safety netting**. If a patient is well and has no end organ involvement, epidemic influenza is usually best managed with supportive care at home. Influenza occurring in pandemics may have a more virulent time course. **Give oseltamivir 75 mg PO twice daily for 5 days**: oseltamivir is normally reserved for patients who are at risk of complications or in pandemic situations. **Admit to a side-room on a general ward for observation, requesting echocaradiogram to rule out myocarditis**: there is no indication to admit this patient to hospital, and protection of healthcare resources should also factor into decisions about self-care. **Discharging to isolate at home with no personal contact allowed** is excessive, as influenza does not require absolute isolation – standard hygiene measures and limiting contact are sufficient. **Keeping in a side-room in ED and informing ICU** is disproportionate without severe symptoms or risk of respiratory failure.

Q456 Breathlessness

Answer 5 – **Tension pneumothorax**. Both **PE** and pneumothorax present with pleuritic chest pain and can cause haemodynamic instability, as in this case. Displacement of the apex beat laterally makes pneumothorax the most likely answer here. Furthermore, tall slim men are at increased risk of developing pneumothoraces.

Asthma exacerbation: asthma typically presents with shortness of breath and wheeze; chest pain would be an unusual presentation. Whilst **pneumonia** can cause chest pain and the observations recorded if associated with sepsis, the onset would be over days rather than minutes. The character of pain experienced during **acute myocardial infarction** is typically described as central heaviness exacerbated by exercise not deep inspiration.

Q457 Lower Respiratory Tract Infection

Answer 3 – **CURB 65 = 3**. CURB 65 is a validated scoring system to predict mortality of patients with pneumonia. This can be used to aid decisions on admission to hospital and the need for oral or intravenous antibiotic therapy. The scoring system allocates one point for each domain. Confusion; Urea > 7 mmol/L; Respiratory Rate ≥ 30;

BP – SBP < 90 DBP ≤ 60 mmHg; Age ≥ **65**. A score of **0–1** points is associated with less than 2.7% mortality and outpatient management is advised. A score of **2** associates with 6.8% 30-day mortality, and inpatient or closely monitored outpatient management is suggested. A score of **3 or more** is associated with 14% 30-day mortality and inpatient admission is advised.

Q458 Pneumothorax

Answer 2 – **Flying is not recommended until 1 week after a chest X-ray demonstrating complete resolution**. This man has a primary spontaneous pneumothorax (PSP) which has been managed conservatively, and prior to discharge he should be given advice about flying. The British Thoracic Society guidelines advise patients should not fly until 7 days after chest X-ray confirmation of full resolution of the pneumothorax, and the reason for waiting 7 days is to exclude early recurrence. The risk of recurrence after a single episode of PSP is 32%. Patients should be aware of this risk and advised to return to the emergency department for review if they develop worsening breathlessness. Other pre-discharge advice should include smoking cessation as smoking increases the risk of recurrence and patients should be aware not to scuba dive unless a surgical pleurectomy has been completed. **Stopping smoking** can reduce the risk of recurrence but does not permit immediate air travel. **Flying 6 weeks after symptom resolution** is excessive; current guidelines recommend 1 week post-clearance on X-ray. **Supplemental oxygen** does not prevent the risk of pneumothorax expansion at altitude. **Surgical pleurectomy** may be considered for recurrent pneumothorax, but it is not a requirement for flying after a single resolved episode.

Q459 Haemoptysis

Answer 1 – **Abnormal clotting**. Spitting blood when cleaning teeth usually indicates an oral or upper airway source, rather than the lungs. He has atrial fibrillation, so is likely to be on anti-coagulants. **Bronchiectasis** is unlikely –though still possible – given his lack of respiratory symptoms and the normal chest X-ray. **Pulmonary emboli** usually present acutely or sub-acutely. If they occur chronically, it would be unusual to have blood just in the mornings. **TB** is unlikely as a cause of bleeding in the absence of respiratory and constitutional symptoms and X-ray signs. **Vasculitis** may cause bleeding from rhinosinus involvement, laryngeal involvement or lung involvement, but would usually be associated with constitutional symptoms and bleed less predictably.

Q460 Acute Bronchitis

Answer 2 – **A history of cystic fibrosis**. This question tests knowledge of indications for antibiotics in acute bronchitis, which is usually caused by respiratory viruses. Management is predominantly supportive in nature. However, NICE guidelines recommend considering offering immediate or delayed antibiotic prescription to patients at high risk of complications. These include those with pre-existing cardiac or respiratory disease (such as cystic fibrosis), those taking immunosuppressants (including higher-dose maintenance steroids), old age, frailty or recent hospital admission. **A history of asthma**: asthma exacerbations are also usually triggered by viruses, so antibiotics not generally indicated. While focal signs such as unilateral crackles on lung auscultation can indicate pneumonia, **crackles/squeaks audible on both lungs** may be present in viral bronchitis. A patient with bilateral bacterial pneumonia would be more unwell than this man. **Repeat SARA-Cov-2 PCR test remains negative after a week**: Covid-19 test doesn't test for the plethora of other respiratory viruses, so a negative test is not an indication for antibiotics.

Sputum remaining purulent for more than 1 week: although data shows that increased sputum colour/purulence makes bacterial infection more likely in those with bronchiectasis or COPD, purulent sputum is seen in those with viral infections. Alone, it is not an indication for antibiotics. However, while viral symptoms can persist for 3–4 weeks, clinical deterioration or development of new sputum purulence may indicate a superadded bacterial infection – and so can be an indication for antibiotics.

Q461 Asthma COPD Overlap Syndrome

Answer 5 – **Treatment including corticosteroid with add-on long-acting beta-agonist**. As per GOLD guidelines, ACOS treatment should be commenced with low-/moderate-dose ICS and LABA. **Adequate controller therapy with ICS but without LABA or LAMA** is inadequate for the obstructive aspect of ACOS. **Inhaled corticosteroid and short-acting beta-agonist when required** do not provide sufficient long-term control. **Specialist referral** may be useful for complex cases, but initial management with ICS and LABA is standard. **Treatment for COPD alone** neglects the inflammatory aspect requiring corticosteroids.

Q462 Bronchiolitis

Answer 1 – **Bronchiolitis**. Bronchiolitis is inflammation of the small airways. This can be seen as a result of infection, can be idiopathic, but can also be seen associated with inflammatory conditions such as rheumatoid arthritis and inflammatory bowel disease.

Upper respiratory tract infections do not affect spirometry or cause slowly worsening breathlessness. **Pulmonary embolism** can cause slowly worsening breathlessness, though it is more often acute or sub-acute. However, it would not alter spirometry. **Pneumonia** is an acute lower respiratory tract infection – i.e. it would not cause slowly worsening breathlessness. It might cause some drop in spirometric measurements (as some alveoli fill with exudate instead of air), but would not cause obstructive spirometry unless there was concurrent airway pathology. **Fibrotic lung disease** causes a restrictive, not obstructive, spirometry result.

Q463 Chronic Obstructive Pulmonary Disease

Answer 3 – **Refer for pulmonary rehabilitation**. This is the correct answer, as the patient has an MRC dyspnoea score of 3 and has COPD, as evidenced by the risk factor, clinical features and obstructive spirometry. **Prescribe a salbutamol nebuliser for use as required**: nebulised salbutamol is not first-line treatment for COPD. **Sending sputum for culture** is not required in the context of recurrent non-purulent sputum with no exacerbations. **Arranging a CT scan of the chest** is not required at this point, as her symptoms are in keeping with her COPD diagnosis and the severity of the airflow obstruction on spirometry. **Start a combined long-acting beta-agonist and inhaled steroid inhaler**: a LABA–LAMA inhaler is recommended first-line treatment in COPD, rather than a LABA–ICS inhaler, unless there are features of atopy or eosinophilia.

Q464 Lung Cancer

Answer 3 – **Non-small cell lung cancer – squamous cell carcinoma.** Squamous cell carcinoma causes a humoral hypercalcaemia, through secretion of a parathyroid hormone-related peptide. This acts like parathyroid hormone and so therefore raises the calcium levels. **Atypical carcinoid** and **typical carcinoid** are neuroendocrine tumours that more commonly cause Cushing's syndrome or carcinoid syndrome rather than hypercalcaemia. **Non-small cell lung cancer – adenocarcinoma** is more associated with malignant pleural effusions or hypertrophic osteoarthropathy. **Small cell lung cancer** is linked with SIADH (hyponatraemia) and ectopic ACTH production rather than hypercalcaemia.

Q465 Occupational Lung Disease

Answer 1 – **CT chest**. This will reveal any early fibrosis as his occupation puts him at risk of asbestosis. An **echocardiogram** might reveal heart failure as an alternative diagnosis, but this is not top of the differential. **Rheumatoid factor** would not help rule a diagnosis in or out. **Spirometry** will be needed for monitoring, but cannot tell whether or not he has fibrosis. **Serial peak flow monitoring** would be indicated to investigate asthma.

Q466 Pulmonary Embolism

Answer 1 – **Bedside echo**. Acute pulmonary hypertension and RV dysfunction would be diagnostic of massive PE and therefore bedside echo would be a useful and rapidly accessible test. The patient is not stable enough to be moved for **CT pulmonary angiogram / V/Q scan**. **ECG** changes are not sensitive or specific for PE. **D-dimer** is not indicated where there is high clinical suspicion of PE / deep vein thrombosis.

Q467 Pulmonary Hypertension

Answer 3 – **Echocardiogram.** The history suggests pulmonary hypertension and the best initial screening test is an echocardiogram. Whilst angina can present with exertional breathlessness and can be painless in the context of diabetes, the examination and ECG findings point away from angina. Whilst her occupational and smoke exposure put her at risk of emphysema, the history and examination findings point towards a cardiac cause of the symptoms. **24-hour ECG recording** is more useful for detecting arrhythmias and would not assess right heart function or pulmonary pressures. **Coronary angiography** is indicated for suspected coronary artery disease, but her symptoms and findings suggest a pulmonary cause. **High-resolution CT chest** can identify interstitial lung disease, but her normal chest X-ray makes this less likely. **Right heart catheterisation** is the gold standard for diagnosing pulmonary hypertension, but it is an invasive test typically performed after echocardiography suggests elevated pulmonary pressures.

Q468 Cough

Answer 3 – **Omeprazole orally.** This man has had a dry cough for some time. The differential is wide, however cancer is felt less likely with no red flag symptoms and a normal CXR. Normal spirometry means asthma and COPD are unlikely and therefore steroids, such as **prednisolone**, and inhalers (e.g. **salbutamol**) are not appropriate. **Amlodipine** is a BP medication and has no impact on the management of respiratory disease. An **ipratropium bromide nasal spray** helps in cases of post-nasal drip but the fact that the cough is dry, worse on bending forwards and when lying flat at night time, is more supportive of a diagnosis of gastro-oesophageal reflux disease. Therefore, omeprazole is an appropriate treatment.

Q469 Cyanosis

Answer 3 – **Pneumonia**. This is a classic presentation of pneumonia with cough, fever and blood-stained sputum. The history is acute, and the patient is febrile with fever and low oxygen saturations. **Lung cancer** rarely presents acutely with fever and cough. It is also most common in older individuals, with the highest rates in those over 70 years of age (British Lung Foundation / Cancer Research UK). **Acute severe asthma** commonly presents with wheeze, cough and severe breathlessness, usually occurring over a relatively short period of minutes to hours. Sometimes there is an identifiable trigger, for example pollen or exercise. Similarly, **pneumothorax** presents very acutely with chest pain and breathlessness. There is no associated haemoptysis and, as for severe asthma, fever is usually absent. **Pulmonary embolism** (PE) could present in this way, but it is less likely than pneumonia as a cause of this presentation. PE presents acutely with severe chest pain and shortness of breath, sometimes accompanied by unilateral leg swelling and pain.

Q470 Pain on Inspiration

Answer 2 – **Chest X-ray**. The most likely diagnosis is pneumothorax. The patient has risk factors for this as he is young, smokes cannabis and has a family history of Marfan's disease, all three of which predispose him to pneumothorax. All the other tests might support this diagnosis, but none alone would allow you to diagnose pneumothorax, apart from a CXR. An **arterial blood gas** might demonstrate hypoxia, but hypoxia can be seen in many respiratory conditions. An **ECG** could show tachycardia, but may be normal, and tachycardia is a non-specific finding in respiratory disease. There are no specific

ECG features associated with pneumothorax. A **D-dimer** would be useful to rule out PE but, if positive, would need a CT pulmonary angiogram or a V/Q scan to confirm the diagnosis. A **troponin** blood test in isolation is not diagnostic of ACS and in this age group ACS would be very unlikely.

Q471 Pleural Effusion

Answer 3 – **Nephrotic syndrome**. All the conditions offered as possible answers could be associated with pleural effusions. However, the short 4-week history, lack of infective signs and significant proteinuria, associated with frothy urine and bilateral leg oedema, makes nephrotic syndrome the most likely diagnosis. None of the other diagnoses would be associated with proteinurea. **Carcinoid syndrome** very rarely presents with pleural involvement. **Mesothelioma** would be very rare in this age group as it is caused by occupational asbestos exposure which is now strictly regulated. A patient with an effusion secondary to **pancreatitis** would be acutely unwell with abdominal pain. **Pulmonary TB** presents with fevers, cough and significant constitutional upset, all of which are absent here.

Q472 Asthma

Answer 1 – **Call for immediate review from the intensive care team**. Intensive care review is the correct answer, because she has developed hypercapnic respiratory failure and so is at imminent risk of respiratory arrest. **Give a salbutamol and ipratropium nebuliser and review in 1 hour**: nebulised bronchodilators are important, but should not delay the review by an intensivist. **Give her nebulised magnesium and intravenous hydrocortisone**: nebulised magnesium is not recommended in the current BTS/SIGN guideline. **Reduce oxygen saturation target to 88–92% and repeat ABG in 1 hour**: reducing oxygen and reassessing is appropriate for a patient with COPD who might experience worsening hypercapnia due to over-oxygenation, but is not appropriate for an acute asthma attack. **Start her on non-invasive ventilation and inform the medical registrar**: NIV is not recommended for asthma outside of an intensive care unit.

Q473 Upper Respiratory Tract Infection

Answer 3 – **No treatment**. The correct answer is no treatment; he has acute rhinosinusitis with no worrisome features and needs nothing more than advice at this point. **Advising OTC antihistamines** would help if there were features suggestive of allergy, but these are not present in the vignette. **Arranging a CT scan of the head and sinuses** or **taking a nasal swab for culture** would only be needed for persistent or recurrent problems. **Prescribe a 5-day course of doxycycline**: antibiotics would only be needed if there were more worrisome features or deterioration.

Q474 Wheeze

Answer 5 – **Oxygen therapy**. This is a young patient with no prior history of respiratory disease with wheeze. This could be asthma, anaphylaxis or aspiration of a foreign body. When assessing any unwell patient, an ABCDE approach is necessary, and structured according to the treatment of the most life-threatening problem first. It appears the airway is safe as there is no swelling of the neck observed so we move to assess 'B' for breathing. Oxygen levels are 92% and the patient is breathless, so it is appropriate to administer oxygen as the first treatment. Performing an **ABG** and **CXR** is appropriate, but these investigations can happen after hypoxia is treated. **Nebulised salbutamol** is appropriate for wheeze, and anaphylaxis treatment with **intramuscular adrenaline** may be necessary, but neither is the most important immediate management step.

Q475 Bronchiectasis

Answer 2 – **Bronchiectasis**. Bronchiectasis is the correct answer because she has a persistent productive cough, chest crackles and finger clubbing. **Asthma** is possible but does not tend to cause this degree of sputum production and she has no atopic features or response to inhaled steroids. **COPD** and **chronic bronchitis** are less likely because she only has 2 pack years of smoking history. **Foreign body inhalation** is a possible cause of chronic cough and bronchiectasis, but no features in the vignette point specifically to this.

Q476 Pneumonia

Answer 4 – **Empyema**. In the context of community-acquired pneumonia, if a patient is not improving clinically despite adequate antibiotic therapy, the presence of empyema (a collection of pus within the pleural cavity) should be considered. (So repeat CXR is indicated.) Empyema is a complication of pneumonia where bacteria invade the pleural space, leading to the accumulation of infected fluid. This condition can cause persistent fever, chest pain and a failure to improve with standard antibiotic treatment. **Acute respiratory distress syndrome (ARDS)** would cause hypoxia and respiratory distress, but the patient's normal respiratory rate and oxygen saturation make this less likely. **Atrial fibrillation** can cause tachycardia but not persistent fever. **Delirium** is not suggested by the history and would not explain persistent fever. **Pleurisy** can cause pleuritic chest pain but not persistent fever and systemic symptoms without associated effusion or empyema.

Rheumatology

17

Q477 Systemic Lupus Erythematosus

Answer 5 – **Systemic lupus erythematosus**. The description is a characteristic presentation of mild lupus. A cause for Raynaud's phenomenon should be sought if it begins after the age of 30 years. The pleurisy which was investigated but without a cause found is likely to be a part of lupus. The family history may represent antiphospholipid syndrome **Giant cell arteritis** presents in people over 50 years of age, with headache, constitutional symptoms and occasionally visual disturbance. **Reactive arthritis** is an inflammatory arthritis that is triggered by an infection elsewhere in the body. It is a condition that self-limits in no more than a few weeks.

Rheumatoid arthritis typically presents as an inflammatory arthritis affecting the small joints. Raynaud's syndrome may be present. Pleurisy occasionally occurs but is not typical. The facial rash described does not occur. There is no association with antiphospholipid syndrome, which in the question is suggested with the family history of pregnancy loss. **Sarcoidosis** most commonly presents with pulmonary symptoms. Arthralgias (joint pain without swelling) and arthritis (joint pain with swelling) may be present, and is commonly bilateral ankle arthritis. Raynaud's syndrome is not seen and there is no association with antiphospholipid syndrome.

Q478 Ankylosing Spondylitis

Answer 1 – **Ankylosing spondylitis**. This is axial spondyloarthritis with psoriasis. In both **cauda equina syndrome** and **lumbar L4/L5 root impingement**, there would be limb neurological abnormalities. Although a **lumbar spinal malignancy** is possible, this is much less likely. **Psoriatic arthritis** presents with limb, rather than axial, symptoms.

Q479 Bursitis

Answer 5 – **Referral to physiotherapy**. This man has subacromial bursitis, likely from occupational overuse. Physiotherapy can help address this through exercises to strengthen the rotator cuff and scapular stabilising muscles. This approach improves the mechanics in the shoulder and helps to prevent future irritation. **Oral gluco-corticoid course for 1 week** and **intraarticular injection of gluco-corticoid** may provide some short-term relief but do not address the underlying cause and are associated with their own adverse effects. **Partial immobilisation with a simple sling** is generally not recommended as it can lead to stiffness and further muscle weakening. **Radiograph of shoulder** is not indicated, given this is a clinical diagnosis without suspicion of other pathology.

Q480 Fibromyalgia

Answer 5 – **Regular slow rhythmic exercise**. Slow rhythmic exercises like Tai Chi and yoga have evidence of restoring function. **A short course of prednisolone** is not indicated in fibromyalgia. **Regular oxycodone, gradually increasing as needed**: opioids are not indicated in any non-specific low back or widespread pain. **2 weeks of complete bed rest**: bed rest is not advised for back pain and may delay recovery. Advice to stay active and continue ordinary activities results in a faster return to work, less chronic disability, and fewer recurrent problems. **3 trigger-point injections with steroids, 1 month apart,** are not indicated in the guidelines. It increases steroid loads with suppression of adreno-pituitary axis, and the help is only for a few days to up to 4 weeks.

Q481 Muscle Pain/Myalgia

Answer 2 – **Atorvastatin**. The most likely cause of her myalgia is her recently started treatment with a statin. **Amlodipine** can cause ankle swelling but does not cause generalised myalgia. The absence of any other symptoms, normal physical examination, and blood tests within normal range except for a high CK level rule out **all other options**.

Q482 Osteoarthritis

Answer 4 – **Plain X-ray of the pelvis**. Hip pathology (e.g. osteoarthritis) often presents as groin pain radiating down the thigh to the knee. Referred knee pain is common in hip osteoarthritis due to the shared nerve supply (obturator nerve). X-ray of the pelvis allows bilateral hip joint evaluation and is the first-line investigation for suspected hip osteoarthritis. **Hip arthrogram** is used for labral tears or hip instability, but not first-line for suspected osteoarthritis. **Lumbar spine X-ray**: lumbar pathology can cause referred pain to the thigh, but hip osteoarthritis is a more likely cause given the history of groin pain and difficulty walking. **Plain X-ray of the left knee**: while knee pain is mentioned, it is likely referred pain from the hip, making pelvic X-ray the priority. **Ultrasound of the pelvis** is not useful for bony pathology and is more appropriate for soft tissue or gynaecological concerns.

Q483 Osteomalacia

Answer 4 – **Low serum phosphate or low serum calcium**. His osteomalacia from insufficient vitamin D is caused by his reduced sun exposure since moving to the UK. This osteomalacia presents with the following serum results: low/normal phosphate, low/normal calcium, high/normal alkaline phosphatase, high parathyroid hormone, low 25-OH vitamin D, and low/normal/high 1,25-OH vitamin D. **All other options** are incorrect.

Q484 Polymyalgia Rheumatica

Answer 3 – **Polymyalgia rheumatica.** PMR is the most appropriate answer as it is common in over-60s, with symmetrical presentation with stiffness in shoulders. In contrast, **infective arthritis** would present more acutely, with swollen joints. **Parkinson's disease** is less likely as no rigidity, tremor or bradykinesia are noted. **Rheumatoid arthritis** is symmetrical but involves small joints in hands and feet. **Polymyositis** causes proximal muscle weakness rather than pain and would show elevated muscle enzymes (e.g. CK). So, the best option is Polymyalgia rheumatica.

Q485 Sarcoidosis

Answer 4 – **Review in clinic with repeat chest X-ray in 3 months**. The triad of arthralgia, bilateral hilar lymphadenopathy and erythema nodosum represents Lofgren's syndrome. If patients have typical findings on a chest X-ray with a typical clinical presentation, then a **high-resolution computed tomography** does not need to be conducted urgently, providing the patient is followed up in clinic with a repeat chest X-ray within 3 months. CT should be conducted sooner if the patient has an atypical history or atypical radiographic findings on CXR. **Fractional exhaled nitric oxide test** (FeNO) is a test for asthma. **Endobronchial ultrasound and biopsy of hilar lymph nodes** is unnecessary initially in a patient with classic Löfgren's syndrome, unless symptoms persist or worsen. **Serum ACE levels** can be elevated in sarcoidosis, but they lack specificity and do not change management in classic, uncomplicated cases.

Q486 Reactive Arthritis

Answer 3 – **reactive arthritis**. This presentation of reactive arthritis is with the triad of acute inflammatory arthritis, conjunctivitis and a likely trigger of asymptomatic genitourinary infection. **Osgood–Schlatter disease** is most common in the peri-pubescent years. **Patellar tendonitis** would have tenderness of the patellar tendon, and there is no association with concurrent conjunctivitis. **Rheumatoid arthritis** is usually a polyarthritis, and symptoms must be present for more than 4–6 weeks to diagnose. Septic arthritis also presents as a monoarthritis, but usually has a high fever.

Q487 Rheumatoid Arthritis

Answer 1 – **Aspirate the affected joint and send for urgent microscopy and culture**. Given the patient has presented with a hot swollen joint and is systemically unwell, the most important thing to attempt to rule out is infection. The best test included here is to aspirate the infected joint and to ask for microscopy and culture. It may be that this is active RA but it is unusual to have a temperature with this; if this man's culture were to be negative, then **checking a serum uric acid** may be considered. If it is thought clinically likely that there is joint sepsis, it would be correct to **commence broad-spectrum intravenous antibiotics**, but only after the synovial aspirate has been taken to prevent a false negative aspirate result. **Discharging home with advice to see his GP if things don't improve** could lead to an untreated septic joint. Gout should be a differential diagnosis in a monoarthritis, and requesting microscopy for crystals would be a good test. **Starting a reducing course of prednisolone** could worsen an infection and should be avoided until septic arthritis is ruled out.

Q488 Idiopathic Arthritis

Answer 1 – **Juvenile idiopathic arthritis (JIA) (oligoarticular subtype)**. JIA is the most likely diagnosis at this stage. **Septic arthritis** usually only affects one joint at presentation, and the time course is more acute. **Transient synovitis** classically affects the hip joint(s) and is more common in males, often preceded by a viral illness. This child presents as 'otherwise well' and with normal observations, making **JIA (systemic subtype)** unlikely. Though five or more joints may become involved later, there is currently only evidence of inflammation in two joints, making **JIA (polyarticular subtype)** a less favourable answer than the oligoarticular subtype.

Q489 Crystal Arthropathy

Answer 1 – **Calcium pyrophosphate dihydrate arthritis**. CPPD arthritis is most common in older people and those with pre-existing osteoarthritis, may be precipitated by another illness, and is more likely given the chondrocalcinosis. **Gout** is a possibility but dramatically less likely as there are no risk factors for gout, other than the intercurrent illness that can cause either crystal arthritis. **Haemarthrosis** is possible as she has a monoarthritis, but it is much rarer and she has no predisposing factors for it. **Rheumatoid arthritis** is a chronic inflammatory polyarthritis rather than an acute monoarthritis. **Septic arthritis** is possible but much less likely given the absence of other risk factors and with the patient being systemically well.

Q490 Acute Joint Pain/Swelling

Answer 5 – **Temporary immobilisation and analgesics**. The most likely diagnosis is a haemarthrosis from a raised INR caused by the recent clarithromycin. **Allopurinol and non-steroidal anti-inflammatories** should not be prescribed with anti-coagulants due to the risk of bleeding. **Colchicine and analgesics** – allopurinol is a long-term, and colchicine an acute, treatment for gout, and the patient's serum urate was recently normal, making gout unlikely. **Reversal of anti-coagulation** is best avoided as his valve gives significant risk of thromboembolism. Joint aspiration is possible (not listed), but as the diagnosis of haemarthrosis is reasonably certain, avoiding interventions, given his valve, is a reasonable approach. **Non-steroidal anti-inflammatory drugs** can be effective for pain but are contraindicated due to the patient's warfarin use, which increases bleeding risk.

Q491 Chronic Joint Pain/Stiffness

Answer 3 – **Osteoarthritis**. The patient has osteoarthritis given the physical findings (including Heberden's and Bouchard's nodes).

Early morning joint stiffness up to 30 minutes is common in OA. Osteoarthritis is usually primary, but the secondary causes should be considered. **Fibromyalgia** gives all four quadrant symptoms but does not give the bony swelling. **Gout** does not have self-limiting episodes and has soft tissue swelling. **Psoriatic arthritis** (PsA) and **RA** both give soft tissue swelling (for both: synovitis; and for PsA: enthesitis).

Q492 Neck Pain/Stiffness

Answer 5 – **Physiotherapy**. The short-term symptoms are most likely to be related to a C6/C7 disc prolapse, and most of these will resolve spontaneously with a conservative approach. **CT scan** will show the bony structures, but not the soft tissues which are causing the symptoms. **MRI** imaging will show the disc prolapse, but is not necessary as most will resolve spontaneously. MRI would be the right answer if the symptoms do not resolve spontaneously. **Nerve conduction studies** would show the position of the lesion, but not the definite cause or, if symptoms were to persist, allow planning for potential surgery. A **neurosurgical opinion** is not required as most causes will resolve spontaneously.

Q493 Osteoporosis

Answer 3 – **Osteoporosis**. The question is pointing to height loss due to one or several vertebral fracture(s). **Bronchial carcinoma** can cause vertebral fracture with bony metastases and occurs in smokers, but is unlikely here both with this disease duration, and because she is otherwise healthy. **Growth hormone deficiency** is a rare cause of childhood failure to grow, and never causes adult height loss. Osteoporosis is much more likely than the others. She has several risk factors (age, early menopause, smoking, low BMI) as well as normal bloods and no sign of the other diseases. **Rickets** is due to childhood vitamin D deficiency causing deficient growth plate mineralization which may cause bowing of the legs. Rickets does not cause adult height loss. **Tuberculosis** can cause vertebral collapse but is not likely in a woman who is otherwise healthy.

Q494 Gonorrhoea

Answer 2 – **Ceftriaxone 1 g intramuscular stat**. This is the best choice as it will provide better cover against more organisms (the history suggests symptoms commencing after the trip to South East Asia and unprotected sex, therefore the infection is likely an Asia–Pacific organism, which may have a different susceptibility profile to those which are locally acquired). It can also be given in the clinical setting so does not rely on the patient being compliant with the course. It has very low risk of causing a cross reaction due to penicillin as it is a third-generation cephalosporin, and the intramuscular delivery is very effective.

The other options provide a narrower spectrum of cover which may not treat a resistant organism. **Azithromycin** is a reasonable second-line option in needle phobia but is inferior to ceftriaxone due to scope of cover. **All the remaining options** require longer courses, which may mean compliance with the regime is compromised, especially if the patient encounters side effects (particularly gastrointestinal upset), which are more common with these medicines.

Q495 Syphilis

Answer 4 – **Secondary**. The patient presents with a typical secondary syphilitic rash, including on the palms and soles. **Primary** syphilis presents with a chancre on a mucosal surface and this is not described in the history. It is not **early latent** syphilis as he is symptomatic. It is not **tertiary** syphilis as he has no cardiovascular, neurological or ophthalmological symptoms. It is not **late latent** syphilis as he has no symptoms and had a negative screen for syphilis 9 months ago.

Q496 Subfertility

Answer 5 – **Supported weight reduction, and sexual intercourse every 2–3 days**.

This advice must be delivered sensitively and with supporting resources where available, e.g. local weight reduction programmes. Women with PCOS will struggle to lose weight as the nature of the condition means that they are insulin resistant. However, the studies suggest that even a 5% weight loss can return ovulation. The patient should also be advised of the future options available to her and the time scale for review to progress to these. These include **metformin** and **clomiphene ovulation induction** or the 2 combined, but they are not first-line in a woman who has only been trying for a month. **ICSI** is not required for this patient. **Semen analysis** may be appropriate if there is no success after 12 months of regular unprotected intercourse, but the focus should initially be on addressing the likely cause (anovulation due to PCOS).

Q497 Trichomonas Vaginalis

Answer 4 – **Posterior fornix**. Trichomoniasis typically presents with scanty, yellow, frothy vaginal discharge and slight dysuria, as described in the patient. The most appropriate area to swab to confirm the diagnosis is the posterior fornix, as Trichomonas vaginalis tends to collect and concentrate in this area. A posterior fornix swab allows for the best chance of detecting the parasite on wet mount microscopy or culture. **Cervical** swabs are more appropriate for Chlamydia and gonorrhoea detection. Swabs of the **low vaginal** area are less sensitive for Trichomonas compared to the posterior fornix. Swabs of the **mid vagina** are also less effective for identifying Trichomonas vaginalis. Swabs of the **urethra** may detect urethral infections but are not the best choice for diagnosing trichomoniasis in women.

Q498 Chlamydia

Answer 2 – **Chlamydia infection**. Postcoital bleeding and yellow vaginal discharge are suggestive of cervicitis, which is commonly caused by Chlamydia trachomatis. Note: long-term partners are sometimes unfaithful. **COCP adverse effect**: the COCP can cause breakthrough bleeding, but it does not cause yellow discharge or cervicitis. Postcoital bleeding is more concerning for infection or cervical pathology. **Cervical cancer** (unlikely but should be considered) can present with postcoital bleeding, but it is less likely in a 25-year-old who has not had previous abnormal smears. A smear test should be performed, but infection should be ruled out first. **Endometrial cancer** (highly unlikely) typically presents with post-menopausal bleeding, not postcoital bleeding in a young woman. **Endometriosis** can cause pelvic pain and abnormal bleeding, but it does not cause yellow vaginal discharge.

Q499 Contraception Request/Advice

Answer 1 – **Combined hormonal contraception (pill, patch or ring)**. Combined hormonal contraception should not be prescribed for women age 35 or over who are also smokers (or within 1 year of quitting) as the risk of venous thromboembolism is significantly increased. The ideal method medically for this individual is the **hormonal intrauterine device** (52 mg versions such as Mirena or Levosert) as it is a treatment for heavy menstrual bleeding in addition to contraception. A reduction in menstrual blood flow may also be achieved with the remaining methods, but irregular bleeding is also a likely side effect. For the **injectable hormonal contraception (sub-cutaneous or intramuscular)** this may reduce with duration of administration, but the patterns with the **subdermal implant** and the **progesterone only pill** are less predictable.

Q500 Erectile Dysfunction

Answer 1 – **He is not receiving sufficient sexual stimulation with his current relationship difficulties**. As with most patients, the picture is a mix of physical and psychological causes. The patient blames his poor relationship for his ED, and this should be explored. His wife is likely to be going through the menopause, which might be affecting her libido. Communication between them does not appear to be good and there is no longer any foreplay. However, there are clues that physical causes also play a part. The 9-month history of deterioration, the lack of morning and night-time erections, his smoking history and sedentary lifestyle, all point to cardiovascular disease being a major contributor to his ED. PDE-5 inhibitors only result in erections if there is normal sexual stimulation. Given the state of their relationship and lack of foreplay, it is likely that this is not happening. **Losing weight and smoking less** will slow progression of his cardiovascular disease and hence his ED but is not the most likely cause of sildenafil not working. **He should have been prescribed tadalafil as requested**: this is incorrect as he does not have one of the qualifying conditions. **The statins he has started** taking are interacting with the sildenafil: this is incorrect as there is no interaction between statins and sildenafil. **There is another organic cause of his erectile dysfunction**: there might be but, from the information given, this is not the most likely cause, plus PDE-5 inhibitors work with a range of organic causes, not just cardiovascular disease.

Q501 Pelvic Inflammatory Disease

Answer 4 – **Ectopic pregnancy**. Ectopic pregnancy can have life-threatening consequences if left undiagnosed and untreated, and can be ruled out with a simple pregnancy test. Pain can present when a pregnancy outside of the uterus grows and eventually ruptures, which poses an immediate or delayed threat to life and possibly other reproductive consequences. **The other answers** are important differentials – however, they are not as likely based on the history and would take further time and investigation to diagnose. Ruling out an ectopic pregnancy may be as simple as a urine sample and 5-minute pregnancy test, and is therefore the most simple and immediate consideration for a young female with lower abdominal pain.

Q502 Loss of Libido

Answer 5 – **Vaginal oestrogen**. This patient has marked vaginal atrophy on examination, which can often contribute towards dyspareunia, coupled with vaginal dryness. Vaginal oestrogen may benefit the patient by providing local oestrogen supplementation. Provided that the patient does not report a peanut allergy, this is safe to prescribe. Systemic absorption of this is minimal and, as such, progestogen is not required. This can be continued long-term if symptoms return upon cessation of the medication. **Check blood hormone status**: NICE Guidelines do not routinely recommend using FSH/LH blood tests to diagnose menopause for otherwise healthy women over 45 years of age. In the UK, the average age of menopause is 51 years, and so it is likely that this patient is already post-menopausal and taking these tests would not provide any further information for the patient. **Mental health review**: the patient does not report low mood. **Oral oestrogen therapy**: the British Menopause Society recommends that if commencing hormone replacement therapy (HRT) over the age of 60 years, it is important to consider the wishes of the patient. However, transdermal routes of application would be preferable as over the age of 60 years there is an increasing risk of venous thromboembolism (VTE) associated with oral oestrogen therapy. Furthermore, this patient is not reported to have had a hysterectomy and, as such, she would also require progesterone for endometrial protection. **Topical testosterone therapy** should only be considered for patients reporting low sexual desire after investigation into other potential causes of this, such as a psychosexual problem or low mood. It would be beneficial to see if vaginal oestrogen helps with this patient's presenting complaint first and then to re-assess any testosterone replacement requirements.

Q503 Painful Sexual Intercourse

Answer 4 – **NAAT (vulvo-vaginal) swab**. This is used for testing for chlamydia and gonorrhoea, whereas **high vaginal swabs** are used to detect bacterial vaginosis, trichomonas vaginalis, candida and GBS. Her presentation and history suggest a sexually transmitted infection may be a cause of her symptoms. **Abdominal CT** is not indicated initially for suspected STIs or PID. **Abdominal ultrasound** might help identify tubo-ovarian abscesses or hydrosalpinx but is less useful for initial diagnosis. **Urinary pregnancy test** is useful if pregnancy is suspected, but the symptoms here are more indicative of an STI or PID.

Q504 Urethral Discharge and Genital Ulcers/Warts

Q504(a) Genital Ulcers

Answer 3 – **Primary herpes simplex infection**. It is primary infection as the lesions are not confined to one dermatome, they are multiple and have a typical description. **Aphthous ulceration** typically occurs intra-orally and rarely presents on the genitals. **Secondary herpes simplex infection** is usually milder, confined to one dermatome and there may be a history of a previous episode. It is painful so **syphilis** is a less likely diagnosis. **Cellulitis** usually has erythema extending out from the ulceration which is hot to touch.

Q504(b) Genital Warts

Answer 1 – **Take a biopsy and treat accordingly**. The symptoms and history are concerning for a diagnosis of vulval intraepithelial neoplasia. **Treating with cryotherapy**, **imiquimod** or **podophyllotoxin** risks progression of disease while waiting to assess response to treatment. **Treating with surgical excision** can be considered once the diagnosis is established. The lesion is large and it will potentially impact her ability to have sex if it is wholly excised with margins, so it needs to be clear that this is necessary treatment before proceeding.

Q504(c) Urethral Discharge

Answer 4 – **Doxycycline 100 mg twice daily for 7 days**. This is first-line treatment for urethritis. **Ceftriaxone 1 gm intramuscular stat** is the first-line treatment for gonorrhoea, for which the patient's symptoms are not typical and gram-negative diplococci would often be seen on microscopy. **Azithromycin 1 gm stat followed by 500 mg daily for a further 48 hours with additional metronidazole 400 mg three times a day for 7 days**: this is incorrect as this is treatment for recurrent urethritis and this is his first presentation. **Azithromycin 1 gm stat followed by 500 mg po daily for a further 48 hours**: azithromycin is a treatment option but is not first line. **Nitrofurantoin MR 500 mg twice daily for 3 days**: this is treatment for a urinary tract infection and this man has a new sexual partner, so an STI is a more likely diagnosis.

Q505 Unwanted Pregnancy and Termination of Pregnancy

Answer 2 – **10 weeks**. Home medical termination (self-managed abortion at home) is approved up to 10 weeks gestation in the UK. This involves taking mifepristone (an antiprogestogen) followed by misoprostol (a prostaglandin), usually 24–48 hours later. Before 10 weeks, medical abortion is considered safe for home use with telephone or virtual consultation, as long as appropriate support is available. Beyond 10 weeks, medical abortion requires in-person medical supervision due to the higher risk of incomplete abortion, excessive bleeding and complications.

Q506 Vaginal Discharge

Answer 3 – **Neisseria gonorrhoea**. The descriptor is leading towards an infective cause for the vaginal discharge. Her risk factors for a sexually transmitted infection are her age, recent change in sexual partner and using no barrier methods for contraception. The presence of gram-negative diplococci is pathognomonic of gonorrhoea. It could be **Chlamydia trachomatis** but the cervical culture suggests an alternative diagnosis; the factors supporting this diagnosis would be change in sexual partner and a cervical discharge. Chlamydia is an obligate intracellular bacterium which is diagnosed using nucleic acid amplification tests not standard microscopy or culture. **Lactobacilli** are the normal vaginal flora and do not produce an offensive vaginal flora. **Staphylococcus aureus** is a common skin flora and is not found in the vagina. **Trichomonas vaginalis** would present with a sore red vagina and in 5% of patients a strawberry cervix may be seen. The change in sexual partner supports it as a possibility as it is an STI, but it is not the correct answer.

Contributors

Joanna Abramik, Tochukwu M. Achonye, Katie Adams, Ifeoluwa Agbeja, Divya Agrawal, Basma Ahmad, Manal Ahmad, Moaz Ahmad, Muhammad S. Ahmad, Umair Ahmad, Ahmed M. G. Ahmed, Toqeer Ahmed, Raza Ali, Louise Alldridge, Omar A. B. AlMasri, Prodromos Anastasiadis, Paul Andrews, Julia Anstey, Natalie Anwyll, Parniya Arooj, Diana Artene, Balpreet Attilia, Tin Htun Aung, Myint Aye, Richard Ayres, Omikunle Babawale, Thomas Badenoch, Amit Badshah, Somnath Bagchi, Alok Bahl, Toby Ball, Alexandra Banner, Hashem Barakat, Ahmad Basma, Adenike R. Bawor-Omatseye, Oliver Beaumont, Sara Belal, Martha Belete, Alina Beltechi, Oliver Bendall, Claire Bethune, Shivam Bhargava, Mohammad Bhat, Shakya Bhattacharjee, Suman Bhattacharyya, Eimear Blunnie, Shruti Bodapati, Simon Bonell, Adam Booth, Neil Bowley, Jessica Braschi, Stewart Brown, Kirsty Brownlie, Martina Bugelli, Amy Burchell, Marta Cabral, Charlotte Cadge, Rosie Campbell, Lauren Carr, Nimisha Chanduka, Kerensa Chapman, Alexandra Childs, John Chilton, Denise Clifford, Hugo Cohen, Paulina Connolly, Hannah Cook, John Corcoran, Connor Cotton, James Coulston, Hannah Courtney, Rory Crowder, Daniel Crowle, Thomas Cuthbert, Anthony Fitzdonald Davies, Drew Davies, Charlie Davis, Kaveh Davoudi, Jacob Day, Mark J. Dayer, William Deeley, David Derry, Alison Dewynter, Indranil Dey, Bipasa Dey, Ashwin Dhanda, Benjamin Diggins, Michael J. Dillon, Leo Donnelly, Hannah Donovan, Gemina Doolub, Edward Doyle, Ilinca Dragusin, Elizabeth J. Drake, Anupreet Dua, Leticia Dujardin, Anushka Ediriweera, Ellie Edlmann, Nick Edmeades, James Edwards, Simon Edwards, Ahmed El-Medany, Lily Evans, Maysa Falah, Anam Fatima, Sophie Fenwick, Hannah Fieldhouse, James Florance, Paul Foster, Caroline Fox, Jonah Fox, Bryher Francis, William Francis-Smith, Kwabena Frimpong-Ansah, William Fullick, Guy O. Furniss, Shafia M. A. Gafoor, Sarah Galloway, Rebecca Garrett, Charlotte Gatenby, Edmund Gerrans, Abel Getachew, Baljeet K. Gholkar, Avik Ghoshal, Rowan Gilmore, Konstantin Glebov, Victoria Goodman, Alexander Gordon, Emma Graham, Megan Griffiths, Ramy Guirguis, Monika Gupta, Louise Gurowich, Nabil Habib, Louis Hainsworth, Sattam A. F. Halaseh,

Shehrazad Halawa, Amy Hanley, Mark Hanson, Natasha A. Hart, Derval Harte, Nourgeihan Hashem, Gemma Hayes, Claire Hein, Pieter van Hensbergen, Ed Herbert, Adele Hill, Thomas C. Hinton, Robert Hirst, Ian Hodgins, Kathryn Hogan, Kate Holyhead, Tim Hookway, Lyndsey Hookway, James Hubbard, Sarah Hudson, Alexandra Hughes, Patrick Hughes, Phil Hughes, Naomi Hulatt, Sarah Huline-Dickens, Catriona Hunter, Lucy Huppler, Katharine Hutchison, Katie Hyde, Alice Inman, Sivani Inparaj, Robert H. James, Martin James, Joanna Jarzabek, Hannah Jenkins, Sarah Johnson, Karen Johnstone, Katherine E. A. Jones, Jennifer Jones, Hugh Jones, Mark Jordan, Caitlin Jordan, Radua Kamal, Venkata M. R. Kanukollu, Aditya Kanwar, Andrew Kelly, Hisham Khalil, Maham Khan, Maryam Khan, Adam Kimble, Zoe King, Rhodri King, Sarah Kingdon, Fiona Kinnarney, Jolanta Kisielewska, Angus Kitchin, Monika Klimczuk, Samantha Knox, Angeliki Kosti, Catherine Krzyzanowska, Hnin L. Y. Kyaw, Sathya Lakpriya, Shashi K. K. Lakshmana, Joshua Lau, Isabella Laws, Claire Lentaigne, Julian Lentaigne, Megan E. Lewis, Kate Liang, Louise Jessica Liyadi, Felicity Lock, Kate F. Lovett, Jonathon Lowe, Jamie Ludgate, Sohaib Mallick, Nehal Mandour, Haritha Maripi, Rachel Marshall-Roberts, Callum Masey, Beth McElroy, Stuart McPhail, Patrick Medd, Nicola Melia, Louise Merker, Sri Vamshi Merugumala, Chloe Milsom, Jonathan Milton, Benjamin Mitchell, Harriet Mitchell-Riall, Devender Mittapalli, Abdul K. Mohammed, Prebashan Moodley, Heather Moore, Ed Morley-Smith, Siobhan M. Moyes, Daniel Mullan, Stephen Mullin, Salman Mushtaq, Nan A. Myint, Hannah Newman, Nikitas Nikitas, Tim Nokes, Malik S. Noor, Bethany Norman, Muhammed A. Noushad, Kieran O'Kane, Andrew O'Leary, Seanan O'Rourke, Ifeoma Offiah, Vicky Ohlsson, Sayaka Okano, Omolola Olamosu, Katie J. Ovens, Joseph Page, Anthony Paluch, Laura Pannell, Jonathan C. Park, Dominique Parslow, Chetan Pataki, Nishchil H. Patel, Ben Patel, Catharine Pearce, Daniel Pearl, Mark Perry, Rory Pinkney, Keith Pohl, Polly Powell, Sherin Prince, Faith Protts, Jamie S. Pruden, Ahmed A. Rahim, Paul Rainsbury, Asef M. Rakin, Vasant Raman, Siobhan M. Rattigan, Hope Raybould, Ross Raymond-Jones, Syed Ali Raza, Jamie Read, Mhairi Reed-Embleton, Qazi Naeem ur Rehman, Timothy Richards, Ann Rigby-Jones, Lucy Robin, Michael Rowe, Holly Roy, Leticia Royo-Dujardin, Victor-Laurian Rusu, Javid Salim, Julia H. Sarginson, Katherine Saunders, Thomas G. Saunders, Mohamed Sayed, David Scott, Francis Screech, Beth Screech, Emma-Tina Segall, Kanch Seneviratne, Rishabha D. Sharma, Vishal Sharma,

Gunjan Sharma, Rishabha D. Sharma, Jonathan Shaw, Emma Shephard, Indy S. Sian, Julia Sieberer, Kimberly Silochan, Alena Sim, Rosie Simson, Ayesha Sithirapathy, Edward Skinner, Will Smith, Jasmine Sofela, Agbolahan Sofela, William Spackman, Aginor Spanoulis, Karran Speakman, Gill Spyer, Robert Stabler, Marios Stavrakas, Katherine Stevenson, Charles Stewart, Jonathan Stone, Lara Strang, Serena R. Strickland, Vrinda Sukumaran, Aaron Sutton, Michael Symes, Jamie Talbot, David Tang, Natalie Taylor, Alexander Taylor, Lindsey Taylor, Muwaffaq Telfah, Shivesh Tewari, Vladimir T. Thaller, Thirupathirajan Thinakararajan, Katie Thomas, Wayne Thomas, Danny Thomas, Graham Thornton, Paul Thorpe, Liberty-Isabelle Todd, Megan Tombling, James S. Tomlinson, Dimitrios Tsiakiris, Zafar Ullah, Waqar Ullah, Akudo Umeh, Marius Vaida, Jonny Varma, Benjamin James Vince, David Waine, Adam Walsh, Stuart Wareham, Helen Watson, Stuart Weatherby, Tom Weatherby, Rui Wei, Ben Whittaker, Nyo P. N. Win, Stephanie Wing, Alexander Witek, Lucy Worlock, Oliver Wright, Shun Yamanaka, Charlotte Yates, Emily Young.

Index